Complex and Revision Shoulder Arthroplasty

Robert Z. Tashjian
Editor

Complex and Revision Shoulder Arthroplasty

An Evidence-Based Approach to Evaluation and Management

Springer

Editor
Robert Z. Tashjian
Department of Orthopedics
University of Utah
Salt Lake City, UT
USA

ISBN 978-3-030-02755-1 ISBN 978-3-030-02756-8 (eBook)
https://doi.org/10.1007/978-3-030-02756-8

Library of Congress Control Number: 2018965740

This Springer imprint is published by the registered company Springer Nature Switzerland AG
The registered company address is: Gewerbestrasse 11, 6330 Cham, Switzerland

Preface

Shoulder arthroplasty has evolved dramatically over the past 50 years and with this evolution so has our ability to treat increasingly complex pathology. Similarly, the tools that the shoulder arthroplasty surgeon can utilize to treat the complex list of problems have also expanded. Choosing the "right size hammer for the correct size nail" and using it appropriately and safely has now become one of the most challenging aspects of shoulder arthroplasty. Lack of knowledge of options or the correct usage of the increasing array of arthroplasty options can have a detrimental effect on the increasing numbers of patients that can be helped by a shoulder replacement. As the numbers of primary shoulder arthroplasties increase, so will the number of revision arthroplasties. The introduction of the reverse shoulder arthroplasty in the United States in the early 2000s has dramatically increased the overall number of primary shoulder arthroplasties performed per year, and as a result revision arthroplasty has also risen dramatically. Strategies and surgical techniques to manage complicated revisions are available in the literature but are not available in one location requiring surgeons to search articles and videos to find appropriate techniques to address some of these most challenging cases. The goal of this book is to put the most up-to-date information on a variety of complicated topics of shoulder arthroplasty in one location.

I am grateful to have recruited a group of experts in the field of shoulder arthroplasty to put together a series of manuscripts outlining the most current treatment strategies for the most complicated situations requiring a primary or revision shoulder arthroplasty. The initial chapters of the book focus on the diagnosis and management of complex primary shoulder arthroplasty including the treatment of severe humeral and glenoid bone loss, the use of computer-assisted planning and patient-specific instrumentation, stemless implants in severe deformity and post-traumatic arthritis. The second section focuses on revision arthroplasty strategies including the workup of a painful arthroplasty, treatment of a failed hemiarthroplasty, anatomic and reverse total shoulder arthroplasty as well as the management of infected or unstable implants. The final section focuses on revision arthroplasty surgical techniques including initial surgical approach, bone grafting techniques, humeral removal techniques and the utility of arthroscopy with failed implants. The authors have synthesized a tremendous amount of material to make clear recommendations regarding the best strategies based upon data as well as including their own personal "pearls of wisdom" as they are all experts in the field. I want to thank each author individually for the time and effort taken to complete this project. I hope the readers will find this book a primary resource of information for managing these complicated and challenging problems.

There are many resources available for strategies to use shoulder arthroplasty to treat simple cases of osteoarthritis, proximal humeral fractures or rotator cuff arthropathy but very few that take the next step. This book is an attempt to take that next step providing an educational foundation for the complex and revision cases. We are complimenting the education in this book with an annual shoulder arthroplasty meeting that will expand on all of the topics in this book including live surgery and video instruction. The first Advanced Shoulder ArthroPlasty (ASAP) Meeting (https://asapmeeting.org) will be held in Park City, Utah, on January 10–12, 2019 and will be held annually or biennially complementing the material in this book. We hope you will decide to attend the meeting or future meetings to further your education, thereby improving the care provided by you to your patients.

Salt Lake City, UT, USA Robert Z. Tashjian, MD

Contents

Contributors

Joseph Albert Abboud, MD The Rothman Institute-Thomas Jefferson University Hospital, Department of Orthopaedics, Philadelphia, PA, USA

William R. Aibinder Department of Orthopedic Surgery, Mayo Clinic, Rochester, MN, USA

Mitch Armstrong Department of Surgery, Queen's University, Kingston Health Sciences Centre, Kingston, ON, Canada

Francesco Ascione Orthopedic Department, Campolongo Hospital, Salerno, Italy

Orthopedic and Traumatolgy Division, Madonna del Buon Consiglio Fatebenefratelli Hospital, Naples, Italy

Bandar Assiry Department of Surgery, Queen's University, Kingston Health Sciences Centre, Kingston, ON, Canada

Ryan T. Bicknell, MD Departments of Surgery and Mechanical and Materials Engineering, Queen's University, Kingston Health Sciences Centre, Kingston, ON, Canada

Peter N. Chalmers, MD Shoulder and Elbow Surgery, Department of Orthopaedic Surgery, University of Utah, Salt Lake City, UT, USA

Aaron Chamberlain, MD Department of Orthopedic Surgery, Washington University, St. Louis, MO, USA

Michael Charles Shoulder/Elbow Surgery and Sports Medicine, Orthopaedic Surgery, UCSF Fresno, Fresno, CA, USA

Christopher Chuinard, MD Great Lakes Orthopaedic Center, Traverse City, MI, USA

Michael C. Cusick Department of Orthopedic Surgery, McGovern Medical School, The University of Texas Health Science Center, Houston, TX, USA

Bassem Elhassan, MD Mayo Clinic, Rochester, MN, USA

Vahid Entezari Department of Orthopaedic Surgery, Rothman Institute at Thomas Jefferson University, Philadelphia, PA, USA

Ryan L. Eschbaugh Orthopaedic and Rheumatologic Institute, Cleveland Clinic, Cleveland, OH, USA

Charles L. Getz, MD Department of Orthopaedic Surgery, Thomas Jefferson University, Philadelphia, PA, USA

Brian F. Grogan Shoulder, Elbow, and Sports Medicine, Department of Orthopedics and Rehabilitation, University of Wisconsin School of Medicine and Public Health, New York, NY, USA

Joseph P. Iannotti, MD, PhD Orthopaedic and Rheumatologic Institute, Cleveland Clinic, Cleveland, OH, USA

Charles M. Jobin, MD Columbia University, Center for Shoulder Elbow and Sports Medicine, New York, NY, USA

Jay D. Keener, MD Shoulder and Elbow Service, Washington University, St. Louis, MO, USA

Jason S. Klein Department of Orthopaedic Surgery, Thomas Jefferson University, Philadelphia, PA, USA

Manesha Lankachandra Department of Orthopaedic Surgery, MedStar Union Memorial Hospital, Baltimore, MD, USA

Julia Lee Mayo Clinic, Rochester, MN, USA

Jonathan Levy, MD Orthopedic Surgery, Holy Cross Orthopedic Institute, Fort Lauderdale, FL, USA

Benjamin J. Lindbloom Shoulder and Elbow Service, Florida Orthopaedic Institute, Tampa, FL, USA

Alexander Martusiewicz Department of Orthopedic Surgery, Washington University, St. Louis, MO, USA

J. Michael Wiater, MD Department of Orthopaedic Surgery, Beaumont Health System, Royal Oak, MI, USA

Mark A. Mighell, MD Shoulder and Elbow Service, Florida Orthopaedic Institute, Tampa, FL, USA

Dragomir Mijic Orthopedic Surgery, The Center for Bone and Joint Disease, Brooksville, FL, USA

Anand M. Murthi, MD Department of Orthopaedic Surgery, MedStar Union Memorial Hospital, Baltimore, MD, USA

Surena Namdari, MD Department of Orthopaedic Surgery, Rothman Institute at Thomas Jefferson University, Philadelphia, PA, USA

Gregory P. Nicholson, MD Department of Orthopedic Surgery, Rush University Medical Center, Chicago, IL, USA

Eric Michael Padegimas The Rothman Institute-Thomas Jefferson University Hospital, Department of Orthopaedics, Philadelphia, PA, USA

Ian A. Power University of Tennessee-Campbell Clinic, Department of Orthopaedic Surgery & Biomedical Engineering, Memphis, TN, USA

Catherine M. Rapp Department of Orthopaedic Surgery, Beaumont Health System, Royal Oak, MI, USA

Eric T. Ricchetti, MD Orthopaedic and Rheumatologic Institute, Cleveland Clinic, Cleveland, OH, USA

Howard D. Routman, MD The Palm Beach Shoulder Service at Atlantis Orthopaedics, Palm Beach Gardens, FL, USA

Joaquin Sanchez-Sotelo, MD Department of Orthopedic Surgery, Mayo Clinic, Rochester, MN, USA

Mayo Clinic and Mayo College of Medicine, Rochester, MN, USA

Jason Scalise, MD The CORE Institute, Phoenix, AZ, USA

Edward J. Shields Department of Orthopaedic Surgery, Beaumont Health System, Royal Oak, MI, USA

Thomas W. Throckmorton, MD University of Tennessee-Campbell Clinic, Department of Orthopaedic Surgery & Biomedical Engineering, Memphis, TN, USA

John Wu Department of Orthopaedic Surgery, Beaumont Health System, Royal Oak, MI, USA

Part I

Complex Primary Shoulder Arthroplasty: Diagnosis and Management

1 Evaluation of Humeral and Glenoid Bone Deformity in Glenohumeral Arthritis

Brian F. Grogan and Charles M. Jobin

Introduction

Glenohumeral arthritis is the sequela of a variety of pathologic shoulder processes, most commonly degenerative osteoarthritis, but may also be secondary to post-traumatic conditions, inflammatory arthritis, rotator cuff tear arthropathy, and postsurgical conditions most commonly post-capsulorrhaphy arthritis. Patients with glenohumeral arthritis commonly demonstrate patterns of bony deformity on the glenoid and humerus that are caused by the etiology of the arthritis. For example, osteoarthritis commonly presents with posterior glenoid wear, secondary glenoid retroversion, and posterior humeral head subluxation, while inflammatory arthritis routinely causes concentric glenoid wear with central glenoid erosion. A thorough history and physical, as well as laboratory and radiographic workup, are keys to understanding the etiology of arthritis and understanding the secondary bony deformity of the glenohumeral joint. Understanding the etiology and pattern of glenoid bone wear helps the surgeon formulate a successful treatment plan and surgical goals to address the pathoanatomy and improve the durability of shoulder arthroplasty. The evaluation of humeral and glenoid bone deformity in glenohumeral arthritis has profound surgical implications and is fundamental to successful shoulder arthroplasty.

B. F. Grogan
Shoulder, Elbow, and Sports Medicine, Department of Orthopedics and Rehabilitation, University of Wisconsin School of Medicine and Public Health, New York, NY, USA

C. M. Jobin (✉)
Columbia University, Center for Shoulder Elbow and Sports Medicine, New York, NY, USA
e-mail: jobin@columbia.edu

Glenoid Deformity in Osteoarthritis

Glenoid deformity and glenohumeral subluxation are commonly seen in the setting of primary osteoarthritis of the glenohumeral joint. The glenoid wear tends to occur posteriorly and may be best viewed on axial radiographs or computed tomography (CT) axial images. Glenoid erosion, as first characterized by Walch, is noted to be either central or posterior, with varying degrees of wear and posterior subluxation of the humerus [1, 2] (Fig. 1.1). The original Walch classification is based on axial CT scan images. Glenoid morphology is classified as Type A1 if the humeral head is centered and glenoid wearing is minimal. A centered humeral head is defined as 45–55% subluxation, where 50% subluxation is defined as a perfectly centered humerus on the glenoid without anterior or posterior subluxation. This subluxation index method of measuring glenohumeral subluxation is useful to define severity of subluxation. Type A2 glenoids feature a humeral head that is centered and glenoid wear significantly medialized. Wear

R. Z. Tashjian (ed.), *Complex and Revision Shoulder Arthroplasty*,
https://doi.org/10.1007/978-3-030-02756-8_1

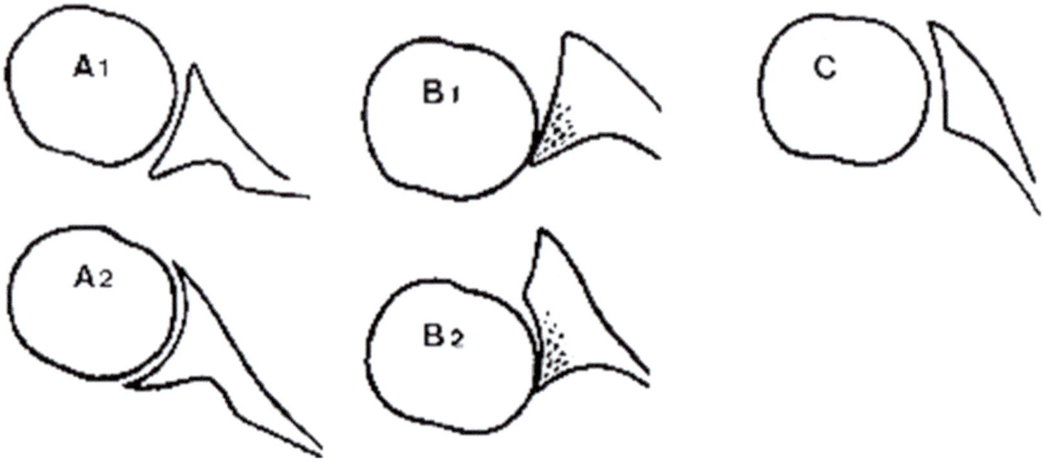

Fig. 1.1 Walch classification of glenoid morphology. Morphologic types of the glenoid in primary glenohumeral osteoarthritis as initially described by Walch. (Adapted from Walch et al. [1])

in A2 glenoids, as compared to A1, is defined as wearing medial to a line connecting the anterior and posterior native glenoid rims that transect the humeral head [3]. Type B1 glenoid wear demonstrates posterior subluxation of the humeral head as well as narrowing of the posterior joint space, subchondral sclerosis, and osteophyte formation. Type B2 morphology is characterized by the biconcave glenoid, with posterior humeral subluxation as well as increased posterior glenoid erosion creating a biconcave appearance of the glenoid on axial CT images. The B2 biconcave glenoid has two glenoid convex surfaces that are termed the neoglenoid which is created from wear of the humeral head and the paleoglenoid that is the native anterior glenoid face that is untouched by the humeral head wear. Walch Type C glenoids are dysplastic and retroverted >25° when using the Friedman method to measure glenoid retroversion where the angle is measured between the centerline of the scapular axis and a line connecting the anterior and posterior glenoid rims (Fig. 1.2) [4]. By definition, Type C glenoid retroversion is not a result of glenoid erosion.

The Walch classification has been modified and expanded to more precisely categorize glenoid wear patterns in order to help guide surgical treatment and predict outcomes. Walch and coauthors have proposed the addition of Types B0, B3, and D [3, 5, 6] (Fig. 1.3). The B0 glenoid is defined by static posterior subluxation of the humeral head before the development of posterior bone erosion of the glenoid. The B0 glenoid has been defined as the pre-osteoarthritic posterior subluxation of the humeral head (PPSHH) [6]. The B3 glenoid as defined by Walch is monoconcave, perhaps the end stage of a B2 glenoid, where progression of neoglenoid wear has eroded thru the anterior paleoglenoid and created a monoconcave neoglenoid ≥15° retroversion and ≥70% posterior humeral subluxation. Measurement of posterior humeral subluxation utilizes the scapular axis method originally described by Kidder measuring the percentage of humeral width that is posterior to the scapular axis line (Fig. 1.4) [3, 4]. This B3 glenoid may represent a progression of the B2 glenoid, featuring an expansion of the neoglenoid surface anteriorly to completely engulf the paleoglenoid to the point where the paleoglenoid is worn away and the glenoid face becomes a monoconcavity with >15° retroversion [5]. With B3 erosion, the humeral head demonstrates posterior subluxation relative to the scapular plane but appears concentric when referenced to the glenoid plane. The D glenoid exhibits any level of glenoid anteversion with humeral head subluxation of less than 40–45%, representing anterior subluxation [3]. Other authors have also added to the initial Walch classification describing B3 and C2 glenoid morphologies. As defined by Iannotti, and based on measurements using 3D CT scans, the

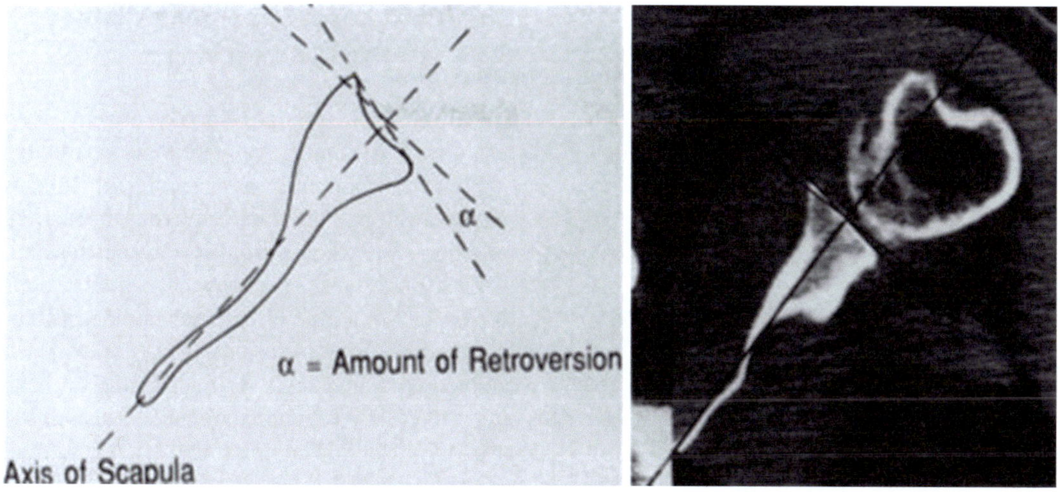

Fig. 1.2 Friedman method to measure glenoid version. The Friedman method utilizes an axial CT image at the mid glenoid with retroversion measured utilizing the angle between the scapular axis and the plane of the glenoid (α). (Adapted from Friedman et al. [4])

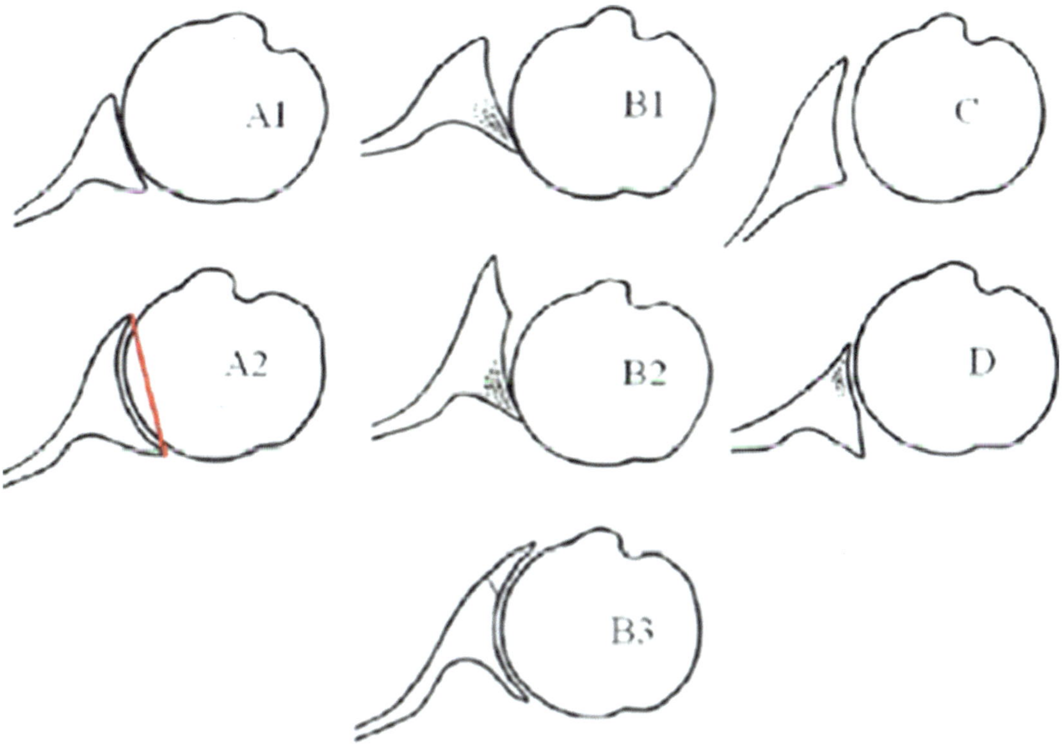

Fig. 1.3 Expanded Walch classification of glenoid morphology. Expanded classification of morphologic types of the glenoid in primary glenohumeral osteoarthritis as described by Walch. (Adapted from Bercik et al. [3])

B3 glenoid has high pathologic retroversion, normal premorbid version, and acquired central and posterior bone loss [8]. Features of the C2 glenoid include dysplasia, high pathologic retroversion, high premorbid retroversion, and acquired posterior bone loss; it may also have a biconcave appearance similar to the traditional Walch B2 glenoid.

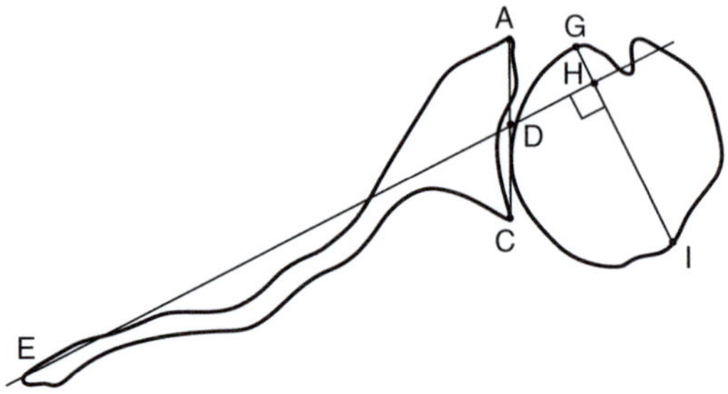

Fig. 1.4 Posterior humeral subluxation. Humeral head subluxation can be assessed as a percentage of the humeral head width that is subluxed posterior to the scapular axis on an axial CT image of the mid-glenoid. A line is drawn from the medial tip of the scapula through the center of the glenoid, also called the Friedman line (line ED). Another line is drawn perpendicular to the Friedman line such that it passes through the widest portion of the humeral head. Humeral head subluxation is then calculated at the percentage of the humeral head that lies posterior to the Friedman line. In this example, the subluxation (HI/GI) is 80%. (Adapted from Mizuno et al. [7])

Glenoid Deformity in Inflammatory Arthropathy

Concentric and central glenoid erosion may result from a number of pathologic conditions but is most commonly associated with inflammatory arthropathies. Characterizing the amount of glenoid joint line medialization secondary to wear is important, as it may have implications to consider anatomic or reverse shoulder arthroplasty and the use of specialized components, augmented components, or bone grafts to make up for the loss of bone stock and to restore the premorbid lateralized joint line. In the setting of rheumatoid arthritis, the Lévigne classification identifies three stages of glenoid wear [9] (Fig. 1.5). On a true anteroposterior radiograph of the shoulder, Stage 1 wear is defined by intact or minimally deformed subchondral bone. Stage

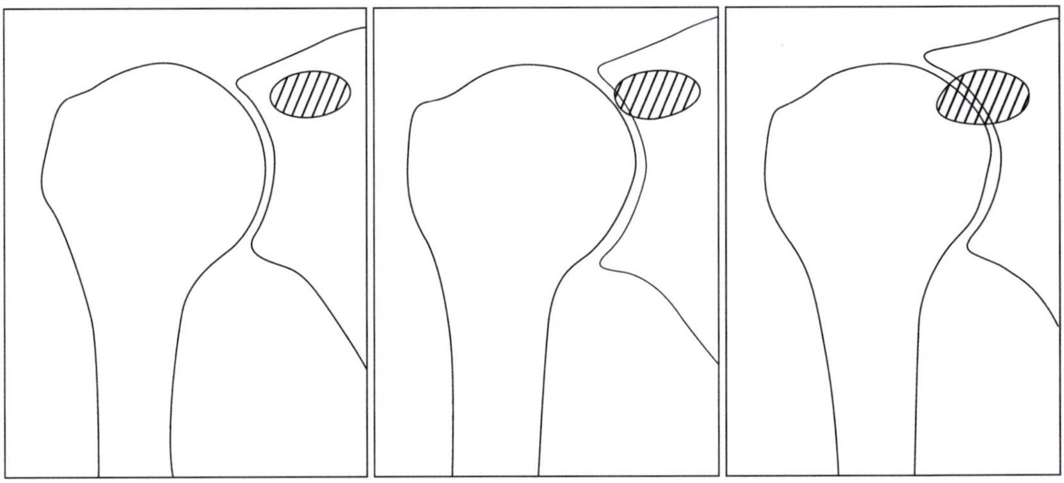

Fig. 1.5 Lévigne classification of glenoid medial wear. Lévigne classification of glenoid medial wear utilizes the AP radiograph and the visible glenohumeral joint line relative to the base or "foot" of the coracoid. Stage 1: subchondral bone intact or minimally deformed. Stage 2: wear reaching the foot of the coracoid. Stage 3: wear beyond the foot of the coracoid. (Adapted from Lévigne and Franceschi [9])

2 wear is present when wearing reaches the foot of the coracoid, and Stage 3 wear is marked by wearing extending medial to the foot of the coracoid.

Glenoid Deformity in Rotator Cuff Tear Arthropathy

Superior glenoid bone loss inflammatory arthropathies are most often seen in the setting of rotator cuff tear arthropathy. The original Favard classification identified four types of erosion but was later expanded with a fifth type (Fig. 1.6) [10]. Type E0 is superior humeral head migration without erosion of the glenoid. Type E1 shows concentric erosion of the glenoid, while Type E2 has erosion of the superior aspect of the glenoid alone. Type E3 is marked by superior erosion extending all the way to the inferior aspect of the glenoid. Finally, Type E4 is inferior wear of the glenoid. An alternative method of classifying osseous abnormalities associated with rotator cuff tear arthropathy was developed by Hamada and later modified by Walch (Fig. 1.7) [11–13]. The Hamada classification of rotator cuff tear arthropathy includes Grade 1 radiographic changes if the acromiohumeral interval (AHI) is maintained. Grade 2 is demonstrated by narrowing of the AHI to ≤5 mm. Grade 3 radiographs show superior migration of the humeral head creating a concavity or acetabularization of the undersurface of the acromion. Walch subdivided Grade 4 into Grade 4A, marked by narrowed glenohumeral joint space without acetabularization of the acromion, and Grade 4B with narrowed glenohumeral joint space as well as acetabularization of the acromion [13]. Grade 5 demonstrates collapse of the humeral head.

Glenoid Deformity in Revision Arthroplasty

In the setting of revision shoulder arthroplasty, significant glenoid bone loss may exist from osteolysis, loose and migrating components, and during the removal of glenoid implants. Residual glenoid defects have been categorized by Cofield based on location and severity [14]. An initial classification determines if the missing bone is primarily central (Type I), peripheral (Type II), or combined central and peripheral (Type III). The glenoid bone loss has then secondarily assigned

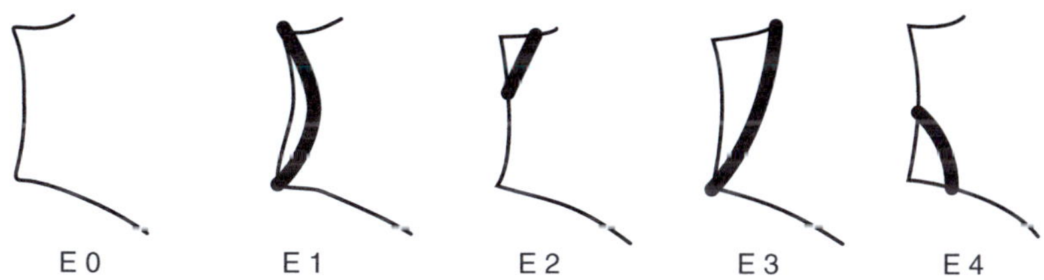

Fig. 1.6 Favard classification of superior-inferior glenoid wear patterns. The type of glenoid erosion according to the Favard classification is characterized by the degree and location of glenoid wear in the sagittal scapular plane. Type E0 is a native glenoid without wear, E1 has central wear, E2 has superior quadrant glenoid wear without wear below the glenoid equator, E3 is a progression of superior E2 wear to include the entire glenoid face, and E4 has inferior glenoid quadrant wear. (Adapted from Lévigne et al. [10])

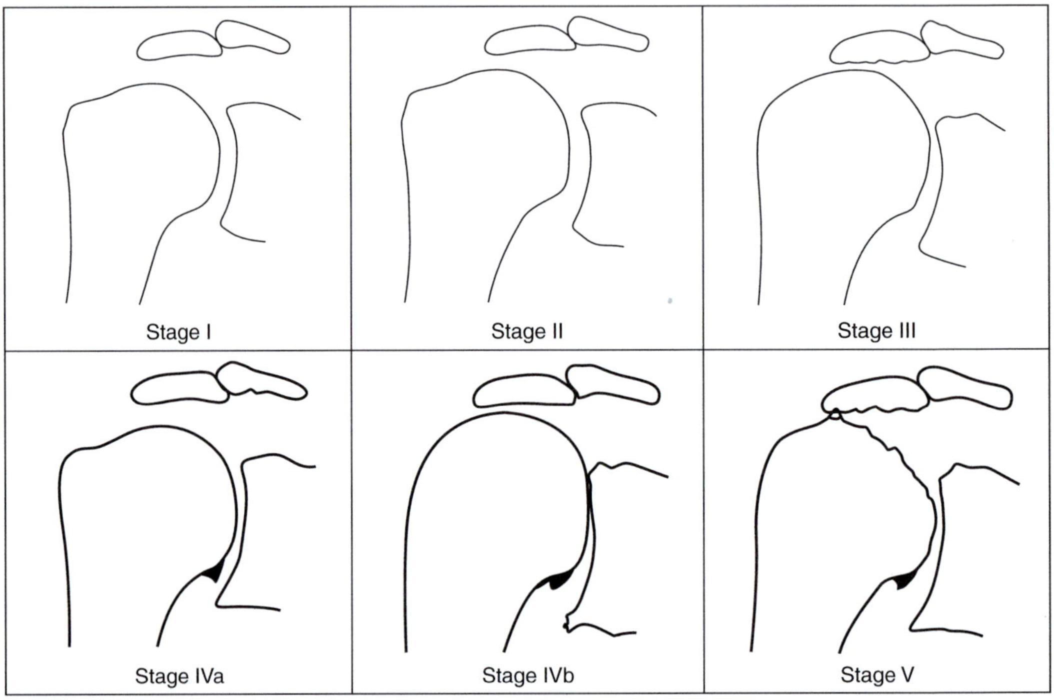

Fig. 1.7 Hamada classification of rotator cuff tear arthropathy. The Hamada classification relies on the development of proximal humeral migration on AP radiographs with the development of acetabularization of the acromion and femoralization of the proximal humerus. (Adapted from https://www.omicsonline.org/OMCRimages/2161-0533-3-159-g004.html)

a severity of mild, moderate, or severe based on the degree of the glenoid surface affected. If only one-third of the glenoid face is affected, then the severity is mild. If two-thirds is affected, then the severity is moderate, and if more than two-thirds, it is severe. This classification was modified by Williams and Iannotti (Fig. 1.8) to communicate whether or not the glenoid vault (V) was contained (V+) or eroded or (V-) in Type I, as well as differentiate symmetric and asymmetric defects in Types II and III [15].

Kocsis described an additional classification of glenoid bone loss in the revision setting [16]. Using anteroposterior (AP) and axial radiographs or corresponding coronal and axial CT scans, three types of glenoid bone loss were described using as reference points the most medial point of the spinoglenoid notch and the most lateral edge of the base of the coracoid. Type I bone loss is characterized by the depth of the glenoid erosion lateral to the base of the coracoid. Type II glenoids erode to a medial location between the lateral edge of the coracoid base and the level of the spinoglenoid notch. Finally, the Type III glenoids have bone loss that extends medial to the level of the spinoglenoid notch.

Measurement of Glenoid Version and Inclination

To supplement the classifications of glenoid wear and bone loss, there are various measurement techniques to quantitate glenoid inclination, glenoid version, glenoid vault depth, and subluxation of the humeral head. Taken together, these descriptive and quantitative measures may assist in predicting prognosis, developing surgical tactics, and anticipating challenges specific to each type of glenoid bone loss. However, it is important when comparing studies to recognize that while they may use similar terms, like glenoid retroversion, the method of measurement may be different between studies in subtle but significant ways.

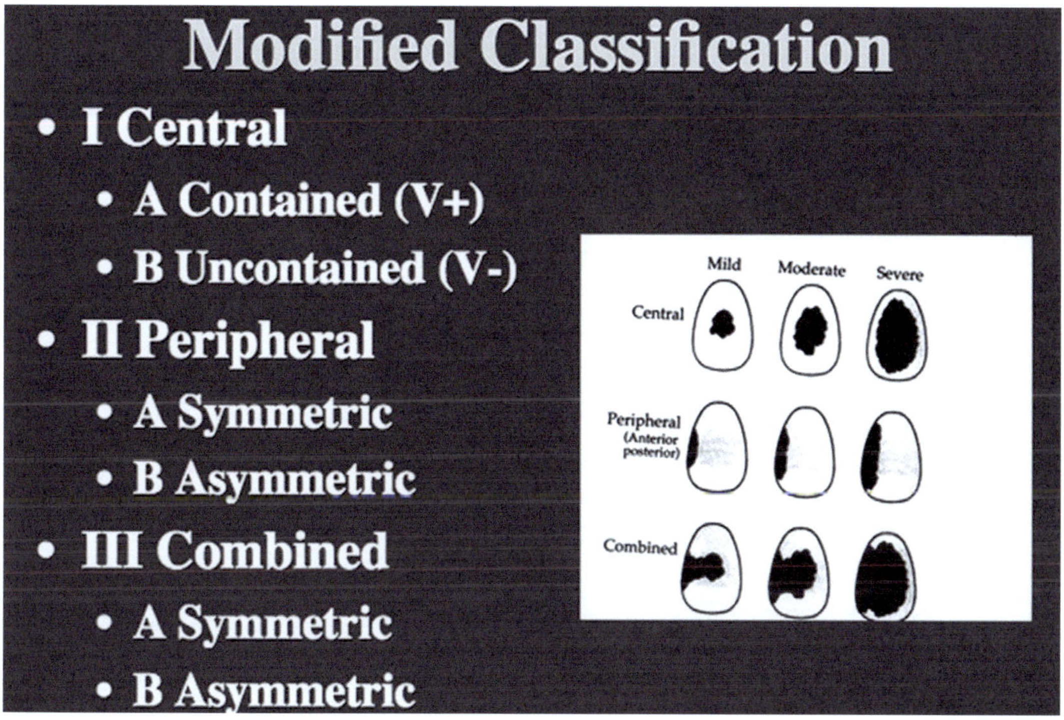

Fig. 1.8 Classification of glenoid bone loss during revision arthroplasty. Modification of Antuna classification of glenoid bone loss as described by Williams and Iannotti. Glenoid bone loss is graded on location (central, peripheral, and combined) and severity (<1/3rd, <2/3rd, >2/3rd), if the loss is symmetric or asymmetric as well as if the glenoid vault (V) is contained (V+) or eroded through (V−). (Adapted from Williams and Iannotti [15])

Perhaps the most commonly used method to measure the version of the glenoid in the axial plane was popularized by Friedman [4]. On the axial cut of a 2D CT scan, a line is drawn between the anterior and posterior margins of the glenoid. A second line, known as Friedman's line, is then drawn from the most medial aspect of the scapula to the midpoint of the glenoid face. Glenoid version is defined as the angular difference between the glenoid line and a line perpendicular to Friedman's line (Fig. 1.2). The biconcave, or Walch B2, glenoid presents a unique challenge to Freidman's method as there are two faces of the glenoid with different versions. To standardize measurement, Walch proposed the term "paleoglenoid" to represent the original glenoid prior to wear, a "neoglenoid" to describe the new concavity caused by posterior erosion, and an "intermediate glenoid" to refer to a combined version of the paleo- and neo-glenoids [17] (Fig. 1.9). By convention, version measurements are most often made using the intermediate glenoid to standardize reporting.

Glenoid version has also been measured utilizing the geometry of the scapular body and vault rather than using Friedman's line. The scapular body line represents the axis of the scapular body, and not the most medial edge of the scapula, viewed on an axial 2D CT scan [18, 19]. Depending on the unique osteology of the individual patient, the scapular body line may or may not run parallel or coincide with Friedman's line. A study comparing these two methods demonstrated a significant difference of −7.3° of retroversion using the scapular body line compared to −10.4° of retroversion using Friedman's line [17]. Hoenecke reported similar findings using the scapular blade axis, which is defined as a line between the medial boarder of the scapula and the most medial aspect of the glenoid vault as seen on axial 2D CT scan images through the middle of the glenoid [20].

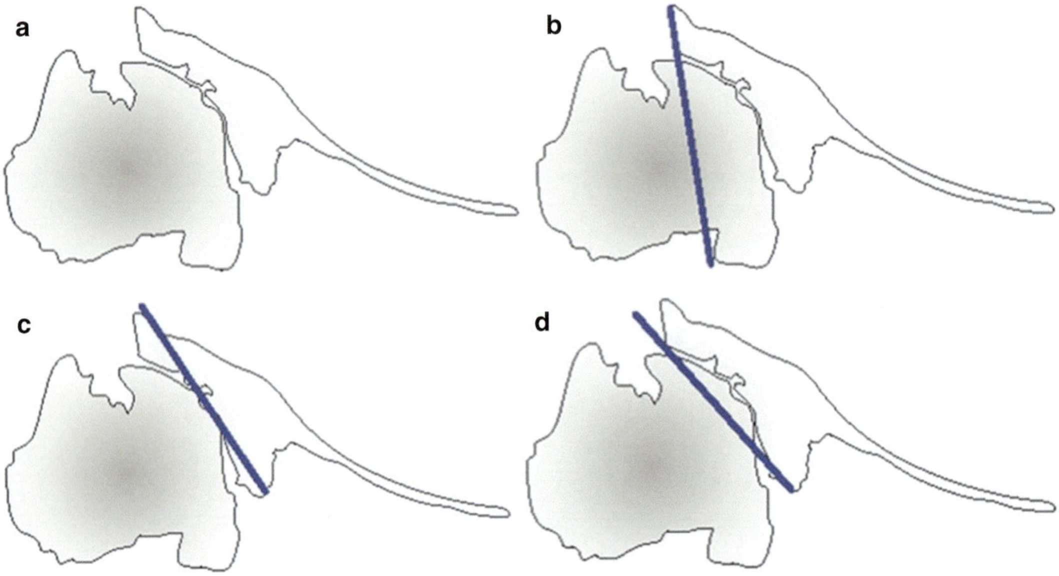

Fig. 1.9 The B2 neoglenoid, paleoglenoid, and intermediate glenoid. The B2 biconcave glenoid (**a**) has two surfaces with differing versions. The paleoglenoid (**b**) can be described as the premorbid glenoid surface prior to wear. The intermediate glenoid (**c**) is the combination of the paleoglenoid and neoglenoid. The neoglenoid (**d**) represents the face of the glenoid created from wear by the humerus. (Adapted from Rouleau et al. [17])

Glenoid inclination may be measured in the coronal plane between the glenoid face and an scapular axis. Churchill measured glenoid inclination using preserved anatomic specimens and a custom jig [21]. He utilized a line passing from the center of the glenoid to the junction of the scapular spine and the medial border of the scapula (a coronal view of Friedman's line). The angle between a line perpendicular to Friedman's line and a line from the superior to inferior glenoid rim was reported as glenoid inclination. Maurer similarly described three angles to define glenoid inclination on AP radiographs and coronal CT scans (Fig. 1.10). The α angle is measured between a line connecting the superior and inferior glenoid rim and a line of the scapular spine. The β angle is measured by the same line connecting the superior and inferior glenoid rim to a line on the floor of the supraspinatus fossa. Angle γ is measured by the same line connecting the superior and inferior glenoid rim to a line on the lateral boarder of the scapula [22]. Angle β was shown to be the most reproducible and resilient to small scapular

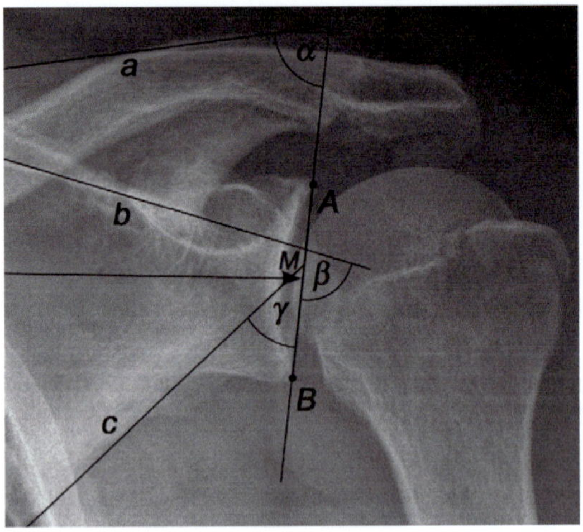

Fig. 1.10 Measurement of glenoid inclination on radiographs. The measurement of glenoid inclination relative to the scapula in an AP radiograph was defined by Maurer et al. The glenoid fossa line (AB) connects the superior and inferior rims of the glenoid. Angle α is between the spine of the scapula (line a) and glenoid fossa line (AB). Angle β is between the floor of the supraspinatus fossa (line b) and the glenoid fossa line (AB). Angle γ is between the lateral margin of the scapula (line c) and the glenoid fossa line (AB). (Adapted from Maurer et al. [22])

rotations commonly seen during clinical practice with variations in patient positioning during x-ray. Daggett, however, demonstrated that the β angle may vary with imaging technique demonstrating the potential need for three-dimensional (3D) CT analysis for reproducible inclination measurements [23]. Using 3D CT software measurement of glenoid inclination as the gold standard, β angle was shown to have a mean variance of 3° on AP radiographs of the shoulder, 10° on unformatted CT scan images in the coronal plane, and 1° on coronal CT scan images reformatted in the plane of the scapula. Another useful coronal measurement of inclination, relative to reverse shoulder placement baseplate positioning, is the "reverse shoulder angle." The reverse shoulder angle is formed by a line along the supraspinatus fossa and a line from the inferior aspect of the glenoid to the point of intersection of the supraspinatus fossa line with the glenoid face [24] (Fig. 1.11).

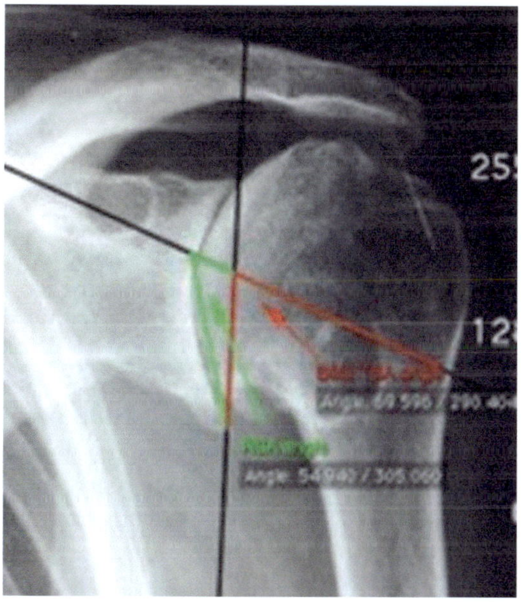

Fig. 1.11 Comparison of the "β Angle" and "reverse shoulder angle." Comparison of glenoid inclination measurement using the β angle (red) and the reverse shoulder angle (green). The reverse shoulder angle accounts for inclination of the area of glenoid (inferior two-thirds) where a baseplate component would be implanted during reverse shoulder replacement. (Adapted from Seidl et al. [24])

The reverse shoulder angle helps assess for superior wear and superior inclination at the inferior two-thirds of the glenoid where a baseplate would commonly be implanted.

Measurement of Glenoid Vault Depth

Glenoid vault depth is measured as an important variable to determine adequate bone stock for successful glenoid component implantation. Glenoid vault depth is defined as the depth of a glenoid face centerline perpendicular to the glenoid face and extending to the medial cortex of the glenoid vault. A cadaveric study by Bicos demonstrated an average glenoid vault depth of 29.3 mm in specimens without significant degenerative changes or glenoid bone loss [25]. Frankle studied the standard centerline as well as a second spine centerline, which begins at the anatomic center of the glenoid and extends medially along the scapular spine [26]. Measurements were taken based on CT scans of normal and abnormal glenoids with subjective erosion. In normal glenoids, the standard centerline depth was 28.6 ± 4.1 mm, and the spine centerline was 42.7 ± 19.1 mm. However, in abnormal glenoids with erosion, the standard centerline and spine centerline depths were significantly decreased at 19.6 ± 9.1 mm and 34.9 ± 17.0 mm, respectively.

Measurement of Humeral Subluxation

Posterior subluxation of the humeral head is commonly noted in cases of glenohumeral joint osteoarthritis. Various methods of measuring the degree of humeral head subluxation have been proposed relative to the scapular axis or glenoid axis. Subluxation posteriorly of the humeral head may be acquired from posterior bone wear or innate to congenital glenoid retroversion. The exact nature of the relationship between glenoid version, glenoid attritional bone loss, and humeral head subluxation remains the subject of debate, but work by Sabesan et al. suggests that glenoid retroversion is more closely correlated with humeral head subluxation relative to the scapula than the subluxation of the humeral head relative to the glenoid [27].

To measure scapulohumeral subluxation, Waters described measurement of posterior subluxation of the humeral head on axial CT images through the middle of the glenoid by taking a linear measurement of the amount of the humeral head anterior to the scapular line (Friedman's line). This distance is then divided by the greatest diameter of the humeral head perpendicular to the scapular line and then multiplied by 100. The resulting number represents the percentage of the humeral head anterior to Friedman's line [28]. Mizuno reported using a very similar technique; however, the measurement was reported as the percentage of the humeral head posterior to Friedman's line, which may be more intuitive when discussing posterior subluxation [7] (Fig. 1.4) and is referred to as the humeral subluxation index [29] or the scapula axis method [8]. Alternatively, the position of the humeral head relative to the scapula can be quantified by measuring the distance from the scapular centerline to the center of rotation of a best-fit sphere imposed upon the humeral head. The distance is reported as the humeral-scapular alignment (HSA) [27].

Several methods have also been described to characterize glenohumeral subluxation. Papilion obtained axial imaging of the glenoid and drew a line from the anterior to posterior glenoid rims. A second perpendicular line bisecting the first line was then extended laterally, and measurement relative to the center of the humeral head was made [30]. This distance is reported as the humeral-glenoid alignment (HGA), and helps adjust for humeral head deformity and osteophytes [27]. Walch used axial CT images and the same perpendicular glenoid face line cited by Papilion, but instead reported the percentage the anteroposterior diameter of the humeral head posterior to this line [1] (Fig. 1.12). This measurement is also analogous to a method reported by Kidder who measured glenohumeral subluxation, referring to it as the Mediatrice method. Comparing humeral subluxation relative to the scapula axis or glenoid axis, the Mediatrice glenoid axis method was shown to have better interobserver and intraobserver reliability [32].

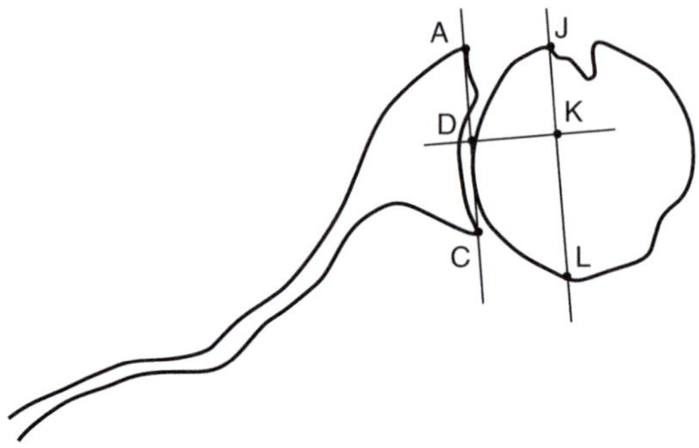

Fig. 1.12 Mediatrice method to measure humeral subluxation. Mediatrice method to measure humeral subluxation, which is the percent of the humeral head posterior to a line (DK) perpendicular to and in the center of the intermediate glenoid (AC). (Adapted from Walch et al. [31])

Conclusion

Assessment of glenoid and humeral bone deformity is critical to understand the pathoanatomy of glenohumeral arthritis. The patterns and types of glenoid wear and the degree of version, inclination, and humeral subluxation likely affect the success of a shoulder arthroplasty and its durability. In general, CT evaluation of glenoid bone deformity is common practice and is superior to x-ray evaluation alone. Likewise, 3D-corrected CT measurements are improved over 2D CT imaging. Better assessment and universal characterization of glenoid deformity will likely assist future research on optimizing outcomes after shoulder replacement.

References

1. Walch G, Badet R, Boulahia A, Khoury A. Morphologic study of the glenoid in primary glenohumeral osteoarthritis. J Arthroplast. 1999;14(6):756–60.
2. Walch G, Boulahia A, Boileau P, Kempf JF. Primary glenohumeral osteoarthritis: clinical and radiographic classification. The Aequalis Group. Acta Orthop Belg. 1998;64(Suppl 2):46–52.

3. Bercik MJ, Kruse K 2nd, Yalizis M, Gauci MO, Chaoui J, Walch G. A modification to the Walch classification of the glenoid in primary glenohumeral osteoarthritis using three-dimensional imaging. J Shoulder Elb Surg. 2016;25(10):1601–6.
4. Friedman RJ, Hawthorne KB, Genez BM. The use of computerized tomography in the measurement of glenoid version. J Bone Joint Surg Am. 1992;74(7):1032–7.
5. Chan K, Knowles NK, Chaoui J, Gauci MO, Ferreira LM, Walch G, et al. Characterization of the Walch B3 glenoid in primary osteoarthritis. J Shoulder Elb Surg. 2017;26(5):909–14.
6. Domos P, Checchia CS, Walch G. Walch B0 glenoid: pre-osteoarthritic posterior subluxation of the humeral head. J Shoulder Elb Surg. 2018;27(1):181–8.
7. Mizuno N, Denard PJ, Raiss P, Walch G. Reverse total shoulder arthroplasty for primary glenohumeral osteoarthritis in patients with a biconcave glenoid. J Bone Joint Surg Am. 2013;95(14):1297–304.
8. Iannotti JP, Jun BJ, Patterson TE, Ricchetti ET. Quantitative measurement of osseous pathology in advanced glenohumeral osteoarthritis. J Bone Joint Surg Am. 2017;99(17):1460–8.
9. Lévigne C, Franceschi JP. Rheumatoid arthritis of the shoulder: radiological presentation and results of arthroplasty. In: Shoulder Arthroplasty. Berlin: Springer; 1999. p. 221–30.
10. Levigne C, Boileau P, Favard L, Garaud P, Mole D, Sirveaux F, et al. Scapular notching in reverse shoulder arthroplasty. J Shoulder Elb Surg. 2008;17(6):925–35.
11. Hamada K, Fukuda H, Mikasa M, Kobayashi Y. Roentgenographic findings in massive rotator cuff tears. A long-term observation. Clin Orthop Relat Res. 1990;254:92–6.
12. Hamada K, Yamanaka K, Uchiyama Y, Mikasa T, Mikasa M. A radiographic classification of massive rotator cuff tear arthritis. Clin Orthop Relat Res. 2011;469(9):2452–60.
13. Walch G, Edwards TB, Boulahia A, Nove-Josserand L, Neyton L, Szabo I. Arthroscopic tenotomy of the long head of the biceps in the treatment of rotator cuff tears: clinical and radiographic results of 307 cases. J Shoulder Elb Surg. 2005;14(3):238–46.
14. Antuna SA, Sperling JW, Cofield RH, Rowland CM. Glenoid revision surgery after total shoulder arthroplasty. J Shoulder Elb Surg. 2001;10(3):217–24.
15. Williams GR Jr, Iannotti JP. Options for glenoid bone loss: composites of prosthetics and biologics. J Shoulder Elb Surg. 2007;16(5 Suppl):S267–72.
16. Kocsis G, Thyagarajan DS, Fairbairn KJ, Wallace WA. A new classification of glenoid bone loss to help plan the implantation of a glenoid component before revision arthroplasty of the shoulder. Bone Joint J. 2016;98-B(3):374–80.
17. Rouleau DM, Kidder JF, Pons-Villanueva J, Dynamidis S, Defranco M, Walch G. Glenoid version: how to measure it? Validity of different methods in two-dimensional computed tomography scans. J Shoulder Elb Surg. 2010;19(8):1230–7.
18. Randelli M, Gambrioli PL. Glenohumeral osteometry by computed tomography in normal and unstable shoulders. Clin Orthop Relat Res. 1986;208:151–6.
19. AK S. Dynamic stability of the glenohumeral joint. Acta Orthop Scand. 1971;42(6):491–505.
20. Hoenecke HR Jr, Tibor LM, D'Lima DD. Glenoid morphology rather than version predicts humeral subluxation: a different perspective on the glenoid in total shoulder arthroplasty. J Shoulder Elb Surg. 2012;21(9):1136–41.
21. Churchill RS, Brems JJ, Kotschi H. Glenoid size, inclination, and version: an anatomic study. J Shoulder Elb Surg. 2001;10(4):327–32.
22. Maurer A, Fucentese SF, Pfirrmann CW, Wirth SH, Djahangiri A, Jost B, et al. Assessment of glenoid inclination on routine clinical radiographs and computed tomography examinations of the shoulder. J Shoulder Elb Surg. 2012;21(8):1096–103.
23. Daggett M, Werner B, Gauci MO, Chaoui J, Walch G. Comparison of glenoid inclination angle using different clinical imaging modalities. J Shoulder Elb Surg. 2016;25(2):180–5.
24. Seidl AJ, Williams GR, Boileau P. Challenges in reverse shoulder arthroplasty: addressing glenoid bone loss. Orthopedics. 2016;39(1):14–23.
25. Bicos J, Mazzocca A, Romeo AA. The glenoid center line. Orthopedics. 2005;28(6):581–5.
26. Frankle MA, Teramoto A, Luo ZP, Levy JC, Pupello D. Glenoid morphology in reverse shoulder arthroplasty: classification and surgical implications. J Shoulder Elb Surg. 2009;18(6):874–85.
27. Sabesan VJ, Callanan M, Youderian A, Iannotti JP. 3D CT assessment of the relationship between humeral head alignment and glenoid retroversion in glenohumeral osteoarthritis. J Bone Joint Surg Am. 2014;96(8):e64.
28. Waters PM, Smith GR, Jaramillo D. Glenohumeral deformity secondary to brachial plexus birth palsy. J Bone Joint Surg Am. 1998;80(5):668–77.
29. Bouacida S, Gauci MO, Coulet B, Lazerges C, Cyteval C, Boileau P, et al. Interest in the glenoid hull method for analyzing humeral subluxation in primary glenohumeral osteoarthritis. J Shoulder Elb Surg. 2017;26(7):1128–36.
30. Papilion JA, Shall LM. Fluoroscopic evaluation for subtle shoulder instability. Am J Sports Med. 1992;20(5):548–52.
31. Walch G, Moraga C, Young A, Castellanos-Rosas J. Results of anatomic nonconstrained prosthesis in primary osteoarthritis with biconcave glenoid. J Shoulder Elbow Surg. 2012;21:1526–33.
32. Kidder JF, Rouleau DM, Pons-Villanueva J, Dynamidis S, DeFranco MJ, Walch G. Humeral head posterior subluxation on CT scan: validation and comparison of 2 methods of measurement. Tech Should Elbow Surg. 2010;11(3):72–6.

2 Computer-Assisted Planning and Patient-Specific Instrumentation (PSI) in Shoulder Arthroplasty

Dragomir Mijic and Jonathan Levy

Over the past several decades, degenerative conditions of the glenohumeral joint have successfully been treated with anatomic and reverse total shoulder arthroplasty, with predictable improvement in pain and functional scores [1–4]. Historically, one of the most challenging aspects of the procedure has been accurate glenoid component insertion. While the ideal position for placement of a glenoid component in anatomic or reverse shoulder arthroplasty has not been clearly established, multiple studies have shown that malposition outside certain parameters leads to increased risk of loosening and/or implant failure [5–11]. There are multiple challenges and variables affecting accurate glenoid component implantation such as patient positioning, body habitus, anatomic variations in native glenoid and scapular morphology, joint contractures, glenoid exposure, glenoid bone erosion, glenoid defect from prior surgery, and loss of reliable anatomic landmarks [12–15]. Functional outcome and implant longevity in shoulder arthroplasty can be significantly influenced by glenoid component position and fixation. Malposition of the glenoid component in anatomic TSA has been reported to be associated with poor function, early loosening, and shoulder instability and is the leading cause of long-term clinical failure [7, 11, 16–18]. Baseplate malpositioning in RSA is associated with instability, decreased impingement-free range of motion, scapular notching, acromion fractures, and in some cases catastrophic failure [19–26].

In anatomic total shoulder arthroplasty, the risk of glenoid component loosening is significantly increased if placed in greater than 10–15° of retroversion [7, 11, 16]. Asymmetric reaming of the anterior "high side" of the glenoid, wedge or stepped augmented glenoid, or bone grafting can be used to correct highly retroverted glenoids to less than 10–15° of retroversion [7, 16, 27–29]. However, the amount of correction can be difficult to judge intraoperatively, and excessive high side reaming can lead to violation of the subchondral bone potentially increasing the risk of glenoid component settling or loosening [30–32]. Glenoid component peg perforation of the glenoid vault is another potential complication of dealing with significant glenoid retroversion and wear, with uncertain consequences [27, 30, 31, 33]. In reverse shoulder arthroplasty, placement of a baseplate with a superior tilt can result in increased baseplate micromotion and loosening, while 20° of superior inclination can block elevation [20–23]. Often the greatest challenges in glenoid component placement during reverse shoulder arthroplasty relate to management of severe glenoid bone deficiencies, where glenoid bone available for secure fixation is limited [34].

D. Mijic
Orthopedic Surgery, The Center for Bone and Joint Disease, Brooksville, FL, USA

J. Levy (✉)
Orthopedic Surgery, Holy Cross Orthopedic Institute, Fort Lauderdale, FL, USA

R. Z. Tashjian (ed.), *Complex and Revision Shoulder Arthroplasty*,
https://doi.org/10.1007/978-3-030-02756-8_2

Accuracy of glenoid component insertion can be improved with proper preoperative and intraoperative assessment of glenoid morphology. For most surgeons, preoperative planning for shoulder arthroplasty begins with detailed evaluation of standard two-dimensional radiographs. The Grashey view is typically used for evaluation of coronal glenoid wear pattern and inclination, while a good quality axillary view can be used for assessment of axial glenoid wear pattern, glenoid version, and humeral head subluxation. Historically measurements of glenoid version were performed using only axillary radiographs. Nyffeler et al. demonstrated that measurement of glenoid version using axillary radiographs had poor intraobserver reliability and, when compared to CT scans, glenoid retroversion was overestimated in 86% of specimens studied [35].

Friedman et al. was the first one to propose a technique for evaluation of glenoid retroversion in patients with glenohumeral osteoarthritis using computed tomography. Friedman's CT technique was an improvement over standard radiographic measurement and became the gold standard for glenoid version measurement; however, several limitations affecting accuracy of measurement remained [36]. Multiple studies have since showed that 2D CT-based version measurements were influenced by orientation of the patient in the scanner, coronal and sagittal orientation of the scapula, orientation of the CT slice in relation to the glenoid surface, and the location of version measurement along the superior-inferior axis of the glenoid [35, 37–42]. Accuracy of 2D CT-based glenoid version and inclination measurement was shown to improve by correcting axial reconstruction images to the plane perpendicular to the plane of the scapula [39, 41]. Further advances in imaging technology allowed for 3D analysis of the scapula as a free body independent of its orientation in the CT scanner, and subsequently 3D measurements of glenoid version and inclination have been shown to have the highest accuracy and greatest intrarater and interrater agreement [38, 40, 43–48]. Additionally, 3D imaging allows for improved evaluation of glenoid bone loss, scapular neck morphology, and estimation of prosthetic fit and facilitates surgical decision-making [43].

The evolution of 3D imaging leads to the development of virtual planning software allowing for simulated 3D implantation of glenoid components. The initial integration of such virtual planning software in shoulder arthroplasty utilized computer-assisted intraoperative navigation [49–53]. While multiple studies demonstrated improvement in accuracy of glenoid component placement in both anatomic and reverse TSA using computer-assisted intraoperative navigation, issues related to increased operative time, cumbersome array setup, additional soft tissue dissection and exposure, iatrogenic fractures related to pins used for array fixation, inaccurate registration of anatomic landmarks, and additional up-front capital cost have led to decreased utilization of navigation until its recent reintroduction [51–54].

Striving toward achieving maximum accuracy of glenoid component placement without the added issues of cost and increased operative time seen with computer navigation, patient-specific instrumentation (PSI) was introduced as an attractive alternative to navigation with similar goals. The placement of a single PSI guide typically requires minimal additional time and no secondary exposures for array placement. Common to all available PSI for shoulder arthroplasty is guided placement of the central axis for the glenoid component. Since all glenoid components, RSA and TSA alike, are implanted with preparation centered on a single axis, creation of a single PSI intraoperative drill guide can help reproduce the virtual plan for component implantation. PSI now allows surgeons to reliably reproduce a preoperative virtual plan during surgery with high levels of accuracy.

Multiple validation studies have tested the ability of PSI to accurately reproduce the 3D preoperative virtual plan and have compared the accuracy of 3D planning and PSI to 2D and 3D planning using standard instrumentation [12, 15, 43, 45–48, 54–65]. There have been several studies evaluating the ability of PSI to accurately reproduce the preoperative 3D virtual plan. Walch et al. evaluated the accuracy of TSA 3D planning and PSI on 18 cadaveric scapulae. Postimplantation CT was used to determine the accuracy of guide pin placement and demonstrated a 1.5 mm entry point error, 1.64° version error, and 1.42° inclination error. Quantitative analysis demonstrated good correlation between preoperative planned and postoperative achieved guide pin position [48]. Levy et al. showed that PSI guides were highly accurate in reproducing the virtual 3D preoperative plan for central drill pathway in reverse shoulder arthroplasty for 14 cadaveric shoulders. The accuracy for entry point was 1.2 mm, inferior tilt 1.2°, and version 2.6° [12]. Dallalana et al. studied the accuracy of PSI in 20 patients (10 TSA patients and 10 RSA patients) using preoperative 3D digital templating with custom-made guides. Final glenoid component position was evaluated using post-op CT scans. Mean glenoid implant deviation in version and inclination were 1.8° and 1.3°, respectively, while mean deviation in anterior-posterior and superior-inferior planes were 0.5 mm and 0.8 mm, respectively [56]. Gauci et al. concluded that the use of 3D preoperative planning and patient-specific instrumentation provided reproducible glenoid component positioning in 17 patients undergoing TSA. Mean deviation in the position of guide wire entry point was <1 mm in both vertical and horizontal planes, while mean errors in inclination and version were 1.8° and 3.4°, respectively [58].

Most recently Berhouet et al. compared accuracy of virtual 3D glenosphere component implantation by uploading 30 shoulder CT scans acquired from patients with primary osteoarthritis or cuff tear arthropathy who were scheduled to undergo shoulder arthroplasty into a virtual planning program. Two surgeons performed "blind 3D surgery" – only being able to visualize glenoid surface, coracoid, and lateral acromion – while one surgeon performed "visible 3D surgery," being able to visualize the entire scapula. Their results were compared for the ability to correct the glenoid version and tilt to neutral angle of 0, achieve at least 50% baseplate contact with the glenoid, position the baseplate as inferiorly as possible on the glenoid, and avoid glenoid vault perforation by the central keel of the baseplate. The ability to use the entire scapula as a reference ("visible 3D surgery") allowed for improved accuracy in achieving near neutral glenoid version and inclination and decreased the incidence of glenoid vault perforation when compared to "blind 3D surgery" [55].

Improved accuracy of 3D planning and PSI over 2D planning and standard instrumentation has been repeatedly demonstrated in clinical and laboratory studies [55]. Hendel et al. evaluated TSA glenoid component placement in 31 patients randomized into 3D/PSI group and conventional 2D CT/standard instrumentation group by comparing desired preoperative implant position and actual postoperative implant position. The average deviation in implant version was 6.9° in the standard 2D group and 4.3° in 3D/PSI group. Utilization of 3D/PSI in patients with retroversion in excess of 16° demonstrated deviation in postoperative implant version of only 1.2° compared to standard 2D group with 10° postoperative implant version [60].

Heylen et al. showed that 3D planning and PSI reduced variability in glenoid component inclination while avoiding extreme inclination errors. Two groups of 18 patients (6 TSA and 12 RSA) were compared – one using 3D planning with PSI and one using standard pre-op planning and standard instrumentation. For patients undergoing TSA, the goal was to place the glenoid component in neutral (0°) of inclination, while 10° of inferior inclination was chosen as optimal inclination for patients undergoing RSA. Pre- and postoperative inclination represented by the beta angle (angle between the floor of the supraspinatus fossa and the line connecting the superior and inferior poles of the glenoid fossa) was measured on AP radiographs by two independent observers. In patients who underwent TSA, the average beta angle was 74° using PSI and 86° for the non-PSI groups. In patients who underwent RSA, the average beta angle was 83° using PSI and 90° for the non-PSI groups. The authors concluded that the risk of extreme glenoid component inclination errors in TSA and RSA was significantly reduced with the use of 3D planning and PSI when compared to standard preoperative planning and instrumentation [61].

Throckmorton et al. performed a multi-surgeon study in 70 cadaveric specimens with radiographic evidence of glenohumeral arthritis assessing accuracy of 3D planning and PSI guides compared to 3D planning and standard instrumentation for anatomic and reverse TSA. Five different surgeons of varying experience levels participated in the study. Thirty-six specimens underwent anatomic TSA (18 with and 18 without PSI), and 34 specimens underwent reverse TSA (17 with and 17 without PSI). All specimens had postoperative CT to evaluate accuracy of glenoid component placement. PSI guides were more accurate than standard instrumentation in TSA group with an average 5-degree deviation in version and 3-degree deviation in inclination when compared to standard instrumentation with 8-degree deviation in version and 7-degree deviation in inclination. There was no statistically significant difference in glenoid position for reverse TSA group when comparing PSI to standard instrumentation [64].

Iannotti et al. showed that the use of 3D planning software and reusable transfer device improved accuracy of guide pin positioning for TSA in nine bone models from patients with glenohumeral arthritis when compared to standard instrumentation alone. The reusable transfer device marked the desired location and trajectory of the guide pin on a plastic model of the patients' glenoid created from the preoperative 3D planning file and replicated that position on the operative glenoid model. Postoperative CT scan was performed with 3D reconstruction to evaluate deviation from the preoperative plan in terms of pin trajectory and location. Clinically, important deviation from the preoperative plan was defined as greater than or equal to a 5-degree deviation in version or inclination or greater than or equal to 3 mm in location (distance from the planned location) [47].

Recently, Lau et al. questioned the accuracy of PSI in shoulder arthroplasty reported in literature. A consecutive series of 11 patients (7 TSA and 4 reverse TSA) underwent implantation of glenoid component using PSI with targeted 0° of glenoid version and inclination in TSA and 10° of inferior tilt in reverse TSA. Post-op CT was used to evaluate accuracy of component placement. Significant variability from target version and inclination was seen in both TSA and reverse TSA groups. For TSA the mean version was 8° +/− 10 retroversion and 1 +/− 4° of inclination, while mean 10 +/− 10° of retroversion and −1 +/− 5° of inclination were seen in reverse TSA group [62]. The validity of this study is questionable considering the overwhelming evidence for improved accuracy with the use of PSI presented in a number of recent studies.

Currently, companies offering 3D glenoid component planning and patient-specific instrumentation options in the United States are DJO Global Match Point System™, Zimmer PSI Shoulder System™, Tornier Blueprint™ 3D Planning and PSI, Zimmer Biomet Signature™ Personalized Patient Care Glenoid System, OrthoVis and DePuy Glenoid Intelligent Reusable Instrument System, and Arthrex Virtual Implant Positioning™ (VIP) System. All of the abovementioned systems except Arthrex utilize a single use 3D-printed guide for central guide pin placement. The Arthrex VIP system utilizes a reusable calibrator device which transfers the desired location and trajectory of the guide pin from a 3D-printed glenoid model to the operative glenoid. Apart from the commercially available PSI guides, Lewis et al. tested a novel custom machined acrylic pin array guide for central guide pin placement with a goal of 5° of glenoid component retroversion and 0° of inclination. The guide consisted of an array of adjustable pins that were set according to 3D preoperative plan and provided replication of planned entry for the central guide pin. Lower version and inclination errors were seen with the use of pin array when compared to standard techniques without the guide [63].

Highlighting the importance of preoperative templating and planning using 3D virtual software, and understanding of 3D glenoid morphology and calling into question the need for a PSI guide in order to achieve the desired implant position, Iannotti et al. showed that there was no significant difference in accuracy of implant placement between groups using 3D planning alone and 3D planning with PSI. In this study, 46 patients with primary glenohumeral arthritis were randomly assigned into 3D CT preoperative templating group with either standard or modular reusable PSI instrumentation and compared this group with non-randomized 17 patients with primary glenohumeral arthritis with 2D imaging and standard instrumentation. The accuracy of postoperative implant position when compared to preoperative plan was assessed via metal suppression CTs in all patients. 3D templating with or without PSI resulted in significant improvement in achieving desired implant position within 5° of inclination or 10° of version when compared to 2D imaging and standard instrumentation. While 3D templating alone improved the accuracy of implant placement for experienced fellowship-trained shoulder surgeons, 3D templating along with PSI may still be of benefit for less experienced surgeons in achieving desired implant position [45].

With increasing severity of glenoid deformity, it becomes more difficult to achieve desired glenoid implant position. In TSA, posterior glenoid wear associated with posterior subluxation and medialization (Walch B2 and B3 glenoids) presents a challenge that requires careful correction of pathologic deformity while avoiding subchondral bone violation and glenoid vault perforation. Intraoperative referencing off of paleoglenoid using standard instrumentation can place the central axis guide pin in native anatomic version; however, the accuracy of this method decreases if there is less than 20% of paleoglenoid remaining [66]. Thus, 3D templating and PSI have a better justified role in these cases of severe glenoid retroversion and bone loss. 3D planning can help to better appreciate the glenoid morphology and appreciate the anatomy of the glenoid vault. It can assist in understanding the ability to completely or partially correct pathologic glenoid version, size glenoid implants, and localize peripheral peg perforation and gain a better understanding of the subchondral bone limits that may occur while reaming and preparing the glenoid [48, 58, 67, 68].

In a randomized clinical trial, Hendel et al. demonstrated that the greatest benefit of 3D preoperative templating and PSI in achieving desired implant position was seen in patients with retroversion in excess of 16° [60]. The use of augmented glenoid components has been suggested in order to correct the glenoid version while minimizing glenoid bone removal, limit the reaming depth, and increase glenoid component support in cases of severe glenoid deformity [69–73]. 3D planning has been considered nearly essential for accurate sizing of the thickness of the augmented glenoid component, which can be a difficult assessment intraoperatively.

The use of 3D planning and PSI can also optimize glenoid baseplate position in reverse shoulder arthroplasty cases with severe glenoid bone loss [12, 55–57]. 3D visualization and templating help in the correction of glenoid version and inclination, identification of optimal glenoid bone stock, calculation of baseplate bone contact onto host bone, estimation of joint-line medialization, need for glenoid bone grafting, determination of optimal screw length and trajectory, and estimation of bony impingement points during ROM [74].

Eraly et al. assessed angular accuracy of glenoid component placement and total baseplate intraosseous screw length with postoperative CTs in ten cadaveric shoulders with maximal glenoid bone loss using 3D planning, patient-specific positioning guides, and custom glenoid baseplates. Five specimens were implanted using patient-specific implanting guide, while the remaining five were implanted without the guide. PSI guide group had significant reduction in baseplate angular deviation from preoperative plan, while average total intraosseous screw length was 89% of the planned in the PSI group compared to 52% in the group without the guide [57].

3D imaging, virtual planning, and PSI allow for improved accuracy of glenoid component positioning for both TSA and reverse TSA when compared to 2D imaging and standard instrumentation. Continued technological innovation will lead to improvement in the ability of PSI to precisely replicate the preoperative virtual plan while controlling many intraoperative variables. In reverse shoulder arthroplasty, the ability to control screw length and position with PSI is critical in avoiding complications associated with suprascapular nerve injury and scapular spine stress fractures. PSI guides which can precisely control the depth and orientation of reaming as well as trajectory and depth of screws in baseplate fixation are currently being trialed. Additionally, advances in templating software will likely facilitate better understanding of impingement-free range of motion and allow for more comprehensive virtual assessment of glenohumeral joint function. Decreasing costs and increasing speed of PSI manufacturing will lead to increased availability and utilization that will hopefully translate to improved accuracy of glenoid component implantation and ultimately improved clinical outcomes of shoulder arthroplasty. Ultimately, utilization of templating software and PSI may be limited by technological errors related to 3D imaging or manufacturing or intraoperative issues related to difficult exposure, PSI guide placement, and other unforeseen circumstances. In such cases where the surgeon does not feel the plan is accurate or properly represents the patient anatomy or where patient anatomy or inadequate exposure makes the use of PSI instruments difficult, intraoperative judgment must be made not to utilize the technology.

Author's Preferred Technique for Surgical Planning

All patients undergoing shoulder arthroplasty have preoperative radiographic evaluation using plain x-rays and computed tomography (CT) scans. All CT scans are ordered with 2D axial, coronal, sagittal, as well as 3D reconstructions. Surgical planning is initiated using these images. This involves measurement of the humeral head diameter on the axial and coronal reconstructions and maximal humeral canal diameter at the distal region of the humeral stem. The projected length of the glenoid vault at the mid-glenoid using axial images is determined, and assessment of overall glenoid wear pattern and humeral head subluxation is performed. This helps to facilitate implant sizing and selection, as well as optimization of implant placement. The decision to use virtual planning software and PSI is generally based on the severity of glenoid wear, patient size (smaller patients in which margin for error is low), or other deformities which may make intraoperative anatomic landmark referencing difficult. In cases of severe glenoid wear, the use of virtual planning and patient-specific instruments (PSI) allows for the anticipation of glenoid component size and optimization of glenoid component position and fixation. Preoperative goals are created prior to initiating virtual planning.

For anatomic total shoulder arthroplasty, the planning goal is achievement of complete glenoid component seating. For concentrically worn glenoids with normal glenoid version, this often requires minimal glenoid reaming. However, in the cases of eccentric glenoid wear or cases of high degrees of retroversion, corrections can be virtually planned. During virtual planning, toggling between 2D axial, coronal, and sagittal images is critical to ensure that subchondral bone is not violated during glenoid preparation. In cases of high degrees of glenoid retroversion, a goal of partial correction to approximately 10° of retroversion is often utilized. The glenoid size, subchondral bone density lines, and degree of version correction all play an important role. In the majority of anatomic TSA cases, only minimal correction of inclination is made in order to avoid excessive superior inclination. Peg placement is also evaluated once the optimal glenoid component position is achieved. When using a peripheral enhanced fixation glenoid (currently author's preferred anatomic glenoid implant), peg perforation is of little concern as the peg design may facilitate bicortical fixation of the glenoid component by capturing the medial glenoid cortex with the peg bristles.

In reverse shoulder arthroplasty, the primary goal of surgical planning is to achieve maximal fixation of the glenoid baseplate with a secondary goal of maximizing impingement-free arc of motion. In cases of normal glenoids or minimal glenoid wear, the anatomic glenoid center line can be used to achieve bicortical fixation with a center screw baseplate. Maximization of impingement-free motion can then be achieved using a lateralized center of rotation glenosphere and proper soft tissue balancing. However, in cases of severe glenoid bone loss, optimal glenoid baseplate fixation may not be possible using the anatomic glenoid center line. In these cases, the alternative center line can be used, anteverting the baseplate, aiming toward the column of the bone where the base of the coracoid and scapular spine unites. The use of a system with a lateralized sphere is recommended if using the alternate center line to avoid impingement. While virtual planning the reaming process, the goal is typically to achieve at least 50% baseplate support on the native glenoid. Humeral head autograft can then be shaped to match the deficiency, and the baseplate peripheral screws can secure the graft. A glenosphere with a lip is selected such that the lip can be rotated to cover the bone graft. By impacting the glenosphere onto the bone graft, compression of the graft is achieved, and load sharing of fixation is enhanced. Virtual planning for RSA facilitates anticipating baseplate support, central screw trajectory, optimal length and orientation of the locking screws, and size and orientation of the graft in order to achieve the best possible baseplate fixation. Since the PSI guide does not control the depth of reaming, screenshots of the virtual appearance of the glenoid during the reaming process are created and printed out for viewing during the procedure.

Challenges to intraoperative PSI use are somewhat system specific. Surgical exposure to facilitate guide placement is critical, as incomplete seating of the PSI guide can result in an inaccurate drill path. The trajectory of the drill path must be unobstructed without touching retractors. In general, apart from additional exposure required for PSI reference, the same principles of glenoid exposure apply whether a PSI is used or not. Glenoid exposure is facilitated by the use of small thin retractors, and when the humeral head obstructs the trajectory of the drill guide, a burr can be used to create a trough in the humeral head along the path of the drill.

DJO Match Point (Austin, TX) is the author's preferred PSI system, and its accuracy has been validated in prior studies. Match Point has a user-friendly virtual planning interface which allows for both TSA and RSA planning. It allows for planning of implant position, orientation, reaming depth, implant seating, peg position, central screw position, peripheral locking screw position and length, bone graft, and glenosphere size and orientation. The PSI guide comes with a 3D glenoid model for reference and additional confirmation of accuracy prior to use. Furthermore, the 3D model can be used to select the portion of the humeral head for bone graft during grafting procedures. Match Point PSI guide is easy to use and can be easily secured to the glenoid face with minimal additional glenoid exposure and a high level of accuracy (Table 2.1).

Table 2.1 Summary of validation studies for PSI

Author	Participants	Type of study	Variation in inclination	Variation in version	Entry point accuracy	Year
Walch [48]	18	Cadaveric	1.42° ± 1.37°	1.64° ± 1.01°	1.05 mm	2015
Levy [12]	14	Cadaveric	1.2° ± 1.2°	2.6° ± 1.7°	1.2 mm	2104
Dallalana [56]	20	In vivo	1.8° ± 1.9°	1.3° ± 1.0°	0.5 ± 0.3 mm (horizontal) 0.8 ± 0.5 mm (vertical)	2016
Gauci [58]	17	In vivo	1.8°	3.4°	0.1 mm (horizontal) 0.8 mm (vertical)	2016
Berhouet [55]	30	Virtual	0.3°	0.1°	not available	2017
Hendel [60]	31	In vivo	2.9°	4.3°	2.4 mm	2012
Throckmorton [64]	70	Cadaveric	3.0° ± 2.8°	5.0° ± 4.5°	2 mm	2015
Iannotti [47]	9	Sawbones	2.8° ± 2.1°	3.1° ± 2.6°	1.2 ± 0.7 mm	2014
Lau [62]	11	In vivo	1° ± 4° (anatomic) 1° ± 5° (reverse)	8° ± 10° (anatomic) 10° ± 10° (reverse)	Not available	2017
Lewis [63]	9	Sawbones	3° ± 2°	3° ± 2°	Not available	2015
Iannotti [45]	46	In vivo	3.1°	4.0°	1.1 mm (horizontal) 0.9 mm (vertical)	2015
Eraly [57]	10	Cadaveric	1.2 ± 1.2	1.8 ± 1.2	1.3 mm	2016

References

1. Deshmukh AV, Koris M, Zurakowski D, Thornhill TS. Total shoulder arthroplasty: long-term survivorship, functional outcome, and quality of life. J Shoulder Elb Surg. 2005;14(5):471–9. https://doi.org/10.1016/j.jse.2005.02.009.
2. Ernstbrunner L, Suter A, Catanzaro S, Rahm S, Gerber C. Reverse total shoulder arthroplasty for massive, irreparable rotator cuff tears before the age of 60 years: long-term results. J Bone Joint Surg Am. 2017;99(20):1721–9. https://doi.org/10.2106/JBJS.17.00095.
3. Guery J, Favard L, Sirveaux F, Oudet D, Mole D, Walch G. Reverse total shoulder arthroplasty. Survivorship analysis of eighty replacements followed for five to ten years. J Bone Joint Surg Am. 2006;88(8):1742–7. https://doi.org/10.2106/JBJS.E.00851.
4. Sowa B, Bochenek M, Bulhoff M, Zeifang F, Loew M, Bruckner T, et al. The medium- and long-term outcome of total shoulder arthroplasty for primary glenohumeral osteoarthritis in middle-aged patients. Bone Joint J. 2017;99-B(7):939–43. https://doi.org/10.1302/0301-620X.99B7.BJJ-2016-1365.R1.
5. Gutierrez S, Greiwe RM, Frankle MA, Siegal S, Lee WE 3rd. Biomechanical comparison of component position and hardware failure in the reverse shoulder prosthesis. J Shoulder Elb Surg. 2007;16(3 Suppl):S9–S12. https://doi.org/10.1016/j.jse.2005.11.008.
6. Gutierrez S, Walker M, Willis M, Pupello DR, Frankle MA. Effects of tilt and glenosphere eccentricity on baseplate/bone interface forces in a computational model, validated by a mechanical model, of reverse shoulder arthroplasty. J Shoulder Elb Surg. 2011;20(5):732–9. https://doi.org/10.1016/j.jse.2010.10.035.
7. Ho JC, Sabesan VJ, Iannotti JP. Glenoid component retroversion is associated with osteolysis. J Bone Joint Surg Am. 2013;95(12):e82. https://doi.org/10.2106/JBJS.L.00336.
8. Hopkins AR, Hansen UN, Amis AA, Emery R. The effects of glenoid component alignment variations on cement mantle stresses in total shoulder arthroplasty. J Shoulder Elb Surg. 2004;13(6):668–75. https://doi.org/10.1016/S1058274604001399.
9. Iannotti JP, Spencer EE, Winter U, Deffenbaugh D, Williams G. Prosthetic positioning in total shoulder arthroplasty. J Shoulder Elbow Surg. 2005;14(1 Suppl S):111S–21S. https://doi.org/10.1016/j.jse.2004.09.026.
10. Nyffeler RW, Sheikh R, Atkinson TS, Jacob HA, Favre P, Gerber C. Effects of glenoid component version on humeral head displacement and joint reaction forces: an experimental study. J Shoulder Elb Surg. 2006;15(5):625–9. https://doi.org/10.1016/j.jse.2005.09.016.
11. Shapiro TA, McGarry MH, Gupta R, Lee YS, Lee TQ. Biomechanical effects of glenoid retroversion in total shoulder arthroplasty. J Shoulder Elb Surg. 2007;16(3 Suppl):S90–5. https://doi.org/10.1016/j.jse.2006.07.010.
12. Levy JC, Everding NG, Frankle MA, Keppler LJ. Accuracy of patient-specific guided glenoid baseplate positioning for reverse shoulder arthroplasty. J Shoulder Elb Surg. 2014;23(10):1563–7. https://doi.org/10.1016/j.jse.2014.01.051.
13. Barrett WP, Franklin JL, Jackins SE, Wyss CR, Matsen FA 3rd. Total shoulder arthroplasty. J Bone Joint Surg Am. 1987;69(6):865–72.
14. Matsen FA 3rd. Early effectiveness of shoulder arthroplasty for patients who have primary glenohumeral degenerative joint disease. J Bone Joint Surg Am. 1996;78(2):260–4.
15. Nowak DD, Bahu MJ, Gardner TR, Dyrszka MD, Levine WN, Bigliani LU, et al. Simulation of surgical glenoid resurfacing using three-dimensional computed tomography of the arthritic glenohumeral joint: the amount of glenoid retroversion that can be corrected. J Shoulder Elb Surg. 2009;18(5):680–8. https://doi.org/10.1016/j.jse.2009.03.019.
16. Farron A, Terrier A, Buchler P. Risks of loosening of a prosthetic glenoid implanted in retroversion. J Shoulder Elb Surg. 2006;15(4):521–6. https://doi.org/10.1016/j.jse.2005.10.003.
17. Gonzalez JF, Alami GB, Baque F, Walch G, Boileau P. Complications of unconstrained shoulder prostheses. J Shoulder Elb Surg. 2011;20(4):666–82. https://doi.org/10.1016/j.jse.2010.11.017.
18. Papadonikolakis A, Neradilek MB, Matsen FA 3rd. Failure of the glenoid component in anatomic total shoulder arthroplasty: a systematic review of the English-language literature between 2006 and 2012. J Bone Joint Surg Am. 2013;95(24):2205–12. https://doi.org/10.2106/JBJS.L.00552.
19. Cheung E, Willis M, Walker M, Clark R, Frankle MA. Complications in reverse total shoulder arthroplasty. J Am Acad Orthop Surg. 2011;19(7):439–49.
20. Favre P, Sussmann PS, Gerber C. The effect of component positioning on intrinsic stability of the reverse shoulder arthroplasty. J Shoulder Elb Surg. 2010;19(4):550–6. https://doi.org/10.1016/j.jse.2009.11.044.
21. Gerber C, Pennington SD, Nyffeler RW. Reverse total shoulder arthroplasty. J Am Acad Orthop Surg. 2009;17(5):284–95.
22. Gutierrez S, Keller TS, Levy JC, Lee WE 3rd, Luo ZP. Hierarchy of stability factors in reverse shoulder arthroplasty. Clin Orthop Relat Res. 2008;466(3):670–6. https://doi.org/10.1007/s11999-007-0096-0.
23. Gutierrez S, Levy JC, Frankle MA, Cuff D, Keller TS, Pupello DR, et al. Evaluation of abduction range of motion and avoidance of inferior scapular impingement in a reverse shoulder model. J Shoulder Elb Surg. 2008;17(4):608–15. https://doi.org/10.1016/j.jse.2007.11.010.
24. Mayne IP, Bell SN, Wright W, Coghlan JA. Acromial and scapular spine fractures after reverse total shoulder arthroplasty. Shoulder Elbow. 2016;8(2):90–100. https://doi.org/10.1177/1758573216628783.

25. Otto RJ, Virani NA, Levy JC, Nigro PT, Cuff DJ, Frankle MA. Scapular fractures after reverse shoulder arthroplasty: evaluation of risk factors and the reliability of a proposed classification. J Shoulder Elb Surg. 2013;22(11):1514–21. https://doi.org/10.1016/j.jse.2013.02.007.
26. Wong MT, Langohr GDG, Athwal GS, Johnson JA. Implant positioning in reverse shoulder arthroplasty has an impact on acromial stresses. J Shoulder Elb Surg. 2016;25(11):1889–95. https://doi.org/10.1016/j.jse.2016.04.011.
27. Iannotti JP, Greeson C, Downing D, Sabesan V, Bryan JA. Effect of glenoid deformity on glenoid component placement in primary shoulder arthroplasty. J Shoulder Elb Surg. 2012;21(1):48–55. https://doi.org/10.1016/j.jse.2011.02.011.
28. Sabesan V, Callanan M, Ho J, Iannotti JP. Clinical and radiographic outcomes of total shoulder arthroplasty with bone graft for osteoarthritis with severe glenoid bone loss. J Bone Joint Surg Am. 2013;95(14):1290–6. https://doi.org/10.2106/JBJS.L.00097.
29. Sears BW, Johnston PS, Ramsey ML, Williams GR. Glenoid bone loss in primary total shoulder arthroplasty: evaluation and management. J Am Acad Orthop Surg. 2012;20(9):604–13. https://doi.org/10.5435/JAAOS-20-09-604.
30. Clavert P, Millett PJ, Warner JJ. Glenoid resurfacing: what are the limits to asymmetric reaming for posterior erosion? J Shoulder Elb Surg. 2007;16(6):843–8. https://doi.org/10.1016/j.jse.2007.03.015.
31. Gillespie R, Lyons R, Lazarus M. Eccentric reaming in total shoulder arthroplasty: a cadaveric study. Orthopedics. 2009;32(1):21.
32. Walch G, Young AA, Boileau P, Loew M, Gazielly D, Mole D. Patterns of loosening of polyethylene keeled glenoid components after shoulder arthroplasty for primary osteoarthritis: results of a multicenter study with more than five years of follow-up. J Bone Joint Surg Am. 2012;94(2):145–50. https://doi.org/10.2106/JBJS.J.00699.
33. Hsu JE, Namdari S, Baron M, Kuntz AF, Abboud JA, Huffman GR, et al. Glenoid perforation with pegged components during total shoulder arthroplasty. Orthopedics. 2014;37(6):e587–91. https://doi.org/10.3928/01477447-20140528-61.
34. Klein SM, Dunning P, Mulieri P, Pupello D, Downes K, Frankle MA. Effects of acquired glenoid bone defects on surgical technique and clinical outcomes in reverse shoulder arthroplasty. J Bone Joint Surg Am. 2010;92(5):1144–54. https://doi.org/10.2106/JBJS.I.00778.
35. Nyffeler RW, Jost B, Pfirrmann CWA, Gerber C. Measurement of glenoid version: conventional radiographs versus computed tomography scans. J Shoulder Elb Surg. 2003;12(5):493–6. https://doi.org/10.1016/s1058-2746(03)00181-2.
36. Friedman RJ, Hawthorne KB, Genez BM. The use of computerized tomography in the measurement of glenoid version. J Bone Joint Surg Am. 1992;74(7):1032–7.
37. Bokor DJ, O'Sullivan MD, Hazan GJ. Variability of measurement of glenoid version on computed tomography scan. J Shoulder Elb Surg. 1999;8(6):595–8.
38. Budge MD, Lewis GS, Schaefer E, Coquia S, Flemming DJ, Armstrong AD. Comparison of standard two-dimensional and three-dimensional corrected glenoid version measurements. J Shoulder Elb Surg. 2011;20(4):577–83. https://doi.org/10.1016/j.jse.2010.11.003.
39. van de Bunt F, Pearl ML, Lee EK, Peng L, Didomenico P. Glenoid version by CT scan: an analysis of clinical measurement error and introduction of a protocol to reduce variability. Skelet Radiol. 2015;44(11):1627–35. https://doi.org/10.1007/s00256-015-2207-4.
40. Hoenecke HR Jr, Hermida JC, Flores-Hernandez C, D'Lima DD. Accuracy of CT-based measurements of glenoid version for total shoulder arthroplasty. J Shoulder Elb Surg. 2010;19(2):166–71. https://doi.org/10.1016/j.jse.2009.08.009.
41. Bryce CD, Davison AC, Lewis GS, Wang L, Flemming DJ, Armstrong AD. Two-dimensional glenoid version measurements vary with coronal and sagittal scapular rotation. J Bone Joint Surg Am. 2010;92(3):692–9. https://doi.org/10.2106/JBJS.I.00177.
42. Lewis GS, Armstrong AD. Glenoid spherical orientation and version. J Shoulder Elb Surg. 2011;20(1):3–11. https://doi.org/10.1016/j.jse.2010.05.012.
43. Scalise JJ, Codsi MJ, Bryan J, Brems JJ, Iannotti JP. The influence of three-dimensional computed tomography images of the shoulder in preoperative planning for total shoulder arthroplasty. J Bone Joint Surg Am. 2008;90(11):2438–45. https://doi.org/10.2106/JBJS.G.01341.
44. Kwon YW, Powell KA, Yum JK, Brems JJ, Iannotti JP. Use of three-dimensional computed tomography for the analysis of the glenoid anatomy. J Shoulder Elb Surg. 2005;14(1):85–90. https://doi.org/10.1016/j.jse.2004.04.011.
45. Iannotti JP, Weiner S, Rodriguez E, Subhas N, Patterson TE, Jun BJ, et al. Three-dimensional imaging and templating improve glenoid implant positioning. J Bone Joint Surg Am. 2015;97(8):651–8. https://doi.org/10.2106/JBJS.N.00493.
46. Iannotti JP, Davidson IU, Ricchetti ET. Three-dimensional preoperative planning and patient-specific instrumentation for total shoulder arthroplasty. Semin Arthroplast. 2017;28(1):25–9. https://doi.org/10.1053/j.sart.2017.05.005.
47. Iannotti J, Baker J, Rodriguez E, Brems J, Ricchetti E, Mesiha M, et al. Three-dimensional preoperative planning software and a novel information transfer technology improve glenoid component positioning. J Bone Joint Surg Am. 2014;96(9):e71. https://doi.org/10.2106/JBJS.L.01346.
48. Walch G, Vezeridis PS, Boileau P, Deransart P, Chaoui J. Three-dimensional planning and use of patient-specific guides improve glenoid component position: an in vitro study. J Shoulder Elb Surg. 2015;24(2):302–9. https://doi.org/10.1016/j.jse.2014.05.029.

49. Verborgt O, De Smedt T, Vanhees M, Clockaerts S, Parizel PM, Van Glabbeek F. Accuracy of placement of the glenoid component in reversed shoulder arthroplasty with and without navigation. J Shoulder Elb Surg. 2011;20(1):21–6. https://doi.org/10.1016/j.jse.2010.07.014.
50. Venne G, Rasquinha BJ, Pichora D, Ellis RE, Bicknell R. Comparing conventional and computer-assisted surgery baseplate and screw placement in reverse shoulder arthroplasty. J Shoulder Elb Surg. 2015;24(7):1112–9. https://doi.org/10.1016/j.jse.2014.10.012.
51. Nguyen D, Ferreira LM, Brownhill JR, King GJ, Drosdowech DS, Faber KJ, et al. Improved accuracy of computer assisted glenoid implantation in total shoulder arthroplasty: an in-vitro randomized controlled trial. J Shoulder Elb Surg. 2009;18(6):907–14. https://doi.org/10.1016/j.jse.2009.02.022.
52. Kircher J, Wiedemann M, Magosch P, Lichtenberg S, Habermeyer P. Improved accuracy of glenoid positioning in total shoulder arthroplasty with intraoperative navigation: a prospective-randomized clinical study. J Shoulder Elb Surg. 2009;18(4):515–20. https://doi.org/10.1016/j.jse.2009.03.014.
53. Edwards TB, Gartsman GM, O'Connor DP, Sarin VK. Safety and utility of computer-aided shoulder arthroplasty. J Shoulder Elb Surg. 2008;17(3):503–8. https://doi.org/10.1016/j.jse.2007.10.005.
54. Suero EM, Citak M, Lo D, Krych AJ, Craig EV, Pearle AD. Use of a custom alignment guide to improve glenoid component position in total shoulder arthroplasty. Knee Surg Sports Traumatol Arthrosc. 2013;21(12):2860–6. https://doi.org/10.1007/s00167-012-2177-1.
55. Berhouet J, Gulotta LV, Dines DM, Craig E, Warren RF, Choi D, et al. Preoperative planning for accurate glenoid component positioning in reverse shoulder arthroplasty. Orthop Traumatol Surg Res. 2017;103(3):407–13. https://doi.org/10.1016/j.otsr.2016.12.019.
56. Dallalana RJ, McMahon RA, East B, Geraghty L. Accuracy of patient-specific instrumentation in anatomic and reverse total shoulder arthroplasty. Int J Shoulder Surg. 2016;10(2):59–66. https://doi.org/10.4103/0973-6042.180717.
57. Eraly K, Stoffelen D, Vander Sloten J, Jonkers I, Debeer P. A patient-specific guide for optimizing custom-made glenoid implantation in cases of severe glenoid defects: an in vitro study. J Shoulder Elb Surg. 2016;25(5):837–45. https://doi.org/10.1016/j.jse.2015.09.034.
58. Gauci MO, Boileau P, Baba M, Chaoui J, Walch G. Patient-specific glenoid guides provide accuracy and reproducibility in total shoulder arthroplasty. Bone Joint J. 2016;98-B(8):1080–5. https://doi.org/10.1302/0301-620X.98B8.37257.
59. Gomes NS. Patient-specific instrumentation for total shoulder arthroplasty. EFORT Open Rev. 2016;1(5):177–82. https://doi.org/10.1302/2058-5241.1.000033.
60. Hendel MD, Bryan JA, Barsoum WK, Rodriguez EJ, Brems JJ, Evans PJ, et al. Comparison of patient-specific instruments with standard surgical instruments in determining glenoid component position: a randomized prospective clinical trial. J Bone Joint Surg Am. 2012;94(23):2167–75. https://doi.org/10.2106/JBJS.K.01209.
61. Heylen S, Van Haver A, Vuylsteke K, Declercq G, Verborgt O. Patient-specific instrument guidance of glenoid component implantation reduces inclination variability in total and reverse shoulder arthroplasty. J Shoulder Elb Surg. 2016;25(2):186–92. https://doi.org/10.1016/j.jse.2015.07.024.
62. Lau SC, Keith PPA. Patient-specific instrumentation for total shoulder arthroplasty: not as accurate as it would seem. J Shoulder Elb Surg. 2018;27(1):90–5. https://doi.org/10.1016/j.jse.2017.07.004.
63. Lewis GS, Stevens NM, Armstrong AD. Testing of a novel pin array guide for accurate three-dimensional glenoid component positioning. J Shoulder Elb Surg. 2015;24(12):1939–47. https://doi.org/10.1016/j.jse.2015.06.022.
64. Throckmorton TW, Gulotta LV, Bonnarens FO, Wright SA, Hartzell JL, Rozzi WB, et al. Patient-specific targeting guides compared with traditional instrumentation for glenoid component placement in shoulder arthroplasty: a multi-surgeon study in 70 arthritic cadaver specimens. J Shoulder Elb Surg. 2015;24(6):965–71. https://doi.org/10.1016/j.jse.2014.10.013.
65. Wylie JD, Tashjian RZ. Planning software and patient-specific instruments in shoulder arthroplasty. Curr Rev Musculoskelet Med. 2016;9(1):1–9. https://doi.org/10.1007/s12178-016-9312-4.
66. Donohue KW, Ricchetti ET, Iannotti JP. Surgical management of the biconcave (B2) glenoid. Curr Rev Musculoskelet Med. 2016;9(1):30–9. https://doi.org/10.1007/s12178-016-9315-1.
67. Scalise JJ, Codsi MJ, Bryan J, Iannotti JP. The three-dimensional glenoid vault model can estimate normal glenoid version in osteoarthritis. J Shoulder Elb Surg. 2008;17(3):487–91. https://doi.org/10.1016/j.jse.2007.09.006.
68. Flurin PH, Janout M, Roche CP, Wright TW, Zuckerman J. Revision of the loose glenoid component in anatomic total shoulder arthroplasty. Bull Hosp Jt Dis. 2013;2013(71 Suppl 2): 68–76.
69. Allred JJ, Flores-Hernandez C, Hoenecke HR Jr, D'Lima DD. Posterior augmented glenoid implants require less bone removal and generate lower stresses: a finite element analysis. J Shoulder Elb Surg. 2016;25(5):823–30. https://doi.org/10.1016/j.jse.2015.10.003.
70. Hermida JC, Flores-Hernandez C, Hoenecke HR, D'Lima DD. Augmented wedge-shaped glenoid component for the correction of glenoid retroversion: a finite element analysis. J Shoulder Elb Surg. 2014;23(3):347–54. https://doi.org/10.1016/j.jse.2013.06.008.

71. Iannotti JP, Lappin KE, Klotz CL, Reber EW, Swope SW. Liftoff resistance of augmented glenoid components during cyclic fatigue loading in the posterior-superior direction. J Shoulder Elb Surg. 2013;22(11):1530–6. https://doi.org/10.1016/j.jse.2013.01.018.
72. Kersten AD, Flores-Hernandez C, Hoenecke HR, D'Lima DD. Posterior augmented glenoid designs preserve more bone in biconcave glenoids. J Shoulder Elb Surg. 2015;24(7):1135–41. https://doi.org/10.1016/j.jse.2014.12.007.
73. Wright TW, Grey SG, Roche CP, Wright L, Flurin PH, Zuckerman JD. Preliminary results of a posterior augmented glenoid compared to an all polyethylene standard glenoid in anatomic total shoulder arthroplasty. Bull Hosp Jt Dis. 2013;2015(73 Suppl 1):S79–85.
74. Werner BS, Chaoui J, Walch G. The influence of humeral neck shaft angle and glenoid lateralization on range of motion in reverse shoulder arthroplasty. J Shoulder Elb Surg. 2017;26(10):1726–31. https://doi.org/10.1016/j.jse.2017.03.032.

3 Stemless Shoulder Arthroplasty in Treating Severe Deformity

Bandar Assiry, Mitch Armstrong, and Ryan T. Bicknell

Advances in Humeral Arthroplasty

Since the development of early shoulder arthroplasty implants, significant advancements have been made in design, materials, indications, and technique. Initial prosthetic options were limited to monoblock stems, which created difficulty in accurately recreating a patient's anatomical variations. With continued development, stemmed implants are now in their fourth generation of design [5], and the development of modularity in these newer stem designs has greatly assisted in improving anatomical restoration. As a result, these implants have provided a satisfactory solution to a variety of glenohumeral pathologies, demonstrating improvements in clinical outcomes, range of motion, and pain [6].

Humeral Complications

Unfortunately, shoulder arthroplasty is not without complications with rates ranging from 0% to 62% [7]. Complications are more frequently encountered on the glenoid side, with loosening being the most commonly reported complication [8]. However, humeral stem-specific complications are also encountered, which include intraoperative fracture, loosening, stress shielding, osteolysis, and traumatic periprosthetic humeral fracture [5, 9]. The rate of intraoperative humeral fracture after anatomic TSA is reported to be 1.5% [10]. Rates of postoperative periprosthetic humeral shaft fracture are reported between 1.6% and 2.4% [11, 12]. Stem-related complications are found particularly in the revision setting and have been shown to result in inferior clinical results [9]. Stem-related problems during revision arthroplasty include stem extraction difficulty, requirement of removal of cement mantle, and intraoperative fracture resulting in proximal humeral bone loss [5]. Difficulty in stemmed humeral implantation resulting in a complication can also occur in primary arthroplasty. Complications are more frequent in complex situations involving distortion of proximal humeral anatomy such as malunion, post-traumatic arthritis, deformity secondary to advanced arthritis, congenital abnormalities, and in situ hardware, such as intramedullary devices or plates/screws [5, 13, 14].

Stemless Arthroplasty

Stemless arthroplasty has arisen in an effort to avoid many of these humeral complications during implantation or removal of a stemmed

B. Assiry · M. Armstrong
Department of Surgery, Queen's University, Kingston Health Sciences Centre, Kingston, ON, Canada

R. T. Bicknell (✉)
Departments of Surgery and Mechanical and Materials Engineering, Queen's University, Kingston Health Sciences Centre, Kingston, ON, Canada

R. Z. Tashjian (ed.), *Complex and Revision Shoulder Arthroplasty*,
https://doi.org/10.1007/978-3-030-02756-8_3

implant. Stemless implants also provide the theoretical advantage of decreased surgical times, less blood loss, and bone preservation [15].

Stemless implants have been available for the past 13 years. The Biomet Total Evolutive Shoulder System (TESS, Biomet, Warsaw, IN, USA) was the first stemless implant available for use in Europe in 2004 (Fig. 3.1.). Since this time, a variety of stemless humeral implants are now available worldwide (Table 3.1). Each implant has specific design features, but the overall stemless design concept is shared.

The stemless design allows for an implant that is entirely contained within the metaphysis, which allows for implant placement irrespective of humeral diaphyseal anatomy [10] or large differences in the humeral shaft-head offset or angles. In the setting of post-traumatic

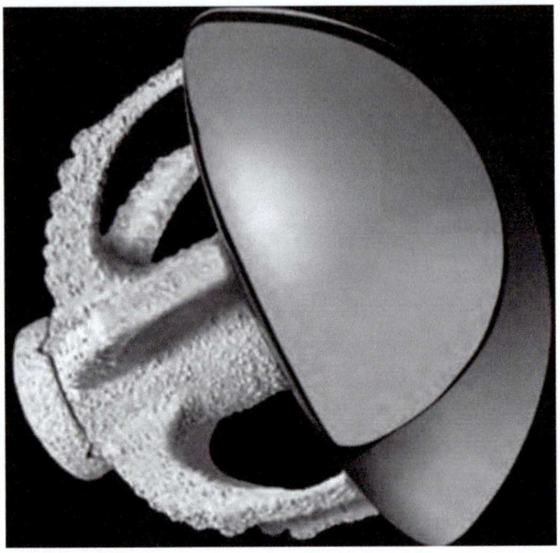

Fig. 3.1 Total Evolutive Shoulder System (Zimmer-Biomet Inc.)

Table 3.1 Stemless shoulder arthroplasty systems currently available

Implant	Type	Outcome
TESS – Biomet Total Evolutive Shoulder System	Anatomic and reverse	31 implants followed over mean of 94.7 months. 93.5% survivorship. Revision rate was 9.7%. All implants showed solid osteointegration of the corolla. Significant improvement in clinical outcome scores. Constant score from 14.7 to 68.8 ($p < 0.001$) [12] 63 implants followed over 3 years. Five cases experienced intraoperative lateral cortex fracture during implantation, all of which healed. No other complications noted. No loosening at final follow-up [9]
Nano – Biomet Comprehensive Nano	Anatomic	No published data on long-term results available
Sidus – Zimmer	Anatomic	No published data on long-term results available
Simplicity – Wright Medical	Anatomic	157 patients followed over 2 years. Reported improvements noted with range of motion, strength, and patient-reported outcome scores. No complications noted with humeral component [5]
Eclipse – Arthrex	Anatomic	43 patients followed prospectively for 9 years. Constant scores improved to 79 ($p < 0.001$). ROM improved ($p < 0.05$). Humeral implant-related complication rate 0%. No loosening noted. Overall humeral-sided complication rate 9.3% (rotator cuff deficiency, resorption of GT, fracture, infection) [13]
Affinis – Mathys Affinis Short	Anatomic	Only system to use a ceramic head. 96 patients in series. Only 12 available at final 2-year follow-up. Improvements noted in ROM and outcome scores. No intraoperative complications noted. No cases of humeral component loosening [14]
SMR – Lima SMR Stemless	Convertible	No published data on long-term results available
Easytech – FX Solutions	Convertible	No published data on long-term results available.
Global Icon – Depuy-Synthes	Anatomic	No published data on long-term results available

proximal humeral deformity, utilizing a stemless implant allows for restoration of the glenohumeral center of rotation independent of the humeral canal position and avoidance of tuberosity osteotomies [13, 15]. Theoretically, a better restoration of the center of rotation may lead to a better proprioceptive feedback of the rotator cuff muscles, but Maier et al. showed that there was no significant proprioceptive difference between the stemless and stemmed design [16].

Indications

Indications for the use of stemless anatomic humeral arthroplasty include the same indications for the use of stemmed humeral implants. These include osteoarthritis, rheumatoid arthritis, post-traumatic arthritis, osteonecrosis, instability arthropathy, and post-infectious arthropathy [10, 17]. Similarly, stemless reverse arthroplasty is indicated for rotator cuff arthropathy and massive irreparable rotator cuff tears with pseudoparalysis in the elderly. These implants are of particular benefit in the setting of proximal humeral deformities as they are placed within the metaphysis independent of diaphyseal position. Similarly, they offer advantages in postfracture canal sclerosis, in situ hardware, and tuberosity malunion by avoiding either the bone or metal [15, 17].

Contraindications

Similar to stemmed shoulder arthroplasty, contraindications include active infection, neuropathic (Charcot) arthropathy, instability, and rotator cuff arthropathy [10, 11, 17]. Contraindications specific to stemless anatomic shoulder arthroplasty include acute proximal humerus fractures, metaphyseal bone loss, osteopenia, osteoporosis, metaphyseal cysts, and metabolic bone disease.

Stemless for Deformity

Shoulder arthroplasty in cases of proximal humeral deformity can be a challenge. In cases of distorted metaphyseal and/or diaphyseal anatomy, inserting a stem may prove impossible due to considerable angulation and narrowing or obstruction of the medullary canal. In some cases, a tuberosity osteotomy can facilitate insertion of a stemmed implant. In one study, a greater tuberosity osteotomy was required in 11–60% of cases, and patients who required a tuberosity osteotomy had poorer results [15, 18]. Therefore, the authors recommended adapting the prosthesis to the distorted anatomy by using a modular prosthesis. But in some cases, the anatomy is altered so much that the modular stemmed implant cannot fit all malunion types. Ballas et al. [15] conducted a retrospective study of 27 patients who had stemless arthroplasty for proximal humerus malunion, with a mean follow-up of 44 months. In all patients, the prosthesis was implanted without the need for tuberosity osteotomy. The Constant score improved from 27 to 62 ($p \leq 0.001$), active anterior elevation from 81° to 129° ($p \leq 0.001$), and external rotation from 5° to 40° ($p \leq 0.001$) with no evidence of radiological loosening. They concluded that the use of a stemless anatomic shoulder arthroplasty avoids the need for tuberosity osteotomy and certain surgical difficulties, even in cases of severe tuberosity malunion, and leads to good functional outcomes in the short term.

Surgical Technique

In the setting of proximal humeral deformity, a complete series of x-rays (true AP, axillary, and lateral), as well as CT scan, is essential. We prefer using CT scans with 3-D reconstructions including humeral subtraction views. This allows for the required preoperative planning and thorough understanding of the deformity.

For an anesthetic, the combination of an interscalene regional block with a general anesthetic is preferred. Appropriate muscle relaxation is required, particularly since deformity cases are often stiff and exposure can be difficult. We secure the patient to the operating room table in a low beach-chair position (approximately 40°) utilizing a pneumatic arm holder for arm positioning.

We use a standard deltopectoral approach as this provides good exposure to both the proximal humerus and glenoid. It is also easily extensile distally if necessary. A tenodesis of the long head of the biceps is performed to the insertional fibers of the pectoralis major. The release of the subscapularis through either a peel or lesser tuberosity osteotomy is used. We prefer to utilize an LT osteotomy in most cases, although care is taken to be minimalistic with the amount of bone osteotomized. This involves using a shallow osteotomy starting at the medial border of the bicipital groove and exiting the LT just lateral to the anatomic neck, so as not to violate the anatomic neck of the humerus. The most medial portion of the subscapularis and capsule is then peeled off. A traditional peel is preferred when the shoulder has an extreme loss of external rotation and when bone quality is in question. Through sequential release of the inferior capsule under tension from the humeral neck and external rotation of the humeral shaft, the humeral head and neck are exposed. Osteophytes are then removed to identify the humeral anatomical neck. It is important to confirm that the rotator cuff muscles are intact if performing an anatomic total shoulder arthroplasty.

The humeral head is dislocated from the glenoid in an anterior direction, and the anatomical neck is carefully marked out. We prefer to perform the humeral osteotomy using a freehand technique, but other options include intramedullary or extramedullary alignment guides. In the setting of proximal humeral deformity, a freehand technique will be used as cut guides are unable to properly account for the deformity. A thorough understanding of the deformity through a review of three-dimensional imaging is imperative at this stage. In general, the anatomic neck osteotomy will recreate the patient's neck-shaft angle as well as version. However, in severe deformity, the anatomic neck axis can be quite distorted. The freedom allotted by a stemless component that does not rely on the humeral canal can enable humeral head replacement while maintaining the greater and lesser tuberosity anatomy, and hence the rotator cuff integrity, despite severe deformity. The osteotomized head or more commonly the cut surface remaining on the proximal humerus after the head is removed can then be used to estimate the size of the humeral head arthroplasty (Fig. 3.2).

An evaluation of the metaphyseal bone is then performed. Churchill et al. {Churchill:2014, JW} described the "thumb test" to provide a guide in making a decision on bone quality. If the metaphyseal bone is easily compressed with thumb pressure, the bone stock may not be sufficient for adequate support of a stemless humeral component (Fig. 3.3).

At this point, if indicated, glenoid preparation and resurfacing are then carried out in the usual manner. Considerable attention toward protection of the osteotomized proximal humerus is

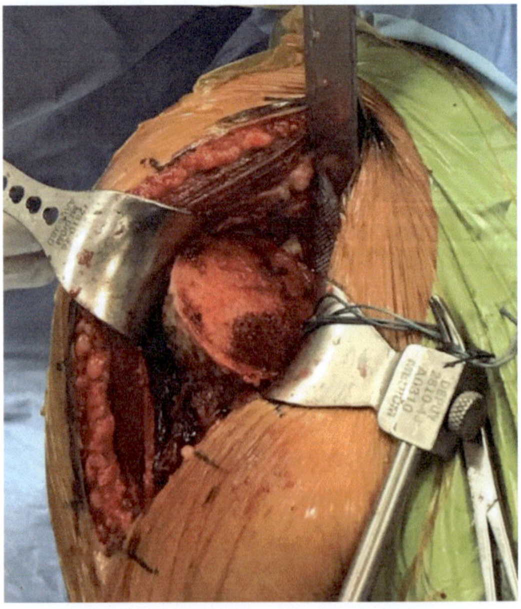

Fig. 3.2 The cut surface remaining on the proximal humerus after the head is removed along the anatomic axis of the humerus

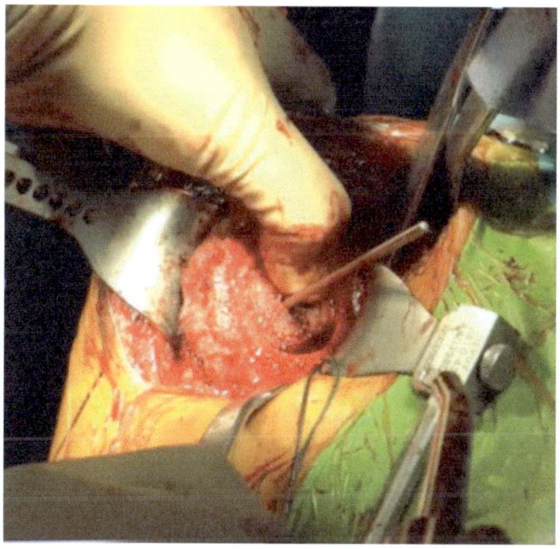

Fig. 3.3 The thumb test, used to provide a guide in making a decision on bone quality

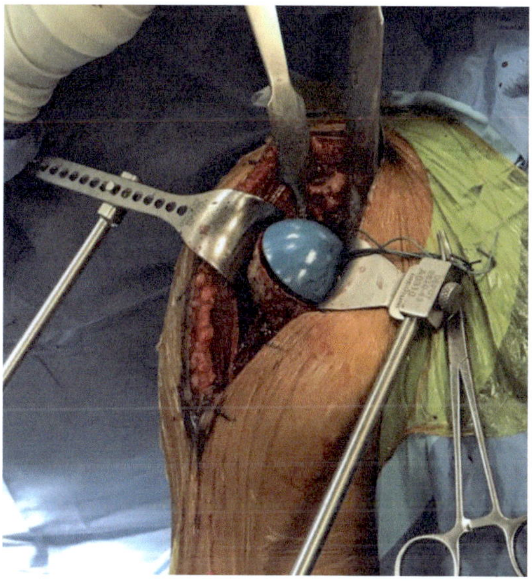

Fig. 3.4 The implant is sized based upon the osteotomized humeral footprint

required as vigorous retraction can damage the more fragile metaphyseal bone, which can be a contraindication to proceeding with a stemless arthroplasty if the implant is unable to maintain circumferential stability within the metaphysis. We find that the use of a broad, malleable posterior glenoid retractor can facilitate retraction of the humeral head and offer adequate protection of the humeral osteotomy as it distributes the "retraction force" over a broad area of the proximal humerus.

For the humeral preparation, there are technical differences depending on the particular implant, but in general the implant is sized based upon the osteotomized humeral footprint (Fig. 3.4). Generally, preference is given to using as large of a humeral implant as possible, in order to engage the more dense cancellous bone toward the periphery of the proximal humerus. Once the size is determined, preparation of the metaphyseal bone is completed in order to accept the stemless implant. This requires a somewhat different exposure than with a traditional stemmed humeral component, since the instruments require insertion perpendicular to the cut anatomic axis of the humeral head, as opposed to being in line with the humeral shaft. This exposure is often facilitated by external rotation, flexion, and adduction of the shoulder.

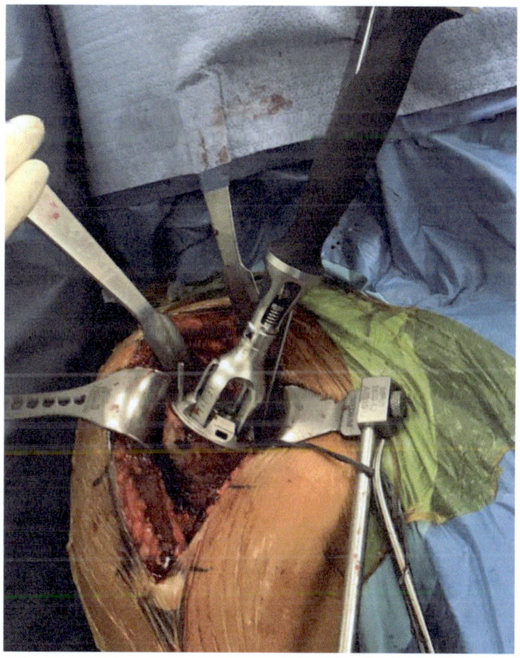

Fig. 3.5 Humeral preparation is often completed with a humeral punch and/or drill

Humeral preparation is often completed with a humeral punch and/or drill (Fig. 3.5). Depending on the design, this punch often does not need to be completely inserted, since the humeral anchor acts as its own punch in many cases. The humeral anchor is then impacted into the prepared metaphyseal bone relying upon a press fit (Fig. 3.6). Trial heads can then be used to determine the appropriate balance and stability. Humeral head orientation (inclination and version) is based entirely on the initial anatomic neck cut, so if that is not accurate, reorienting the humeral head position is not possible. Head size can be adjusted similarly to stemmed humeral arthroplasty. Soft tissue tension can be adjusted through the use of different head sizes, but offset heads are not available in most systems. These are not thought to be necessary, since the humeral anchor can be placed at the center of rotation of the humeral head, as it is constrained by the humeral canal as in stemmed humeral arthroplasty. The final humeral head implant is then secured to the base plate through impaction of a Morse taper (Fig. 3.7). We do not typically use intraoperative fluoroscopy, if the anatomy is clearly visible. However, in severe deformity, this can be helpful.

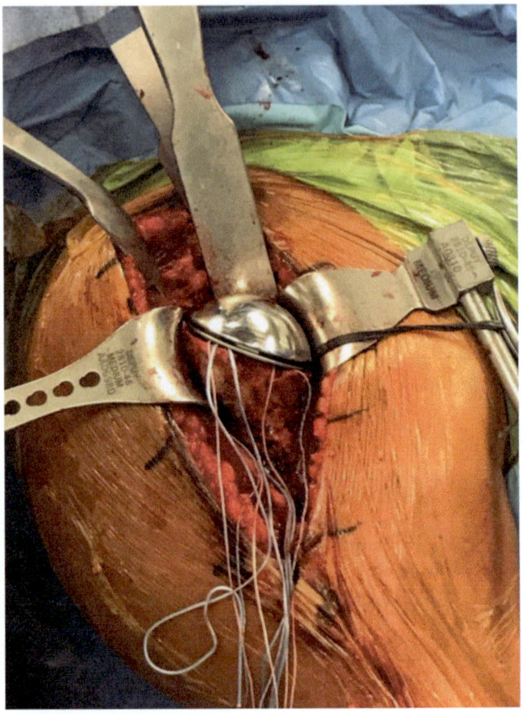

Fig. 3.7 The final humeral head implant is then secured to the base plate through impaction of a Morse taper

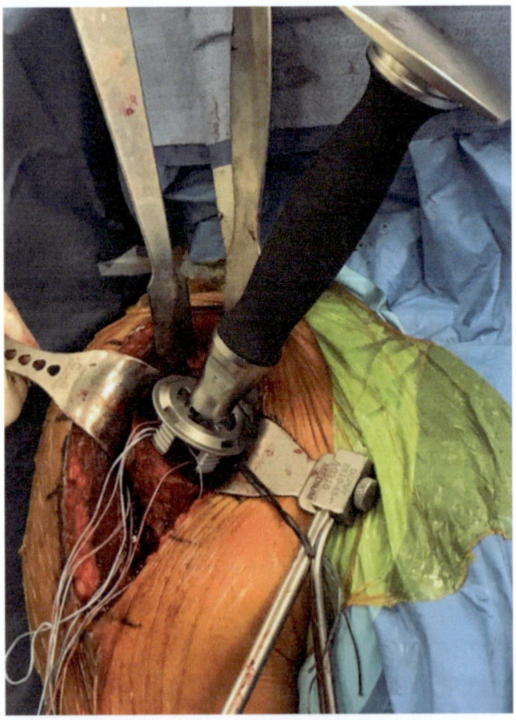

Fig. 3.6 The humeral anchor is then impacted into the prepared metaphyseal bone relying upon a press fit

The glenohumeral joint is then thoroughly irrigated and the subscapularis is repaired. When managing the subscapularis repair, it is necessary to pre-drill and pass sutures prior to impacting the stemless implant. We place transosseous sutures through bone tunnels that start laterally in the dense bone of the bicipital groove and exit through the humeral head anatomic neck cut surface. In some designs, these sutures can even be placed through slots in the humeral anchor. This typically involves use of four bone tunnels, with a double stranded #5 high strength suture through the second-from-top tunnel, which goes around the thickest middle portion of the LT osteotomy and is tied with a Nice knot. The remaining three tunnels utilize #2 high strength sutures tied with modified Mason-Allen stitches. We also place an additional #2 high strength suture to repair the lateral aspect of the rotator interval between the upper subscapularis and the anterior supraspinatus. In the setting of stemless reverse shoulder arthroplasty, we only repair the subscapularis if there is appropriate length available for this. We do not typically utilize a subdeltoid hemovac drain. Postoperative rehabilitation is similar to that used for a stemmed implant.

Outcomes

Recent literature comparing stemless to stemmed humeral implants for anatomic arthroplasty, including mid- to long-term follow-up, has shown equivocal clinical outcomes, pain control, ROM, and revision rates, raising the question of the necessity of the humeral stem [2, 13, 19, 20]. Churchill et al. [21] reported a prospective multicenter study of 157 patients who underwent stemless arthroplasty followed for a minimum of 2 years. All shoulder outcome measures significantly improved at the 3-, 6-, 12-, and 24-month intervals, compared with baseline. At 2 years, the mean adjusted Constant, SST, and ASES scores improved from 56% to 104% ($p < 0.0001$), from 4 points to 11 points ($p < 0.0001$), and from 38 points to 92 points ($p < 0.0001$), respectively. The mean forward elevation improved from 103 ± 27 to 147 ± 24 ($p < 0.0001$) and the mean external rotation from 31 ± 20 to 56 ± 15 ($p < 0.0001$). The mean strength in elevation improved from 5.7 to 7.1 kg ($p < 0.0001$), and the mean visual analog scale pain score decreased from 5.9 to 0.5 ($p < 0.0001$). Collin et al. [6] reported a prospective study of stemless TSA in 47 patients. At a mean follow-up of 35 months, the mean Constant score was 69 points (mean gain of 36 points), and the mean anterior flexion was 131° (mean gain of 48°). In four cases, the primary fixation was deemed insufficient for a stemless implant intraoperatively. Radiographic assessment showed no signs of early migration or loosening at 4 years. However, periprosthetic radiolucent lines were observed at the upper zones in 17 shoulders. However, CT scans were performed on eight patients, and none revealed signs of loosening. Hawi et al. [13] evaluated clinical outcomes in 49 shoulders, 9 years after stemless shoulder arthroplasty. The Constant score improved from 52% to 79% ($p < 0.0001$). The active range of motion also increased for flexion from 101° to 118° ($p = 0.022$), for abduction from 79° to 105° ($p = 0.02$), and for external rotation from 21° to 43° ($p < 0.0001$). No revisions due to loosening or countersinking of the humeral implant were observed. Habermeyer et al. [22] prospectively evaluated stemless shoulder arthroplasties in 78 patients with a mean age of 58 years at a mean follow-up of 72 months. The Constant score improved from 38% to 75% ($p < 0.0001$). Active range of motion improved for flexion from 114° to 141°, abduction from 74° to 130°, and external rotation from 25° to 44° ($p < 0.0001$). The overall complication rate was 12.8%, with an overall revision rate of 9%. None of the stemless implants were revised for loosening.

Several studies have compared outcomes of a stemless implant with those of a conventional stemmed implant after anatomic arthroplasty. Uschok et al. [20] evaluated 40 patients with primary osteoarthritis of the shoulder in a prospective randomized trial. Group 1 included 20 patients who received a stemless total shoulder arthroplasty and group 2 included 20 patients who received a stemmed total shoulder arthroplasty. The Constant score improved in both groups from 54 and 26, respectively, to 66 and 66, respectively, at 2 years and improved to 73 and 70, respectively, at 5 years. The Constant score improved at 2 years and 5 years in both groups, with no difference between groups. No humeral implant complications were observed in group 1 (stemless). In group 2 (stemmed), a fracture of the greater tuberosity resulted in traumatic loosening of the humeral implant. Razmjou et al. [23] conducted a prospective longitudinal study of 74 patients, comparing three different implants: the Neer II, Bigliani-Flatow, and stemless TESS. No difference was seen in clinical outcome scores, satisfaction, or strength. The ASES score improved from the baseline score of 29 to 86 (Neer II), 34 to 82 (Bigliani-Flatow), and 41 to 82 (TESS) at 2-year follow-up. No humeral radiolucent lines were seen in the TESS group, compared with 18% [24] of the Neer II group and 8% [24] of the Bigliani-Flatow group. Berth et al. [25] randomized 82 patients to either a standard stemmed or a stemless anatomic shoulder arthroplasty. Both groups yielded significant improvements over preoperative values. There was no difference between groups with respect to the Constant score, DASH score, and active range of motion. As well, the mean hospital stay after surgery did not differ between groups. In contrast, the mean operative time ($p < 0.002$) and blood loss ($p < 0.026$) were significantly higher in the stemmed than in the stemless group. One humeral-sided complication, consisting of a greater tuberosity fracture, was seen in the stemmed group and no complications occurred in the stemless group.

Stemless Reverse Shoulder Arthroplasty

Reverse shoulder arthroplasty has changed the treatment of a variety of shoulder pathologies, including severe deformity. Similar to anatomic shoulder arthroplasty, reverse shoulder arthroplasty has evolved, and stemless implants are available, potentially offering similar benefits (Fig. 3.8). However, it is unclear whether the promising short- and midterm outcomes of stemless anatomic arthroplasty can be extrapolated to stemless reverse shoulder arthroplasty, since the differences in design, force directions, and magnitudes are drastically different in reverse shoulder arthroplasty.

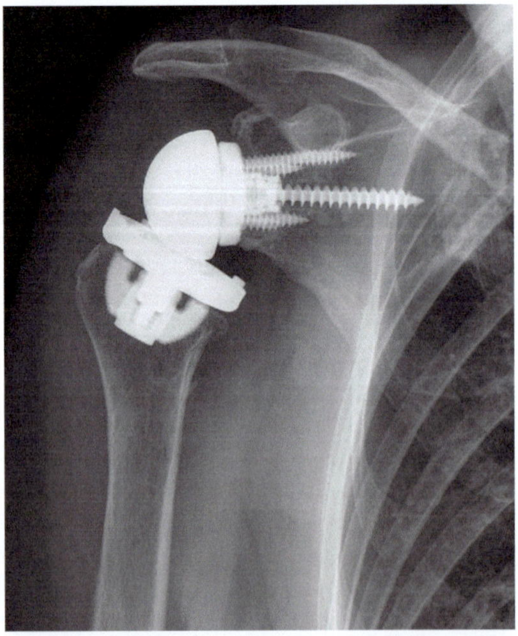

Fig. 3.8 A stemless reverse shoulder arthroplasty (Comprehensive Nano, Zimmer-Biomet Inc.)

Ballas and Beguin reported on 56 stemless reverse implants with a mean 59 months follow-up [26]. They found improvements in outcome scores (Constant and Oxford shoulder) and range of motion. They reported no incidence of humeral component loosening, but one patient required conversion to a conventional stemmed reverse prosthesis for recurrent instability. Another patient developed significant osteolysis around the greater tuberosity although displacement of the humeral component did not occur. Teissier et al. reported a prospective series of 91 stemless reverse implants with a mean follow-up of 41 months [27]. Patient satisfaction was reported as good or excellent in 96%. They also showed good improvement in outcome scores (Constant and ASES) and range of motion. There were no cases of humeral component loosening. Engelhardt et al. reported a series of 67 reverse implants, 56 of which were stemless, with a short-term mean follow-up of 17 months [28]. The outcome scores (Constant and DASH) were reported as good, however were not separated into stemmed and stemless. They found no cases of humeral loosening in the cuff tear arthropathy group (58 cases) but 1 case of stemless humeral loosening in the revision surgery group (9 cases). Although, the revision group was underrepresented, the authors cautioned against using a stemless reverse implant in revision cases where metaphyseal bone could be compromised. Kadum et al. reported 17 stemless reverse implants with a short-term mean follow-up of 14 months [29]. Their outcomes were not stratified by implant type (stemmed, stemless, anatomic, and reverse). They reported one case of failure of a stemless humeral implant, which was converted to a stemmed implant. No other humeral components had any evidence of radiolucent lines or loosening. Kadum et al. reported 40 shoulders followed for an average of 39 months [30]. Although there were large inequalities in the groups and relatively low numbers, the outcomes between stemmed and stemless implants were similar. However, they noted two early revisions in the stemless group due to displacement of the humeral implant. Moroder et al. published [31] a case-control series of 24 patients with cuff tear arthropathy treated with a stemless reverse arthroplasty, who were matched against 24 controls treated with a stemmed reverse arthroplasty. Follow-up was an average 35 months. No significant difference was found in outcome score (Constant, ASES, pain), satisfaction, range of motion, or strength. No cases of humeral component loosening were noted in either group.

Overall, the literature shows promising results in the short to midterm with a stemless reverse arthroplasty. There are more reported failures of this type of humeral implant compared to the stemmed version, but studies are limited, and no studies have elucidated specific indications or risks for failure. There have been no randomized stemmed vs. stemless studies for a reverse arthroplasty. Therefore, although early results seem promising, there is much work to be done in this area before a stemless reverse shoulder arthroplasty can be deemed to be safe and reliable with predictable outcomes.

Conclusions

Stemless shoulder arthroplasty offers many potential advantages including greater versatility in matching native anatomy, bone preservation, and less difficult revision surgery. These advantages may offer particular benefits in the setting of severe proximal humeral deformity. The currently available short- to midterm results are promising but much more research is needed to determine long-term survival. For stemless reverse arthroplasty, the limited reported outcomes appear similar to the stemmed reverse implants. However, there may be a higher failure rate, and the specific indications and risks for failure have not been identified.

References

1. Churchill RS. Stemless shoulder arthroplasty: current status. J Shoulder Elb Surg. 2014;23(9):1409–14.
2. Collin P, Matsukawa T, Boileau P, Brunner U, Walch G. Is the humeral stem useful in anatomic total shoulder arthroplasty? Int Orthop (SICOT). 2017;41(5):1035–9.
3. Bohsali KI, Wirth MA, Rockwood CA. Complications of total shoulder arthroplasty. J Bone Joint Surg Am. 2006;88(10):2279–92.
4. Gonzalez J-F, Alami GB, Baque F, Walch G, Boileau P. Complications of unconstrained shoulder prostheses. J Shoulder Elb Surg. 2011;20(4):666–82.
5. Churchill RS, Athwal GS. Stemless shoulder arthroplasty-current results and designs. Curr Rev Musculoskelet Med. 2016;9(1):10–6.
6. Athwal GS, Sperling JW, Rispoli DM, Cofield RH. Periprosthetic humeral fractures during shoulder arthroplasty. J Bone Joint Surg Am. 2009;91(3):594–603.
7. Boyd AD, Thornhill TS, Barnes CL. Fractures adjacent to humeral prostheses. J Bone Joint Surg Am. 1992;74(10):1498–504.
8. Worland RL, Kim DY, Arredondo J. Periprosthetic humeral fractures: management and classification. J Shoulder Elb Surg. 1999;8(6):590–4.
9. Huguet D, Declercq G, Rio B, Teissier J, Zipoli B, TESS Group. Results of a new stemless shoulder prosthesis: radiologic proof of maintained fixation and stability after a minimum of three years' follow-up. J Shoulder Elb Surg. 2010;19(6):847–52.
10. Petriccioli D, Bertone C, Marchi G. Stemless shoulder arthroplasty: a literature review. Joints. 2015;3(1):38–41.
11. Athwal GS. Spare the canal: stemless shoulder arthroplasty is finally here: commentary on an article by R. Sean Churchill, MD, et al.: "clinical and radiographic outcomes of the simpliciti canal-sparing shoulder arthroplasty system. A prospective two-year multicenter study". J Bone Joint Surg Am. 2016;98(7):e28.
12. Beck S, Beck V, Wegner A, Dudda M, Patsalis T, Jäger M. Long-term survivorship of stemless anatomical shoulder replacement. Int Orthop (SICOT). 2018.
13. Hawi N, Magosch P, Tauber M, Lichtenberg S, Habermeyer P. Nine-year outcome after anatomic stemless shoulder prosthesis: clinical and radiologic results. J Shoulder Elb Surg. 2017;26(9):1609–15.
14. Bell SN, Coghlan JA. Short stem shoulder replacement. Int J Shoulder Surg. 2014;8(3):72–5.
15. Ballas R, Teissier P, Teissier J. Stemless shoulder prosthesis for treatment of proximal humeral malunion does not require tuberosity osteotomy. Int Orthop (SICOT). 2016;40(7):1473–9.
16. Maier MW, Lauer S, Klotz MC, Bülhoff M, Spranz D, Zeifang F. Are there differences between stemless and conventional stemmed shoulder prostheses in the treatment of glenohumeral osteoarthritis? BMC Musculoskelet Disord. 2015;16(1):275.
17. Cruickshank DW, Bicknell RT. Stemless shoulder replacement: a new concept for shoulder arthritis. Curr Orthop Pract. 2017;28(2):153–0.
18. Boileau P, Trojani C, Walch G, Krishnan SG, Romeo A, Sinnerton R. Shoulder arthroplasty for the treatment of the sequelae of fractures of the proximal humerus. J Shoulder Elb Surg. 2001;10(4):299–308.

19. Mariotti U, Motta P, Stucchi A, di Sant'Angelo FP. Stemmed versus stemless total shoulder arthroplasty: a preliminary report and short-term results. Musculoskelet Surg. 2014;98(3):195–200.
20. Uschok S, Magosch P, Moe M, Lichtenberg S, Habermeyer P. Is the stemless humeral head replacement clinically and radiographically a secure equivalent to standard stem humeral head replacement in the long-term follow-up? A prospective randomized trial. J Shoulder Elb Surg. 2017;26(2):225–32.
21. Churchill RS, Chuinard C, Wiater JM, Friedman R, Freehill M, Jacobson S, et al. Clinical and radiographic outcomes of the simpliciti canal-sparing shoulder arthroplasty system: a prospective two-year multicenter study. J Bone Joint Surg Am. 2016;98(7):552–60.
22. Habermeyer P, Lichtenberg S, Tauber M, Magosch P. Midterm results of stemless shoulder arthroplasty: a prospective study. J Shoulder Elb Surg. 2015;24(9):1463–72.
23. Razmjou H, Holtby R, Christakis M, Axelrod T, Richards R. Impact of prosthetic design on clinical and radiologic outcomes of total shoulder arthroplasty: a prospective study. J Shoulder Elb Surg. 2013;22(2):206–14.
24. Neer CS. The classic: articular replacement for the humeral head 1955. Clin Orthop Relat Res. 2011;469:2409–21.
25. Berth A, Pap G. Stemless shoulder prosthesis versus conventional anatomic shoulder prosthesis in patients with osteoarthritis: a comparison of the functional outcome after a minimum of two years follow-up. J Orthop Traumatol. 2013;14(1):31–7.
26. Ballas R, Béguin L. Results of a stemless reverse shoulder prosthesis at more than 58 months mean without loosening. J Shoulder Elb Surg. 2013;22(9):e1–6.
27. Teissier P, Teissier J, Kouyoumdjian P, Asencio G. The TESS reverse shoulder arthroplasty without a stem in the treatment of cuff-deficient shoulder conditions: clinical and radiographic results. J Shoulder Elb Surg. 2015;24(1):45–51.
28. Engelhardt v LV, Manzke M, Filler TJ, Jerosch J. Short-term results of the reverse Total Evolutive Shoulder System (TESS) in cuff tear arthropathy and revision arthroplasty cases. Arch Orthop Trauma Surg. 2015;135(7):897–904.
29. Kadum B, Hassany H, Wadsten M, Sayed-Noor A, Sjödén G. Geometrical analysis of stemless shoulder arthroplasty: a radiological study of seventy TESS total shoulder prostheses. Int Orthop (SICOT). 2016;40(4):751–8.
30. Kadum B, Mukka S, Englund E, Sayed-Noor A, Sjödén G. Clinical and radiological outcome of the Total Evolutive Shoulder System (TESS®) reverse shoulder arthroplasty: a prospective comparative non-randomised study. Int Orthop (SICOT). 2014;38(5):1001–6.
31. Moroder P, Ernstbrunner L, Zweiger C, Schatz M, Seitlinger G, Skursky R, et al. Short to mid-term results of stemless reverse shoulder arthroplasty in a selected patient population compared to a matched control group with stem. Int Orthop (SICOT). 2016;40(10):2115–20.

4 Anatomic Shoulder Arthroplasty in the Setting of Glenoid Bony Erosion (Walch B2-, B3-, and C-Type Glenoids)

Jay D. Keener

Introduction

Anatomic total shoulder arthroplasty (TSA) has been shown to be a reliable surgery for pain relief, improvement of shoulder function, and quality of life. The presence of biconcave glenoid deformity poses a significant reconstructive challenge for a shoulder surgeon as this deformity has been associated with poorer clinical outcomes and a higher rate of complications. Reconstructive options are largely dictated by the severity of the glenoid deformity and the degree of preoperative humeral head subluxation; however, other factors such as patient age and activity level and rotator cuff muscle health must be considered in choosing the optimal treatment option for these patients.

Recent research has better defined the morphologic changes seen in these shoulders including adaptive bony changes. The role of computerized tomography (CT) scans has been extensively studied in attempts to better define these deformities. Additionally, software programs, which reformat CT scan images, can generate three-dimensional bony reconstructions, now allowing real-time computer simulation of surgery with generation of patient-specific instrumentation when needed. This chapter will review the relevant pathologic anatomic considerations, diagnostic imaging options, and anatomic TSA reconstructive options for shoulders with biconcave glenoid deformities.

J. D. Keener (✉)
Shoulder and Elbow Service, Washington University, St. Louis, MO, USA
e-mail: keener@wudosis.wustl.edu

Etiology and Incidence

Walch et al. originally classified glenoid morphology based on the pattern of glenoid bone wear and the presence or absence of humeral head subluxation [1]. Arthritis with a posteriorly subluxated humeral head was designated as a B-type glenoid and further classified as B1 or B2 deformity based on the degree on bone erosion (Fig. 4.1). In his original series of 113 subjects, 32% of arthritic shoulders were classified as B type. Type B1 deformities (17% incidence) were associated with posterior humeral head subluxation and posterior joint space narrowing. Type B2 deformities (15%) demonstrated posterior glenoid bone erosion producing a posterior cupula and a resultant biconcave appearance of the glenoid. Type C deformities were originally classified as a retroversion deformity of greater than 25° as measured by the Friedman method, not caused from glenoid erosion. Type C glenoids were felt to be dysplastic in origin. The authors noted increased retroversion of B-type shoulders (mean 18°) but did not feel that retroversion explained the biconcavity of the glenoid. CT scan analysis of the same cohort suggested that subluxation was responsible for glenoid erosive changes [2]. The authors concluded that posterior

R. Z. Tashjian (ed.), *Complex and Revision Shoulder Arthroplasty*,
https://doi.org/10.1007/978-3-030-02756-8_4

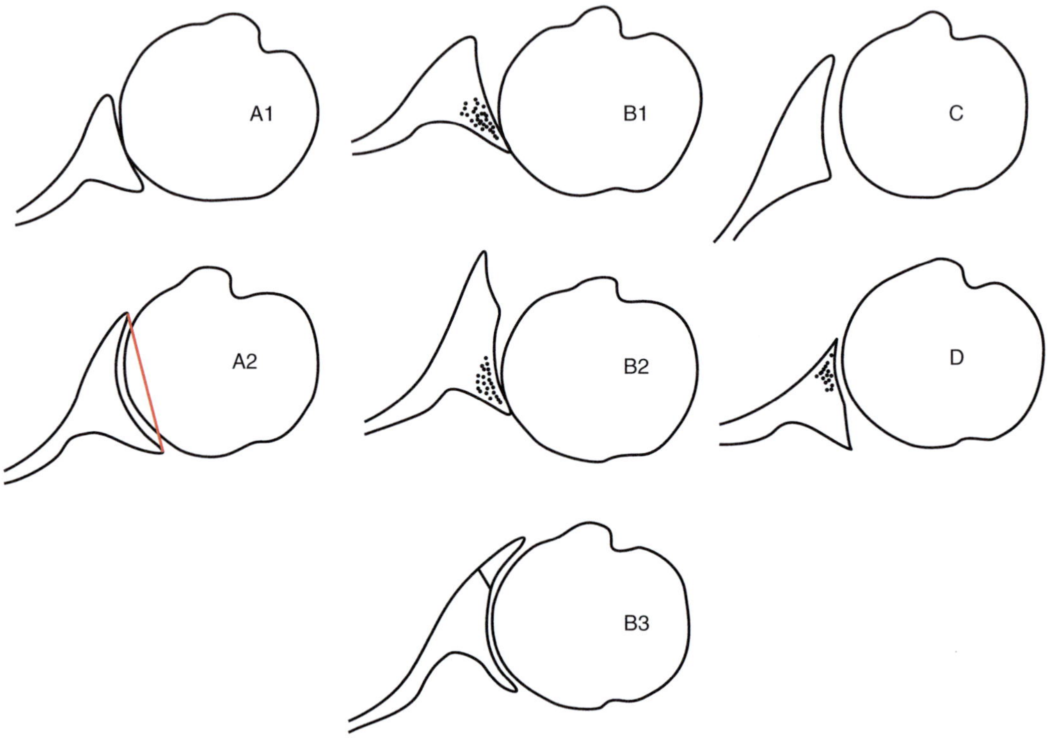

Fig. 4.1 Modified Walch classification of glenoid morphology in primary glenohumeral osteoarthritis. (**a**) Schematic representation of the modified Walch classification of glenoid morphology. The B-type glenoids are associated with posterior subluxation and variable amounts of posterior glenoid erosion. (Reference: Bercik et al. [27]. Fig. 2, page 1602)

subluxation did not correlate with glenoid retroversion.

The incidence of posterior glenoid erosion is in the range of 30–40% of shoulders with primary osteoarthritis [1, 3]. The etiology of posterior glenoid erosion in the setting of primary osteoarthritis is unknown. Multiple authors have noted a lack of correlation between glenoid retroversion and the degree of humeral head subluxation and subsequent glenoid wear [1, 4, 5]. This suggests that retroversion does not create subluxation but rather results from subluxation and the subsequent abnormal wear over time. Ricchetti et al. using the glenoid vault model demonstrated the premorbid glenoid version of osteoarthritic shoulders was similar to normal controls [6, 7]. The concept of abnormal premorbid glenoid version for B2 shoulder is debated, however. Knowles et al. showed the native version of the paleoglenoid region in B2 arthritic shoulders was more retroverted (mean 14°) compared to normal controls (mean 5°), suggesting these shoulders may possess an intrinsic predisposition toward posterior subluxation [8]. Walch described the pathologic condition of static posterior humeral head subluxation as a precursor to the development of arthritis with a posterior glenoid wear pattern [9]. This condition is felt to be distinct from acquired posterior instability or glenoid dysplasia but is rather acquired over time. It has been theorized that the static posterior humeral head subluxation that precedes the development of posterior glenoid wear is a result of various static and dynamic soft tissue parameters that have yet to be elucidated [10].

Evaluation

The clinical evaluation begins with assessment of shoulder active and passive range of motion (ROM) and rotator cuff strength. Standard radiographs are generally adequate to both determine the severity of arthritis and properly classify the glenoid morphology. These include a standard shoulder series including an anteroposterior view, true anteroposterior view, scapular Y, and axillary views. The axillary view is important to identify posterior humeral head subluxation and identify abnormal patterns of glenoid wear but is not accurate in quantifying the glenoid version and inclination angles.

For shoulders with significant glenoid wear secondary to osteoarthritis, a CT scan is recommended. CT scans allow for detailed analysis of glenoid deformity and humeral head subluxation and also allow assessment of fatty muscle infiltration and atrophy of the rotator cuff musculature. Fine cuts (1 mm or less) are recommended to allow for three-dimensional rendering of the bony anatomy. If possible, the scanning protocol should include the entire scapula. Because the gantry angle of the CT is oriented in reference to the body, the gantry is off axis in relation to the glenohumeral joint. Several studies have demonstrated improved accuracy in measuring glenoid version and inclination of three-dimensional CT scan images compared to two-dimensional images [11–14]. One study demonstrated that uncorrected two-dimensional images overestimate glenoid retroversion by 2–5° and glenoid inclination by a mean of 21° compared to two-dimensional images with a corrected gantry angle [12]. Using corrected two-dimensional images, the glenoid version is assessed by the Friedman method on axial images either using the intermediate glenoid line (a line connecting the anterior paleoglenoid to the posterior neoglenoid edges) or the neoglenoid surface (Fig. 4.2). The percent

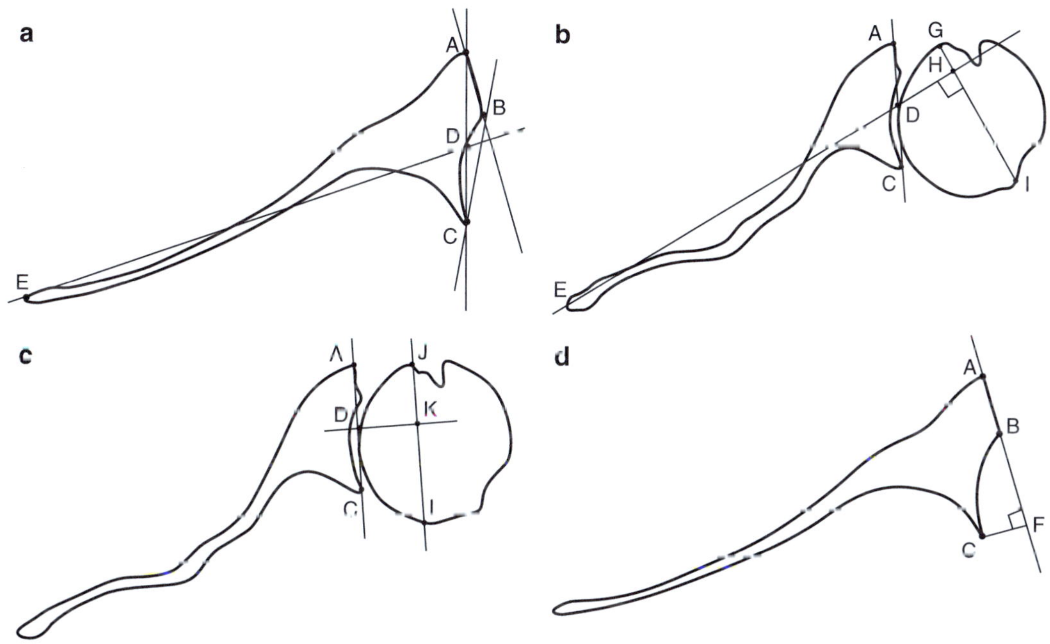

Fig. 4.2 Definitions of glenoid radiographic measures for the biconcave glenoid. Axial view (CT scan) of the shoulder. (**a**) Retroversion according to the Friedman line (ED): AB represents the paleoglenoid, BC represents the neoglenoid, and AC is the intermediate glenoid. (**b**) Subluxation with regard to the scapular body (scapular axis) or Friedman line (ED): the percentage of humeral head posterior to that line (HI/GI) is assessed at the longest anteroposterior diameter of the head on a line perpendicular to the scapular axis. (**c**) Subluxation with regard to the glenoid axis (mediatrice line) defined as DK, drawn as a perpendicular line to the intermediate glenoid (AC) passing in its middle (subluxation/glenoid): the percentage of humeral head posterior to that line is measured at the largest anteroposterior diameter (KL/JL). (**d**) Depth of glenoid erosion: CF depth magnitude (mm) corresponds to the perpendicular distance between the posterior border of the glenoid erosion and the paleoglenoid reference line (AF). (Reference: Walch et al. [38]. Fig. 1, page 1527)

humeral head subluxation is usually expressed in relation to the scapular plane, which is an extension of the Friedman scapular line across the humeral head using the axial image with the largest diameter of the humeral head.

In recent years, automated software programs have become increasingly more popular to quantify glenoid bony deformity. These programs will generate a three-dimensional model of the scapula and humeral head. The computer will then calculate a mean glenoid version and percent humeral head subluxation based upon the bony anatomy in reference to the scapular plane (Fig. 4.3). The majority of these programs also allow simulation of surgery by superimposing prosthetic components onto the bony anatomy. These programs allow precise calculation of implant size and seating based on variable amounts of glenoid version correction and reaming. When needed, patient-specific instrumentation (PSI) guides can be generated and implemented in the operating room in an attempt to recreate the surgical plan executed with the computer software. The use of CT scan in the setting glenohumeral osteoarthritis has greatly improved our understanding of complex bony deformities. One study showed significantly improved accuracy in recreating the optimal implant placement following templating with 3D CT scan imaging compared to 2D imaging [15]. The addition of PSI has been shown to further improve the accuracy of ideal glenoid implant positioning [16–18]. Randomized clinical trials have demonstrated improved accuracy of glenoid component placement and version corrected with the use of PSI in glenoids with variable deformities compared to standard surgical techniques [19, 20].

Characteristic Features: B2/B3 Glenoid

There are several characteristic features that define the deformity associated with biconcave (B2) glenoid arthritic shoulders. Asymmetric cartilage wear due to posterior humeral head subluxation occurs initially. Over time the posterior glenoid bone erodes producing the classic biconcave glenoid deformity consisting of the anterior (paleoglenoid) and posterior (neoglenoid) glenoid surfaces (Fig. 4.4). The acquired glenoid retroversion abnormality produced is highly variable with mean values in most series between 16° and 23° [1, 3, 6, 7]. The pattern of glenoid wear occurs in the posteroinferior direction rather than straight posterior [3, 21, 22]. Knowles et al. demonstrated the direction of the line of glenoid erosion was toward the 8 o'clock position for a right shoulder oriented a mean of 28° from the superoinferior axis and was remarkably consistent across deformity severities [21]. In a review of 55 shoulders,

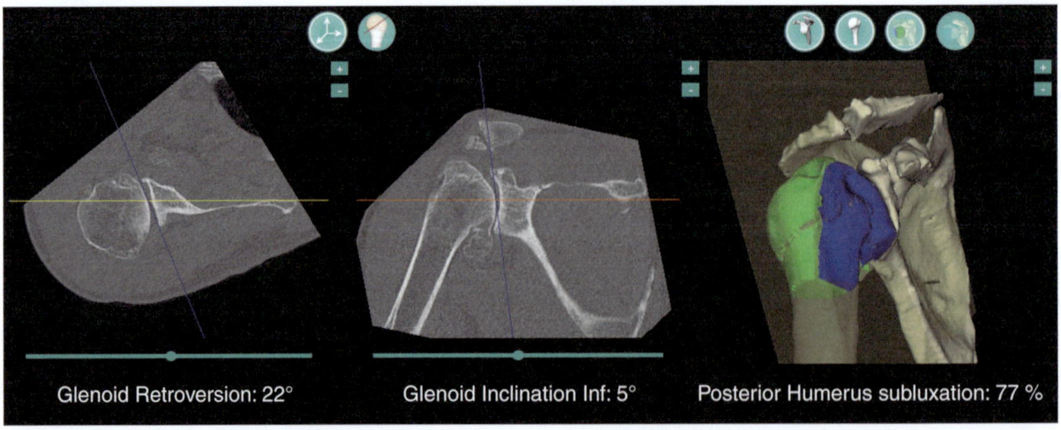

Fig. 4.3 3D reconstruction of a right shoulder with automated calculation of glenoid variables. Proprietary software 3D reconstruction of B2 glenoid with automated calculation of glenoid version, glenoid inclination, and glenoid subluxation. The humeral head in green represents the amount of head posterior to the defined scapular axis; the humeral head in blue represents the amount of head anterior to the scapular axis

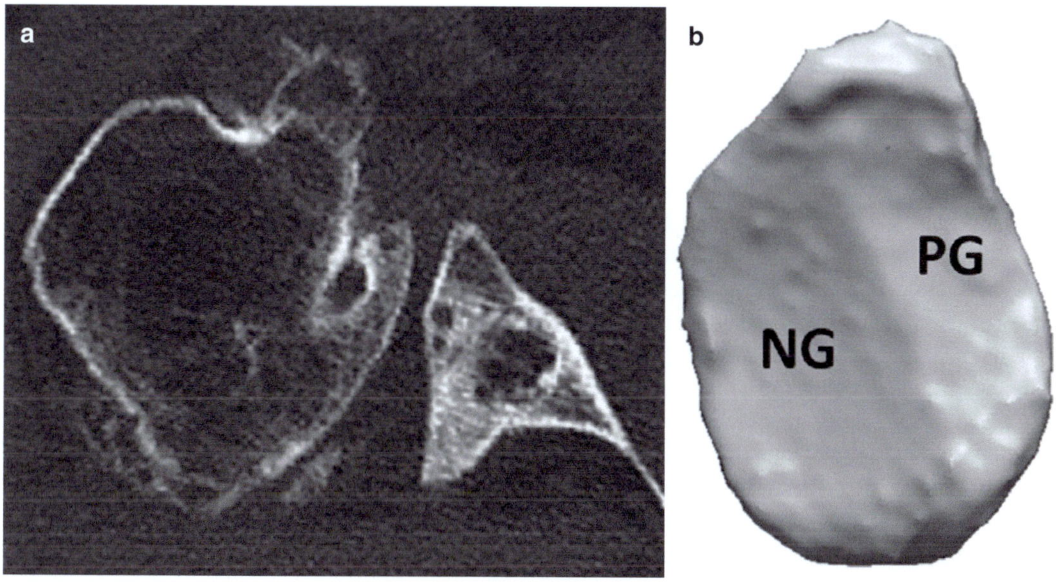

Fig. 4.4 Orientation of the glenoid wear pattern in biconcave glenoid deformities. (**a**) A 2D axial CT scan view of a right shoulder demonstrating an asymmetric type B2 glenoid. (**b**) Sagittal view of a 3D reconstruction demonstrating a B2 glenoid with posteroinferior erosion. The neoglenoid (NG) and paleoglenoid (PG) are depicted. (Reference: Knowles et al. [21]. Fig. 1, page 504)

the proportionate size of the neoglenoid was quite variable and occupied a mean of 44% of the glenoid surface area. The biconcave deformity and resultant posterior bone erosion will vary based on the severity of the deformity; however, the severity of maximal bone erosion is consistently directed to the posteroinferior glenoid (Fig. 4.4). The erosion depth has been shown to be a mean of 4–5 mm in both radiographic and clinical studies [3, 22, 23]. Adaptive changes to the glenoid and humeral head surface features and bone density are common. The radius of curvature of the neoglenoid (mean 37 mm) has been shown to be flatter than the paleoglenoid (mean 34 mm), both of which are greater than the humeral head (mean 32 mm) [21]. Knowles et al. demonstrated significantly greater bone density and less subchondral bone porosity in the neoglenoid compared to the paleoglenoid [24]. This was distinctly different than the uniform bone density changes that were seen in arthritic shoulders with symmetric erosion.

The severity of humeral subluxation in shoulders with a B2/B3 deformity is variable and has been described in a variety of manners. This variability is a result of both deformity severity and the reported methods of subluxation calculation. Subluxation values will depend if the humeral head position is referenced from the scapular plane (humeroscapular) or perpendicular to the glenoid center (humeroglenoid) (Fig. 4.2). Furthermore, variable morphology of the glenoscapular anatomy (the orientation and shape of the glenoid vault in relation to the scapular body) has been shown to affect calculated version and subluxation measurements [4]. Sabesan et al. demonstrated that humeroscapular subluxation values were significantly different than glenoscapular subluxation values in arthritic shoulders [25]. In this series, there was a strong correlation between glenoid retroversion deformity and humeral head subluxation in relation to the centerline of the scapula (humeroscapular relationship). When utilizing the glenoscapular plane, there was variable correlation between glenoid version and subluxation. For the B3 glenoid, progressive erosion results in a humeral head that is consistently centered in the glenoid plane but remains posteriorly subluxated in reference to the scapular plane [26].

Recently, the type B3 glenoid has been described (Fig. 4.1). With this wear pattern, the posterior glenoid is progressively worn to a monoconcave pattern. Bercik et al. stated these shoulders possessed a retroversion of at least 15° or least 70% posterior humeral head subluxation in the presence of significant posterior glenoid wear [27]. Chan et al. in a CT scan analysis of B3 glenoids noted a mean retroversion angle of 24°, a mean superior inclination of 8°, and a mean posterior subluxation of 80% in reference to the scapular plane [26]. These authors noted the joint line to be medialized a mean of 14 mm further suggesting that the B3 glenoid represents a continuum of the B2 glenoid as a result of further glenoid erosion. With progressive erosion the native paleoglenoid disappears as the neoglenoid enlarges. Interestingly, the humeral head appears to become more centered with the B3 deformity. Recentering of the humeral head can be misleading in this situation however, as it is seen primarily in reference to the glenoid plane and not the scapular plane [7, 26]. Iannotti et al., further describing the B3 glenoid using the vault model, suggested the premorbid version of the glenoid to be within normal range and also demonstrated increased medial wear of the joint line compared to B2 deformities [7].

Adaptive changes to the arthritic humeral head are common. Marginal osteophytosis along the anatomic neck is frequently seen and varies in size. Over time the humeral head flattens, and the subchondral bone becomes more dense. Flattening of the humeral head results in an increased diameter without a significant change in head thickness. Knowles et al. demonstrated an increase in the radius of curvature of arthritic humeral heads (mean 59 mm) compared to normal controls (mean 49 mm) [28]. Unlike the glenoid, adaptive changes to the humeral head were similar across all Walch glenoid types.

Treatment Options

Defining Surgical Goals

Placement of an anatomic shoulder arthroplasty in the setting of a glenoid deformity is challenging and requires precise understanding of the type and magnitude of deformity, which will vary greatly between shoulders. The goals of surgery in this setting are to place the prosthetic components in an anatomic manner that will provide adequate implant seating and good joint stability in a durable fashion [29]. Because of the adaptive soft tissue and bony changes seen in these shoulders, soft tissue balancing must be combined with reorientation of the abnormal glenoid version to an acceptable degree. In general, the goals of glenoid implant placement are to correct pathologic glenoid version to within 10° of neutral version, achieve a minimum glenoid implant face support of 80%, and avoid implant perforation at the medial glenoid vault. Correction of version is based upon theoretical concerns of the effects of excessive eccentric loading upon glenoid fixation [30–34], malalignment-induced cement mantle fatigue [31, 35, 36], as well as limited clinical data, suggesting increased risk of the development of radiographic lucencies [37, 38] with excessively retroverted glenoid implants.

On the humeral side, the version angle of the humeral osteotomy should either recreate the native humeral version or perform a slight anteversion correction (to 20–30°). It should be noted that humeral anteversion correction has not been shown to improve prosthetic implant stability in the setting of experimental posterior glenoid loss [29, 39]. The methods chosen to achieve these stated goals will depend upon the magnitude of the glenoid deformity, the severity of humeral head subluxation, patient-related factors (age, activity level, and shoulder range of motion), and surgeon preferences.

Partial Glenoid Version Correction (High-Side Reaming)

Partial correction of excessive glenoid retroversion in the setting of B2 glenoid through high-side reaming has long been an accepted method of treating these deformities. The goal of this surgery is to reorient the glenoid into an acceptable version angle. The potential benefits of high-side reaming relate to its simplicity by avoiding the use of augmented components or bone grafting. However, given the limited bone stock of the glenoid vault and the magnitude of deformities often encountered, there are limits to the severity of glenoid deformities that can be treated with this technique. The potential negative consequences of high-side reaming are significant. Excessive reaming will medialize the joint line and affect soft tissue tension, rotator cuff function, and glenohumeral stability. Currently, it is unknown what effect glenoid version correction has upon the adaptive soft tissue changes that have occurred in these shoulders. Additionally, clinical data is lacking regarding the ideal glenoid component position for proper soft tissue balancing in shoulders with glenoid erosion. Reaming will violate variable amounts of glenoid cortical bone and expose the weaker trabecular bone depending on the severity of the deformity [3, 36, 40, 41]. Reaming may also require downsizing the glenoid component to match the size of the glenoid face and risks perforation of the medial glenoid vault with the pegs/keels [42, 43]. This latter risk is somewhat dependent on the shape and morphology of the glenoid implant design (peripheral versus in-line pegs).

Partial correction through high-side reaming is most accurately performed after surgical planning using CT software. The challenge for the surgeon is to execute the surgical plan with accuracy at the time of surgery. Iannotti et al. have shown that even when a deformity is within correctable limits, it is not always technically possible even in the hands of an experienced surgeon [44]. When necessary, the use of PSI instruments can properly orient and guide the glenoid preparation based upon bony landmarks. Given the shape and dimensions of the glenoid, one can predict the amount of glenoid version correction achievable with reaming. In general, 1 mm of anterior high-side glenoid reaming anteverts the glenoid by 2°. Chen demonstrated that for every 5° angular reaming correction increment, the mean reaming depth increased by 1.4 mm [41]. The limits of reaming are debatable and dictated somewhat by the size of the glenoid and available bone stock and the willingness to breach cortical bone. Cadaveric studies have suggested the maximal amount of corrective reaming of the glenoid to be 10–15° before excessive bone loss and/or medial implant perforation occurs when attempting to correct to neutral version [42, 43, 45]. For these reasons, acquired retroversion deformity greater than 20–25° represent the upper limit of deformity that can be corrected with high-side reaming alone if the acceptance of some degree of residual retroversion is tolerable. Breaching the anterior glenoid surface cortical bone is common with corrective reaming, which will compromise the quality of the remaining bone. Chen et al. showed significantly decreased remaining bone quality (approximately 15–20% decreased bone density) of the anterior glenoid after corrective reaming of 10° and 15° compared to 0° and 5° reaming [41]. Another clinical study examined corrective reaming of B2 glenoids (mean retroversion 18°, range 8–43°) in vivo with the goals of partial correction to achieve a minimum of 80% glenoid component support and a version angle to within 10° of the paleoglenoid [3]. In this series, 47% of the glenoids were not able to be 100% seated, and compromise of more than 50% of the subchondral cortical bone was necessary in 30% of shoulders to achieve adequate support. A biomechanical study by Wang et al. compared the performance of cemented all-polyethylene glenoid placed with eccentric reaming to a wedge-shaped augmented glenoid component [46]. A 12° posterior glenoid defect was created. An 8° augmented implant was compared to a standard glenoid placed with eccentric reaming to neutral version. The standard implant had less micromotion and catastrophic fixation failure after cyclical loading compared to the augmented component.

Figure 4.5 illustrates a case of corrective high-side reaming for a severe B2 glenoid deformity (29° intermediate glenoid line retroversion on corrected 2D CT scan axial slice at the mid-glenoid) performed with a freehand technique in a 52-year-old female. Exposure to the glenoid is facilitated by removal of anterior glenoid osteophytes and/or the anterior glenoid rim. The geometric center of the glenoid is marked with cautery. The junction of the anterior glenoid vault and the scapular body is palpated to determine

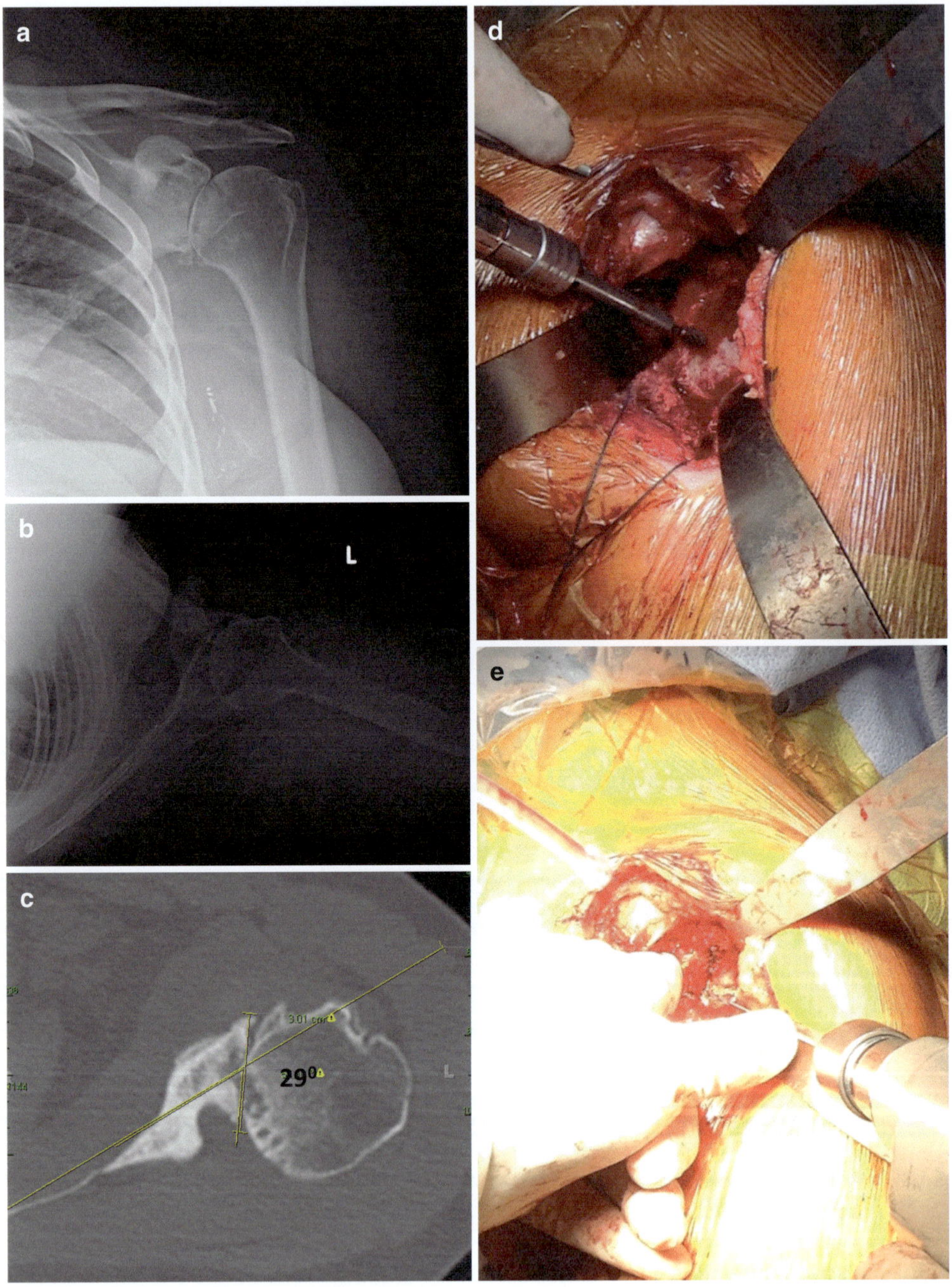

Fig. 4.5 Stepwise performance of partial glenoid version correction with high-side reaming. (**a**) True AP view of the left shoulder of a 52-year-old with glenohumeral arthritis. (**b**) Axillary view demonstrating posterior glenoid wear and humeral head subluxation. (**c**) Two-dimensional axial CT slice in which the gantry angle has been corrected to the plane of the scapula. The patient has a type B3 glenoid. Glenoid retroversion measures 29°. (**d**) Intraoperative view of the same shoulder. A burr is used to remove some anterior glenoid osteophyte and improve exposure. (**e**) A 2.0 mm drill is used to sound the depth of the glenoid vault at the desired version correction angle which is facilitated by palpating the junction of the anterior glenoid and scapular body. (**f**) The central peg tunnel is drilled at the desired version correction angle. (**g**) A glenoid reamer is used to ream the high (anterior) glenoid bone to the desired version angle. Approximately 5–6 mm of bone is removed anteriorly. (**h**) The anterior glenoid is reamed medially at the same angle until there is support of a minimum of 80% of the glenoid face. (**i**) The glenoid is cemented once the desired seating is determined. (**j**) True AP view of the same shoulder 2 years postoperatively. Nonprogressive radiolucent line is seen around the inferior peg. (**k**) Axillary view of the same shoulder. The humeral head is well-centered

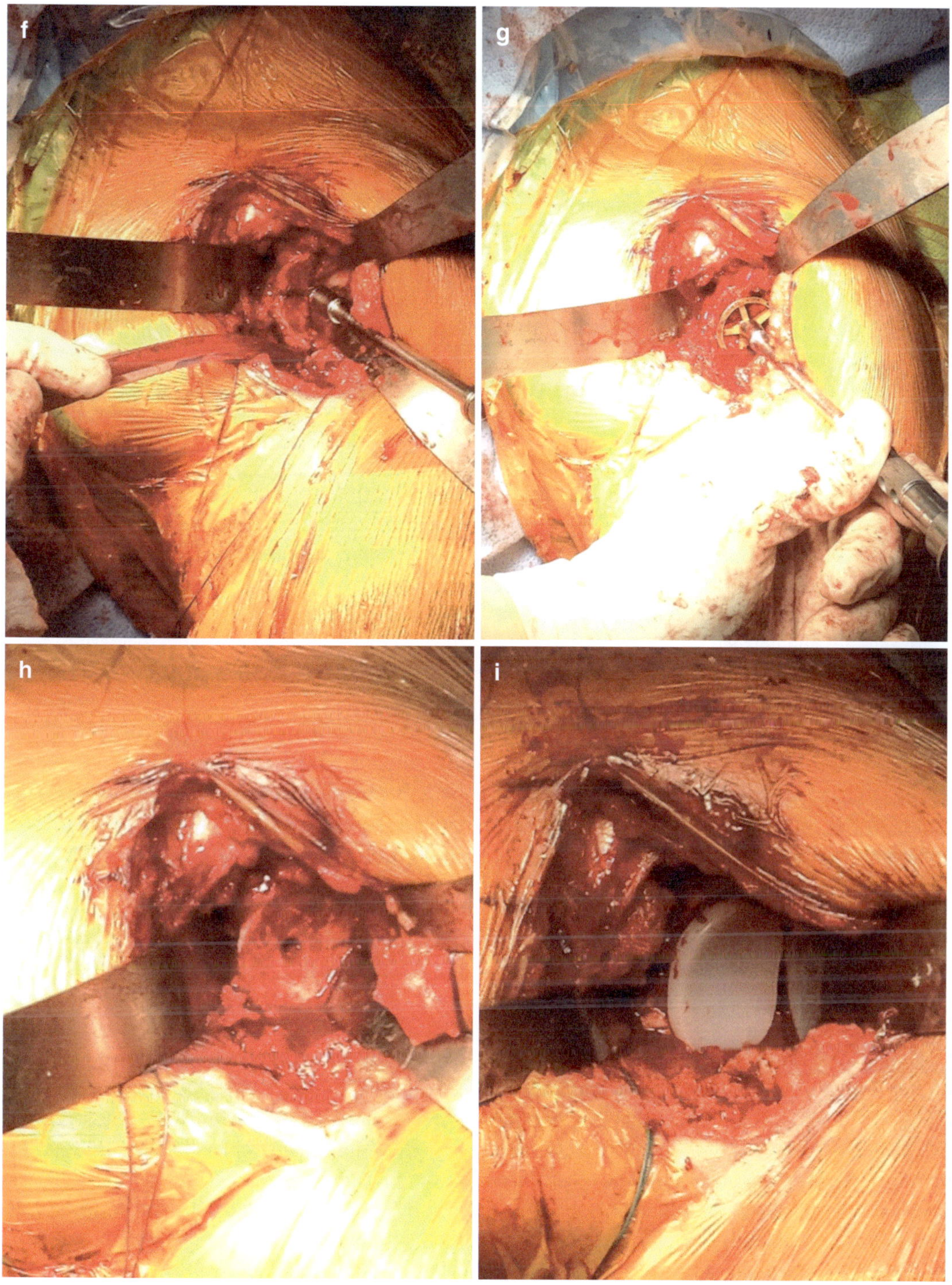

Fig. 4.5 (continued)

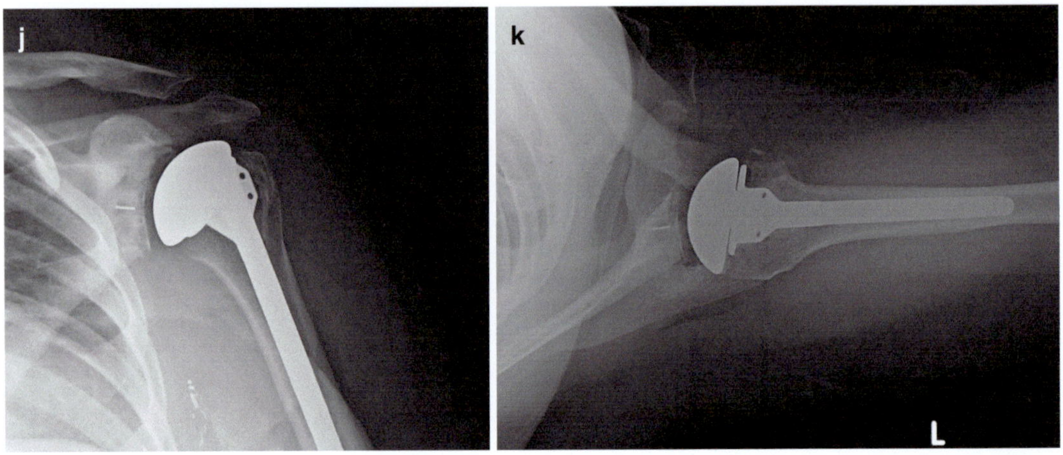

Fig. 4.5 (continued)

the position of the maximum glenoid vault depth. A 2 mm drill is used to sound the glenoid vault depth at the desired version correction angle (in this case approximately 15° or 6–7 mm high-side reaming). The central tunnel is drilled at the same starting point and correction angle as determined by the sounding drill. The glenoid face is reamed until roughly 80–90% glenoid implant face support is achieved. Alternatively, glenoid reaming can be performed over a central guide pin placed either freehand or with the aid of a PSI guide. In this case, the cortical bone is breached anteriorly to achieve adequate seating at the desired correction angle. This case illustrates the upper limits of deformity that can be treated with corrective high-side reaming alone.

One goal of anatomic shoulder arthroplasty is to achieve a well-centered humeral head. In some cases, due to joint line medialization, excessive posterior subluxation of the humeral head is seen during intraoperative trialing. It is important in these shoulders to emphasize stability trailing with various head size options after placement of the glenoid component to avoid postoperative instability. Options to augment stability are to upsize the humeral head size or thickness, placement of plication sutures in the posterior capsule or to dial an eccentric humeral head to an anterior offset position. The latter technique has been shown to increase the resistance to posterior humeral head translation and improve joint loading in cadaveric shoulders with simulated glenoid retroversion deformities (Fig. 4.6) [47]. With this technique, restoration of the normal head to tuberosity relationship is important to optimize rotator cuff function. A clinical study of 33 shoulder arthroplasties showed significant improvement in humeral head centering (referenced from the glenoid center) compared to preoperative radiographs (mean 10.4% preoperative vs. 0.9% postoperative subluxation) utilizing anterior eccentric humeral head placement [48]. A potential downside of a reversed offset humeral head is the potential for increased pressure on the subscapularis repair from the anterior overhang of the humeral head. However, the single published series related to this technique noted no instances of subscapularis clinical failure postoperatively [48].

Posterior Glenoid Bone Grafting

Another option for managing posterior glenoid bone loss during anatomic shoulder arthroplasty is the placement of structural bone graft. Bone grafting is generally indicated in patients with more severe acquired retroversion deformities (20–30°) where high-side reaming alone to achieve the desired goal of version correction is either not sufficient or not desired. Because of the increased popularity of reverse shoulder arthroplasty in these situations, posterior bone grafting is usually recommended for patients that are con-

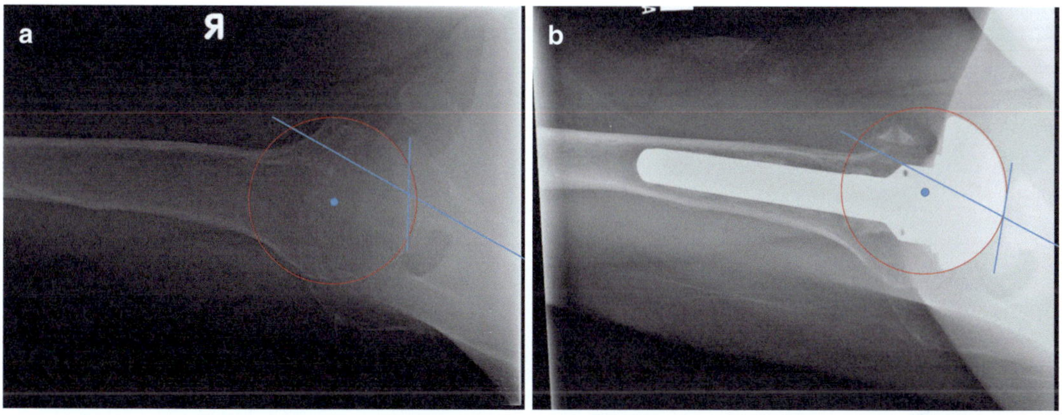

Fig. 4.6 Reverse offset humeral head. (**a**) Axillary view of the right shoulder with a B3 glenoid deformity. Note the significant posterior subluxation of the humerus in relation to the scapular plane as defined by the Friedman line. (**b**) Axillary view following anatomic shoulder arthroplasty with a reverse (anterior) offset humeral head and partial corrective anterior glenoid reaming. Note the improved alignment of the prosthetic humeral head in relation to the scapular plane

sidered either too young or active for RSA. The potential benefits of bone grafting are restoration of an acceptable version angle without excessive reaming and medialization of the joint line. This will potentially augment glenohumeral stability and rotator cuff function. Limitations of this procedure are related to concerns for lack of bone graft incorporation or graft resorption. Additionally, technical expertise is required for this procedure.

Ideally autologous bone graft from the humeral head is commonly utilized. The articular surface of the humeral head mates well with the radius of curvature of the neoglenoid. The appropriate size and thickness are determined following partial reaming of the native glenoid (Fig. 4.7). The neoglenoid cortical bone is perforated at several points with a small drill or pin to facilitate healing of the graft. The graft is fixated with small screws (2.4 or 2.7 mm) which are countersunk under the trabecular surface. Multiple screws provide increased compression and fixation of the graft. Final reaming of the grafted surface is performed prior to implant placement.

Figure 4.7 illustrates a technique of partial glenoid version correction with high-side reaming combined with placement of a posterior glenoid autologous bone graft. In this case severe B2 deformity with glenoid retroversion of 38° and posterior humeral head subluxation of 93% is seen in this 51-year-old male. Initially corrective high-side reaming of the anterior glenoid is performed free hand with an estimated correction of 15–20°. After reaming, the posterior third of the glenoid remains unsupported. To prevent further medialization and bone loss from reaming, a bone graft is placed in the posterior glenoid. The graft is fashioned from the resected humeral. Generally, the radius of curvature of the anterior humeral head matches that of the posterior neoglenoid. The graft is reduced and held in place with two K-wires. The graft is then fixated with three 2.4 mm screws with small heads. The screws are countersunk into the graft surface, and the graft is gently reamed flush with the central and anterior glenoid-reamed surface. The postoperative radiographs show good graft placement and recentering of the humeral head. In this case, the eccentric humeral head is dialed into an anterior or reversed offset position to counterbalance posterior humeral subluxation.

Augmented Glenoid Implants

Much like glenoid bone grafting, augmented glenoid implants are indicated for deformities considered too large for corrective reaming to obtain the desired

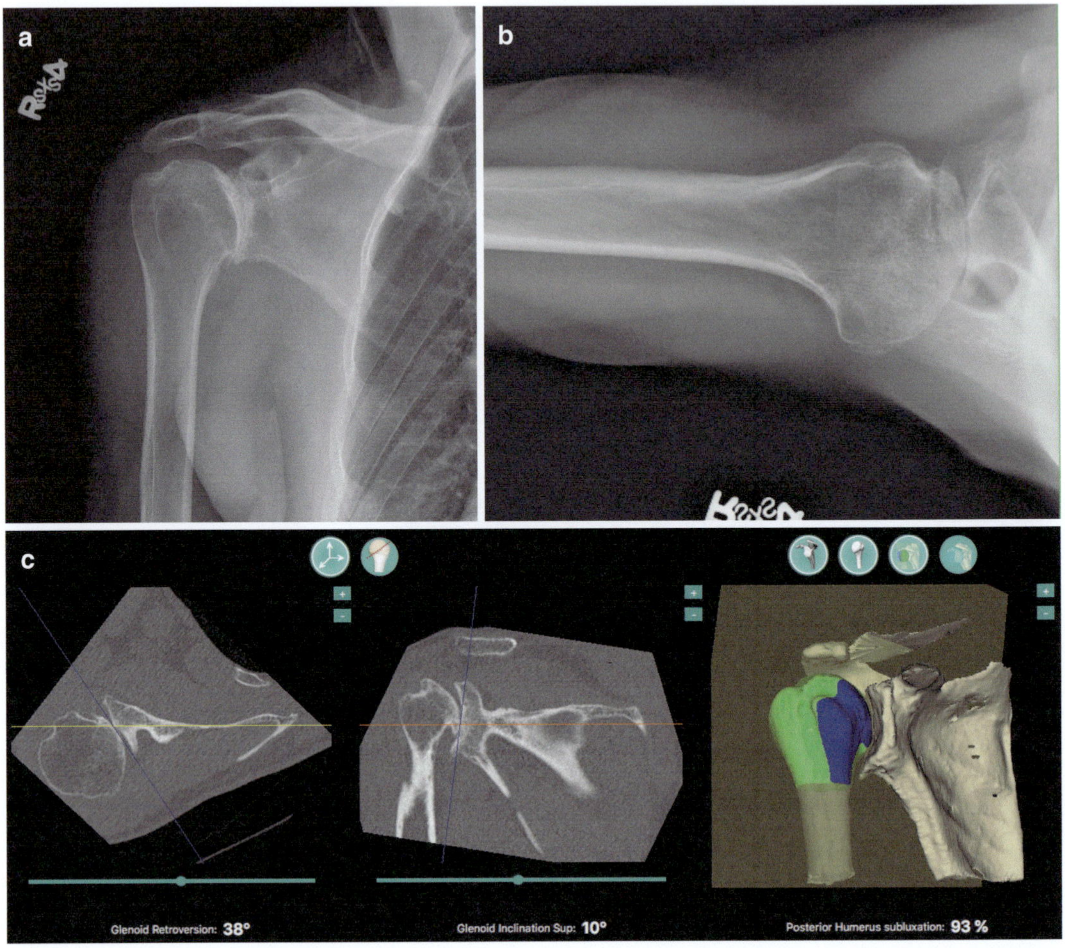

Fig. 4.7 B2 glenoid managed with posterior glenoid bone graft. (**a**) True AP view of the right shoulder of a 57-year-old male with advanced glenohumeral osteoarthritis. (**b**) Axillary view of the same shoulder demonstrating severe posterior humeral head subluxation and a biconcave glenoid (B2 deformity). (**c**) Three-dimensional software analysis of a CT scan of the same shoulder. Glenoid retroversion measures 38°. (**d**) Intraoperative picture of the same shoulder. Placement of an autologous bone graft from the humeral head fashioned to the size of the defect. (**e**) The graft has been fixation with screws buried under the surface of the bone. Final glenoid reaming has been performed for adequate seating of the implant. (**f**) Postoperative true AP film of the same shoulder demonstrating fixation of the graft. (**g**) Postoperative axillary view demonstrating full seating of the glenoid implant and improved position of the humeral head

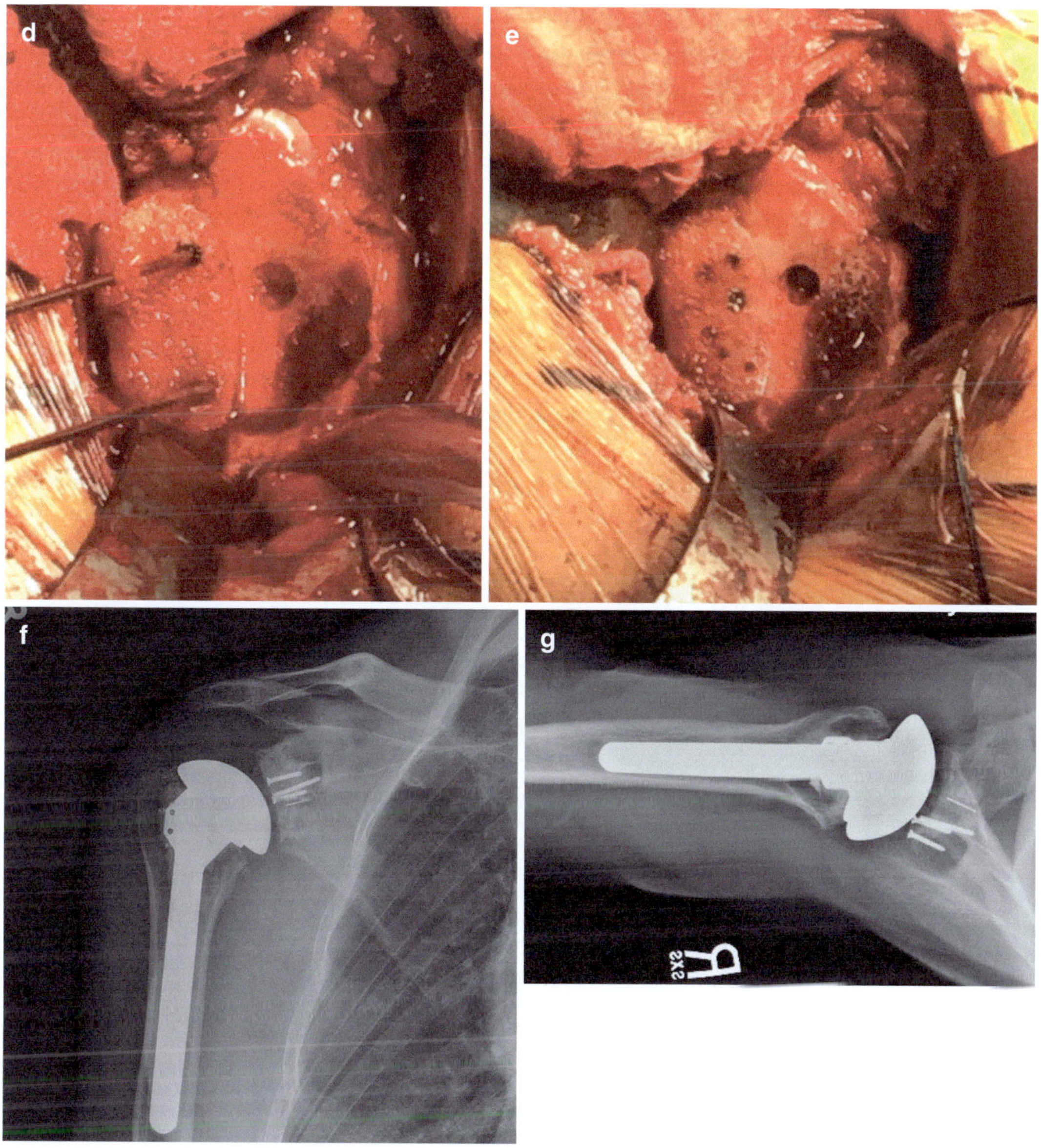

Fig. 4.7 (continued)

glenoid version. The use of augmented glenoids can also be utilized in smaller deformities if corrective reaming is not preferred. The advantages of augments include the ability to correct glenoid version with minimal reaming and without medialization of the joint line. This will optimize glenohumeral stability and rotator cuff function and maximize the size of the articular surface.

Augmented polyethylene glenoid implants have become increasingly popular in recent years, and early clinical results are promising. However, the available clinical data is only short term, and longevity compared to standard implants is unknown. Additionally, depending on the shape and size of the augment and the desired final version, variable amounts of bone must be removed to accommodate the implant. Basic science data have revealed several relative advantages of various augment designs. Computer modeling demonstrated less bone resection with a posterior wedge-shaped augment compared to a full-wedge and posterior-step augment with better bone density in the residual glenoid for B2 deformities (Fig. 4.8) [49]. Another study compared the volume of bone removed with computer simulated corrective reaming and placement of a standard, full-wedge and posterior-step augmented glenoids [50]. In this series of B2 glenoids, the mean retroversion angle was 21°, and the mean area of the neoglenoid was 65% of the glenoid surface. The authors noted the least volumetric and linear bone resection with a full-

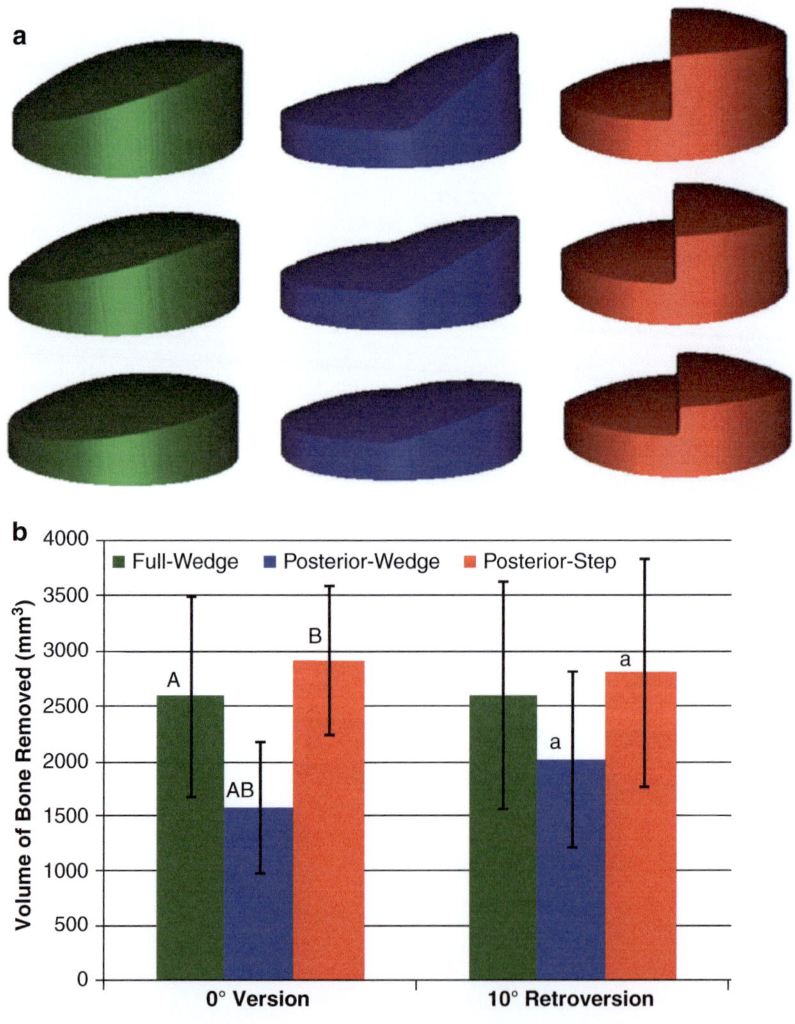

Fig. 4.8 Quantitative measurement of bone removal with various augmented designs. (**a**) Models of three specific posterior glenoid augment designs. Green = full-wedge, blue = posterior-wedge, and red = stepped design implant. Each design is available in different dimensions allowing correction of variable deformity severities. (**b**) The volume of the bone removed with a posterior-wedge implant was significantly less than the other designs at correction to 0° version. (Reference: Knowles et al. [49]. Fig. 1 (page 1219) and Fig. 5A (page 1222))

wedge-shaped augment. The standard glenoid implant removed the most bone and left the highest percent of trabecular bone supporting the implant surface. Sabesan et al. compared standard glenoid to augmented implants in a computer simulation model of 29 shoulders with acquired posterior glenoid loss (mean retroversion of 21°, range 4.5° to 43°) where pathologic version was corrected to neutral [23]. They found that a greater amount of correction could be obtained with less reaming and medialization with augmented (mean 3.8 mm) components compared to standard glenoids (mean 8.3 mm).

In addition to lower amounts of bone resection, augmented glenoids have been shown to reduce the volume of residual bone with excessive strain compared to standard implants placed with corrective reaming in a finite element model [51]. Another study comparing standard glenoid and augmented implants placed in varying degrees of retroversion reported greater bone stress when implants were placed in greater retroversion and the least stress with augmented wedged implants [52]. Additionally, the fatigue life of the cement was best in neutrally implanted glenoids. Posterior-step augments have compared favorably biomechanically to wedge augments and standard implants with compressive posterior loading producing less lift-off of the anterior aspect of the implant [53].

Outcomes

There are multiple studies examining the outcomes of anatomic shoulder arthroplasty in patients with a B2 or posteriorly eroded glenoid. It is generally felt that these shoulders have an inferior outcome and higher rate of complications than shoulders without advanced glenoid wear or with a concentric wear pattern. In their classic study, Iannotti and Norris noted lower ASES scores, greater pain, and decreased external rotation ROM in shoulders with posterior subluxation following anatomic TSA [54] with conventional implants. More recently, an analysis of the long-term survivorship of pegged glenoid implants found severe glenoid erosion patterns (A2, B2, and C) to be associated with a higher rate of glenoid loosening [55].

Partial Glenoid Version Correction

Partial glenoid version correction via high-side reaming has produced good outcomes at short-term follow-up, but this technique should be limited to mild to moderate glenoid deformities. As mentioned previously, one of the primary goals of surgery is to correct glenoid version to within 10° of neutral to minimize eccentric loading and cement stress across the glenoid implant. Gerber et al. reported the results of 23 shoulders (mean age of 60 years) with static posterior subluxation of the humeral head [5]. Nine shoulders were classified as B1, five as B2, and nine as type C glenoids. The mean preoperative glenoid retroversion was 18° (range 8–40°), and posterior subluxation as defined from the glenoid center was 71% (range 65–81%). Attempts were made to correct version to within 10° of neutral version with high-side reaming alone. In 21 of 23 shoulders, the humeral head was considered recentered at a mean of 42 months follow-up. The corrected glenoid retroversion was between 0° and 15° (mean 9°) in 20 of 23 shoulders determined by CT scan. Increased preoperative version correlated with poorer postoperative shoulder functional scores; however, postoperative version was not correlated to outcomes. There were no reported complications in this series. Habermeyer also reported that posterior humeral head subluxation could be corrected with eccentric reaming and TSA [56]. The authors defined humeral head subluxation as a head center more than 5 mm from the glenoid center on axillary radiographs. In their series, 22 of 49 shoulders with a Walch B-type glenoid had posterior decentering that was corrected in all cases with eccentric glenoid reaming at a mean of 2 years follow-up. Similar to other studies, postoperative shoulder function (Constant score) was lower for shoulders with preoperative humeral subluxation compared to those with concentric wear.

A recent study compared the results of anatomic TSAs placed with the glenoid component placed in less than 15° of retroversion to those placed at 15° or greater retroversion [57]. The authors used a minimalistic bone preserving technique where the glenoid was reamed only to create a concentric surface rather than to correct version to a desired degree. Intraoperative stability was augmented with anterior offset of the humeral head and soft tissue procedures when needed. The authors noted similar clinical outcomes (SST score), similar rates of glenoid lucencies, and no differences in humeral head centering at short-term follow-up (mean 2.5 years). Contrary to these findings, Ho et al. reported a series of 66 anatomic TSAs treated with corrective reaming and placement of a hybrid bone ingrowth polyethylene glenoid [37]. Preoperative imaging allowed characterization of glenoid retroversion into three groups (<15°, between 15° and 25°, and >25°). At a mean of 3.8 years follow-up, the authors noted good clinical results. Radiographic glenoid lucencies correlated with length of follow-up, preoperative glenoid retroversion, and the severity of residual glenoid component retroversion. After controlling for length of follow-up, only postoperative glenoid retroversion of >15° correlated with and increased risk of progressive central peg lucencies which were seen in 30% of the cohort. A recent study by Orvets et al. examined the outcomes of 59 arthritic shoulders with a Walch B2 glenoid deformity managed with eccentric glenoid reaming and placement of a cemented pegged glenoid component [58]. The mean preoperative glenoid retroversion was 18° (range −1° to 36°), and the mean posterior humeral subluxation was 67%. At a mean follow-up of 50 months, the mean ASES, VAS pain, and SST scores were 84, 1.4, and 9.1, respectively. There were no revisions due postoperative instability or glenoid loosening. Radiographic follow-up at a mean of 31 months demonstrated 38 shoulders with no glenoid lucencies, 13 with grade 1, 1 with grade 2, and 5 with grade 3 lucencies. No glenoids were considered radiographically loose. The progression of radiolucencies was not different between shoulders with a preoperative glenoid version of 20° or less compared to more than 20°.

A series by Walch et al. has described some of the limitations and pitfalls of eccentric reaming for arthritic glenoids with a biconcave deformity [38]. In a series of 92 anatomic TSAs followed for mean of 77 (14–180 months), there were significant complications which correlated with the severity of the glenoid deformity. In this series, attempts were made to asymmetrically ream the glenoid to within 10° of neutral version, and in seven cases posterior glenoid bone grafting was performed. Revision surgery was required in 16% of shoulders, and 21% of the glenoids had radiographic loosening. Prosthetic instability was correlated with neoglenoid retroversion (33° vs. 25°) and posterior humeral subluxation (>80%) as defined by the scapular plane. Radiographic loosening was correlated with the duration of follow-up and higher intermediate glenoid retroversion. Overall, complications were correlated with a greater degree of neoglenoid retroversion, the authors designating a value of 27° of higher to be clinically significant. This subgroup accounted for 73% of the total complications in this cohort, and when the deformity was above this threshold, the risk for complications was 44%.

Posterior Glenoid Bone Grafting

Glenoid bone grafting has long been advocated as a treatment option for shoulders with severe posterior glenoid wear; however, the popularity of this surgery has been limited by variable reports of successful incorporation of bone grafts. Short-time results have been encouraging; however, longer follow-up has shown some concern for glenoid survivorship. Neer reported the use of large structural autografts was needed in approximately 4% of shoulder arthroplasties when severe glenoid defects were noted [59]. At a mean of 4.4 years follow-up, 17 of 19 shoulders had satisfactory or good clinical results, and none of the glenoid implants were felt to be clinically loose. The Mayo Clinic experience showed reasonable results at midterm follow-up (mean 5.3 years) with the use of autologous bone grafting in 28 anatomic shoulder arthroplasties [60]. In this series, all but three glenoid components were either cemented metal-backed implants (n = 15) or uncemented metal ingrowth (n = 8) implants. Good to satisfactory clinical results using Neer's criteria were seen in 23 of 28 shoulders. Radiographic loosening was noted in three shoulders; however, 15 additional shoulders had either incomplete (n = 11) or complete (n = 4) radiolucencies. Another study from the same institution reported the results of 25 shoulders followed up for a mean of 7.6 years [61] treated with autologous bone grafting from the humeral head. Half of the implants were metal-backed, and the others were all-polyethylene. Twenty-three of 25 shoulders had good or satisfactory clinical results. Ten glenoid implants were at risk for loosening including six shoulders with glenoid subsidence and six with graft resorption or failure of healing.

Sabesan et al. reported the results of 12 shoulders with severe posterior glenoid bone loss (mean retroversion of 44°) managed with TSA and autologous bone grafting [62]. Ten of 12 patients had good or excellent Penn scores at a mean of 53 months follow-up. Ten shoulders had complete graft incorporation, two had partial graft resorption, and two were revised (one from failure of graft fixation and another due to infection). Recently, Nicholson reported good clinical results in 28 shoulders with severe posterior glenoid erosion treated with anatomic TSA and an autologous bone graft from the humeral head [63]. Glenoid retroversion and subluxation were analyzed with radiographs only. The mean version of 28° was corrected to 4° following surgery, and the humeral head was recentered in all cases. The mean ASES score improved from 39 to 90 points at a mean of 4 years follow-up. The graft was fully incorporated in all shoulders, and three shoulders had at least one broken screw. No progressive radiolucencies were noted, and two shoulders had radiolucency around a single glenoid peg.

Augmented Glenoid Implants

In recent years the use of augmented implants has grown in popularity as a method of correcting abnormal glenoid version without significant reaming and medialization of the glenoid. Initial designs showed relatively high rates of radiographic complications [64] and low component survivorship [65]. Recent studies, with only short periods of follow-up, have produced encouraging early clinical and radiographic results. A recent study reported the results of 21 arthritic shoulders with posterior glenoid bone loss treated with a stepped design augmented glenoid component [66]. The mean preoperative version was 20.8° (range 12–37°), and mean posterior bone loss was 4.7 mm. At a minimum of 2-year follow-up, good clinical results were seen with no complications or revisions. The corrected glenoid retroversion angle was a mean of 9° (range 0–32°). Humeral subluxation was reliably corrected on plain radiographs. Twenty-four percent of the glenoids had low-grade radiolucent lines, but none were progressive. Another study reported the results of the same stepped design posterior augment in 22 shoulders followed for a mean of 36 months [67]. The mean preoperative retroversion was 23.5° (range 16–37°). Significant improvements in shoulder ROM and clinical scores were noted. Radiographically, the mean Lazarus glenoid lucency score was 0.5 with 12 shoulders demonstrating complete osseous integration of the central peg fins and only 1 shoulder with progressive lucency around the central peg. In this series, two shoulders developed postoperative instability. Wright et al. compared the results of a standard polyethylene glenoid component (n = 24) to age- and gender-matched arthritic shoulders (n = 24) with posterior bone erosion treated with a wedge-shaped augmented implant [68]. At 2 years follow-up, both groups showed improvements in shoulder function scores that were not statistically different. Sixty percent of the augmented glenoid had a radiolucent line with a mean total radiolucency score of 1.1, whereas 33% of the nonaugmented group had a radiolucent line with a mean radiolucency score of 0.44. One augmented glenoid was considered radiographically loose. There were no shoulders with posterior subluxation in the augmented group.

Authors Preferred Method of Treatment

The factors important for the choice of surgical technique and/or implants to manage an arthritic shoulder with posterior glenoid wear include the glenoid type, the severity of retroversion deformity (and resultant bone loss), the severity of posterior humeral head subluxation, the age of the patient, and preoperative active range of motion of the shoulder. All shoulders with posterior glenoid erosion receive a preoperative CT scan to quantify the bony anatomy and for surgical planning. The author believes that the majority of B2-type glenoids with an intermediate glenoid retroversion of 20° or less can be managed with high-side reaming alone with a goal of correcting with 10° of neutral version. In these cases, an intraoperative determination of the need for posterior capsule plication and/or reverse offset of the humeral head is performed individually. These shoulders can also be managed with posterior augmented glenoids based on surgeon preference. Occasionally, more severe deformities can be managed with high-side reaming alone, but this technique is reserved for very young patients (< age 55). In more severe-type B2/B3 shoulders with a retroversion deformity between 20° and 30°, or in B3 shoulders in which more severe medialization is noted, alternative techniques are utilized. If the patient is over 65 or has active elevation of 90° or less, the author prefers to place a reverse shoulder arthroplasty. If the patient is under 60–65 years of age and has greater than 90° of elevation, the authors prefer a technique of partial correction with limited high-side reaming (to prevent excessive medialization and bone loss) combined with placement of an autologous glenoid autograft. Alternatively, these shoulders can be managed with a larger posterior augment.

Conclusions

Anatomic TSA remains a successful treatment options for arthritic shoulders with posterior glenoid wear. The development of a successful treatment strategy depends on an accurate assessment and quantification of the bony deformity. Recent advances in CT scan software allow accurate assessment of magnitude of bony deformity and associated humeral head subluxation and real-time recreation of surgical planning. The general goals of surgery are to correct pathologic glenoid retroversion to within 10° of neutral, obtain at least 80% glenoid component seating, and recenter the humeral head in the transverse plane. The correction of severe deformities may be aided by the selective use of patient-specific instrumentation. The primary options for anatomic TSA should be based upon the severity of glenoid retroversion and associated bone loss and include partial glenoid version correction, placement of the posterior glenoid bone graft, or the use of a posterior augmented glenoid. Each of these strategies has relative advantages and disadvantages. Given the limits of partial glenoid version correction, clinicians should become familiar with adjunct techniques to treat more severe glenoid deformities. Further research is needed to define the success and durability of these treatments over time.

References

1. Walch G, Badet R, Boulahia A, Khoury A. Morphologic study of the glenoid in primary glenohumeral osteoarthritis. J Arthroplast. 1999;14(6):756–60.
2. Badet R, Walch G, Boulahia A. Computed tomography in primary glenohumeral osteoarthritis without humeral head elevation. Rev Rhum Engl Ed. 1998;65(3):187–94.
3. Churchill RS, Spencer EE Jr, Fehringer EV. Quantification of B2 glenoid morphology in total shoulder arthroplasty. J Shoulder Elbow Surg/American Shoulder and Elbow Surgeons [et al]. 2015;24(8):1212–7.
4. Hoenecke HR Jr, Tibor LM, D'Lima DD. Glenoid morphology rather than version predicts humeral subluxation: a different perspective on the glenoid in total shoulder arthroplasty. J Shoulder Elbow Surg/American Shoulder and Elbow Surgeons [et al]. 2012;21(9):1136–41.
5. Gerber C, Costouros JG, Sukthankar A, Fucentese SF. Static posterior humeral head subluxation and total shoulder arthroplasty. J Shoulder Elbow Surg/American Shoulder and Elbow Surgeons [et al]. 2009;18(4):505–10.

6. Ricchetti ET, Hendel MD, Collins DN, Iannotti JP. Is premorbid glenoid anatomy altered in patients with glenohumeral osteoarthritis? Clin Orthop Relat Res. 2013;471(9):2932–9.
7. Iannotti JP, Jun BJ, Patterson TE, Ricchetti ET. Quantitative measurement of osseous pathology in advanced glenohumeral osteoarthritis. J Bone Joint Surg Am. 2017;99(17):1460–8.
8. Knowles NK, Ferreira LM, Athwal GS. Premorbid retroversion is significantly greater in type B2 glenoids. J Shoulder Elbow Surg/American Shoulder and Elbow Surgeons [et al]. 2016;25(7):1064–8.
9. Walch G, Ascani C, Boulahia A, Nove-Josserand L, Edwards TB. Static posterior subluxation of the humeral head: an unrecognized entity responsible for glenohumeral osteoarthritis in the young adult. J Shoulder Elbow Surg/American Shoulder and Elbow Surgeons [et al]. 2002;11(4):309–14.
10. Domos P, Checchia CS, Walch G. Walch B0 glenoid: pre-osteoarthritic posterior subluxation of the humeral head. J Shoulder Elbow Surg/American Shoulder and Elbow Surgeons [et al]. 2018;27(1):181–8.
11. Bryce CD, Davison AC, Lewis GS, Wang L, Flemming DJ, Armstrong AD. Two-dimensional glenoid version measurements vary with coronal and sagittal scapular rotation. J Bone Joint Surg Am. 2010;92(3):692–9.
12. Chalmers PN, Salazar D, Chamberlain A, Keener JD. Radiographic characterization of the B2 glenoid: the effect of computed tomographic axis orientation. J Shoulder Elbow Surg/American Shoulder and Elbow Surgeons [et al]. 2017;26(2):258–64.
13. Budge MD, Lewis GS, Schaefer E, Coquia S, Flemming DJ, Armstrong AD. Comparison of standard two-dimensional and three-dimensional corrected glenoid version measurements. J Shoulder Elbow Surg/American Shoulder and Elbow Surgeons [et al]. 2011;20(4):577–83.
14. Hoenecke HR Jr, Hermida JC, Flores-Hernandez C, D'Lima DD. Accuracy of CT-based measurements of glenoid version for total shoulder arthroplasty. J Shoulder Elbow Surg/American Shoulder and Elbow Surgeons [et al]. 2010;19(2):166–71.
15. Iannotti JP, Weiner S, Rodriguez E, Subhas N, Patterson TE, Jun BJ, et al. Three-dimensional imaging and templating improve glenoid implant positioning. J Bone Joint Surg Am. 2015;97(8):651–8.
16. Walch G, Vezeridis PS, Boileau P, Deransart P, Chaoui J. Three-dimensional planning and use of patient-specific guides improve glenoid component position: an in vitro study. J Shoulder Elbow Surg/American Shoulder and Elbow Surgeons [et al]. 2015;24(2):302–9.
17. Throckmorton TW, Gulotta LV, Bonnarens FO, Wright SA, Hartzell JL, Rozzi WB, et al. Patient-specific targeting guides compared with traditional instrumentation for glenoid component placement in shoulder arthroplasty: a multi-surgeon study in 70 arthritic cadaver specimens. J Shoulder Elbow Surg/American Shoulder and Elbow Surgeons [et al]. 2015;24(6):965–71.
18. Iannotti J, Baker J, Rodriguez E, Brems J, Ricchetti E, Mesiha M, et al. Three-dimensional preoperative planning software and a novel information transfer technology improve glenoid component positioning. J Bone Joint Surg Am. 2014;96(9):e71.
19. Hendel MD, Bryan JA, Barsoum WK, Rodriguez EJ, Brems JJ, Evans PJ, et al. Comparison of patient-specific instruments with standard surgical instruments in determining glenoid component position: a randomized prospective clinical trial. J Bone Joint Surg Am. 2012;94(23):2167–75.
20. Kircher J, Wiedemann M, Magosch P, Lichtenberg S, Habermeyer P. Improved accuracy of glenoid positioning in total shoulder arthroplasty with intra-operative navigation: a prospective-randomized clinical study. J Shoulder Elbow Surg/American Shoulder and Elbow Surgeons [et al]. 2009;18(4):515–20.
21. Knowles NK, Keener JD, Ferreira LM, Athwal GS. Quantification of the position, orientation, and surface area of bone loss in type B2 glenoids. J Shoulder Elbow Surg/American Shoulder and Elbow Surgeons [et al]. 2015;24(4):503–10.
22. Beuckelaers E, Jacxsens M, Van Tongel A, De Wilde LF. Three-dimensional computed tomography scan evaluation of the pattern of erosion in type B glenoids. J Shoulder Elbow Surg/American Shoulder and Elbow Surgeons [et al]. 2014;23(1):109–16.
23. Sabesan V, Callanan M, Sharma V, Iannotti JP. Correction of acquired glenoid bone loss in osteoarthritis with a standard versus an augmented glenoid component. J Shoulder Elbow Surg/American Shoulder and Elbow Surgeons [et al]. 2014;23(7):964–73.
24. Knowles NK, Athwal GS, Keener JD, Ferreira LM. Regional bone density variations in osteoarthritic glenoids: a comparison of symmetric to asymmetric (type B2) erosion patterns. J Shoulder Elbow Surg/American Shoulder and Elbow Surgeons [et al]. 2015;24(3):425–32.
25. Sabesan VJ, Callanan M, Youderian A, Iannotti JP. 3D CT assessment of the relationship between humeral head alignment and glenoid retroversion in glenohumeral osteoarthritis. J Bone Joint Surg Am. 2014;96(8):e64.
26. Chan K, Knowles NK, Chaoui J, Gauci MO, Ferreira LM, Walch G, et al. Characterization of the Walch B3 glenoid in primary osteoarthritis. J Shoulder Elbow Surg/American Shoulder and Elbow Surgeons [et al]. 2017;26(5):909–14.
27. Bercik MJ, Kruse K 2nd, Yalizis M, Gauci MO, Chaoui J, Walch G. A modification to the Walch classification of the glenoid in primary glenohumeral osteoarthritis using three-dimensional imaging. J Shoulder Elbow Surg/American Shoulder and Elbow Surgeons [et al]. 2016;25(10):1601–6.
28. Knowles NK, Carroll MJ, Keener JD, Ferreira LM, Athwal GS. A comparison of normal and osteoarthritic humeral head size and morphology. J Shoulder

Elbow Surg/American Shoulder and Elbow Surgeons [et al]. 2016;25(3):502–9.
29. Iannotti JP, Spencer EE, Winter U, Deffenbaugh D, Williams G. Prosthetic positioning in total shoulder arthroplasty. J Shoulder Elbow Surg/American Shoulder and Elbow Surgeons [et al]. 2005;14(1 Suppl S):111S–21S.
30. Shapiro TA, McGarry MH, Gupta R, Lee YS, Lee TQ. Biomechanical effects of glenoid retroversion in total shoulder arthroplasty. J Shoulder Elbow Surg/American Shoulder and Elbow Surgeons [et al]. 2007;16(3 Suppl):S90–5.
31. Farron A, Terrier A, Buchler P. Risks of loosening of a prosthetic glenoid implanted in retroversion. J Shoulder Elbow Surg/American Shoulder and Elbow Surgeons [et al]. 2006;15(4):521–6.
32. Nyffeler RW, Sheikh R, Atkinson TS, Jacob HA, Favre P, Gerber C. Effects of glenoid component version on humeral head displacement and joint reaction forces: an experimental study. J Shoulder Elbow Surg/American Shoulder and Elbow Surgeons [et al]. 2006;15(5):625–9.
33. Terrier A, Buchler P, Farron A. Influence of glenohumeral conformity on glenoid stresses after total shoulder arthroplasty. J Shoulder Elbow Surg/American Shoulder and Elbow Surgeons [et al]. 2006;15(4):515–20.
34. Mansat P, Briot J, Mansat M, Swider P. Evaluation of the glenoid implant survival using a biomechanical finite element analysis: influence of the implant design, bone properties, and loading location. J Shoulder Elbow Surg/American Shoulder and Elbow Surgeons [et al]. 2007;16(3 Suppl):S79–83.
35. Hopkins AR, Hansen UN, Amis AA, Emery R. The effects of glenoid component alignment variations on cement mantle stresses in total shoulder arthroplasty. J Shoulder Elbow Surg/American Shoulder and Elbow Surgeons [et al]. 2004;13(6):668–75.
36. Yongpravat C, Kim HM, Gardner TR, Bigliani LU, Levine WN, Ahmad CS. Glenoid implant orientation and cement failure in total shoulder arthroplasty: a finite element analysis. J Shoulder Elbow Surg/American Shoulder and Elbow Surgeons [et al]. 2013;22(7):940–7.
37. Ho JC, Sabesan VJ, Iannotti JP. Glenoid component retroversion is associated with osteolysis. J Bone Joint Surg Am. 2013;95(12):e82.
38. Walch G, Moraga C, Young A, Castellanos-Rosas J. Results of anatomic nonconstrained prosthesis in primary osteoarthritis with biconcave glenoid. J Shoulder Elbow Surg/American Shoulder and Elbow Surgeons [et al]. 2012;21(11):1526–33.
39. Spencer EE Jr, Valdevit A, Kambic H, Brems JJ, Iannotti JP. The effect of humeral component anteversion on shoulder stability with glenoid component retroversion. J Bone Joint Surg Am. 2005;87(4):808–14.
40. Yongpravat C, Lester JD, Saifi C, Trubelja A, Greiwe RM, Bigliani LU, et al. Glenoid morphology after reaming in computer-simulated total shoulder arthroplasty. J Shoulder Elbow Surg/American Shoulder and Elbow Surgeons [et al]. 2013;22(1):122–8.
41. Chen X, Reddy AS, Kontaxis A, Choi DS, Wright T, Dines DM, et al. Version correction via eccentric reaming compromises remaining bone quality in B2 glenoids: a computational study. Clin Orthop Relat Res. 2017;475(12):3090–9.
42. Clavert P, Millett PJ, Warner JJ. Glenoid resurfacing: what are the limits to asymmetric reaming for posterior erosion? J Shoulder Elbow Surg/American Shoulder and Elbow Surgeons [et al]. 2007;16(6):843–8.
43. Gillespie R, Lyons R, Lazarus M. Eccentric reaming in total shoulder arthroplasty: a cadaveric study. Orthopedics. 2009;32(1):21.
44. Iannotti JP, Greeson C, Downing D, Sabesan V, Bryan JA. Effect of glenoid deformity on glenoid component placement in primary shoulder arthroplasty. J Shoulder Elbow Surg/American Shoulder and Elbow Surgeons [et al]. 2012;21(1):48–55.
45. Nowak DD, Bahu MJ, Gardner TR, Dyrszka MD, Levine WN, Bigliani LU, et al. Simulation of surgical glenoid resurfacing using three-dimensional computed tomography of the arthritic glenohumeral joint: the amount of glenoid retroversion that can be corrected. J Shoulder Elbow Surg/American Shoulder and Elbow Surgeons [et al]. 2009;18(5):680–8.
46. Wang T, Abrams GD, Behn AW, Lindsey D, Giori N, Cheung EV. Posterior glenoid wear in total shoulder arthroplasty: eccentric anterior reaming is superior to posterior augment. Clin Orthop Relat Res. 2015;473(12):3928–36.
47. Kim HM, Chacon AC, Andrews SH, Roush EP, Cho E, Conaway WK, et al. Biomechanical benefits of anterior offsetting of humeral head component in posteriorly unstable total shoulder arthroplasty: a cadaveric study. J Orthop Res. 2016;34(4):666–74.
48. Hsu JE, Gee AO, Lucas RM, Somerson JS, Warme WJ, Matsen FA 3rd. Management of intraoperative posterior decentering in shoulder arthroplasty using anteriorly eccentric humeral head components. J Shoulder Elbow Surg/American Shoulder and Elbow Surgeons [et al]. 2016;25(12):1980–8.
49. Knowles NK, Ferreira LM, Athwal GS. Augmented glenoid component designs for type B2 erosions: a computational comparison by volume of bone removal and quality of remaining bone. J Shoulder Elbow Surg/American Shoulder and Elbow Surgeons [et al]. 2015;24(8):1218–26.
50. Kersten AD, Flores-Hernandez C, Hoenecke HR, D'Lima DD. Posterior augmented glenoid designs preserve more bone in biconcave glenoids. J Shoulder Elbow Surg/American Shoulder and Elbow Surgeons [et al]. 2015;24(7):1135–41.
51. Allred JJ, Flores-Hernandez C, Hoenecke HR Jr, D'Lima DD. Posterior augmented glenoid implants require less bone removal and generate lower stresses: a finite element analysis. J Shoulder Elbow Surg/American Shoulder and Elbow Surgeons [et al]. 2016;25(5):823–30.

52. Hermida JC, Flores-Hernandez C, Hoenecke HR, D'Lima DD. Augmented wedge-shaped glenoid component for the correction of glenoid retroversion: a finite element analysis. J Shoulder Elbow Surg/ American Shoulder and Elbow Surgeons [et al]. 2014;23(3):347–54.
53. Iannotti JP, Lappin KE, Klotz CL, Reber EW, Swope SW. Liftoff resistance of augmented glenoid components during cyclic fatigue loading in the posterior-superior direction. J Shoulder Elbow Surg/ American Shoulder and Elbow Surgeons [et al]. 2013;22(11):1530–6.
54. Iannotti JP, Norris TR. Influence of preoperative factors on outcome of shoulder arthroplasty for glenohumeral osteoarthritis. J Bone Joint Surg Am. 2003;85-A(2):251–8.
55. McLendon PB, Schoch BS, Sperling JW, Sanchez-Sotelo J, Schleck CD, Cofield RH. Survival of the pegged glenoid component in shoulder arthroplasty: part II. J Shoulder Elbow Surg/American Shoulder and Elbow Surgeons [et al]. 2017;26(8): 1469–76.
56. Habermeyer P, Magosch P, Lichtenberg S. Recentering the humeral head for glenoid deficiency in total shoulder arthroplasty. Clin Orthop Relat Res. 2007;457:124–32.
57. Service BC, Hsu JE, Somerson JS, Russ SM, Matsen FA 3rd. Does postoperative glenoid retroversion affect the 2-year clinical and radiographic outcomes for total shoulder arthroplasty? Clin Orthop Relat Res. 2017;475(11):2726–39.
58. Orvets ND, Chamberlain AM, Patterson BM, Chalmers PN, Gosselin M, Salazar D, et al. Total shoulder arthroplasty in patients with a B2 glenoid addressed with corrective reaming. J Shoulder Elbow Surg/American Shoulder and Elbow Surgeons [et al]. 2018;27(6S):S58–64.
59. Neer CS 2nd, Morrison DS. Glenoid bone-grafting in total shoulder arthroplasty. J Bone Joint Surg Am. 1988;70(8):1154–62.
60. Steinmann SP, Cofield RH. Bone grafting for glenoid deficiency in total shoulder replacement. J Shoulder Elbow Surg/American Shoulder and Elbow Surgeons [et al]. 2000;9(5):361–7.
61. Klika BJ, Wooten CW, Sperling JW, Steinmann SP, Schleck CD, Harmsen WS, et al. Structural bone grafting for glenoid deficiency in primary total shoulder arthroplasty. J Shoulder Elbow Surg/ American Shoulder and Elbow Surgeons [et al]. 2014;23(7):1066–72.
62. Sabesan V, Callanan M, Ho J, Iannotti JP. Clinical and radiographic outcomes of total shoulder arthroplasty with bone graft for osteoarthritis with severe glenoid bone loss. J Bone Joint Surg Am. 2013;95(14):1290–6.
63. Nicholson GP, Cvetanovich GL, Rao AJ, O'Donnell P. Posterior glenoid bone grafting in total shoulder arthroplasty for osteoarthritis with severe posterior glenoid wear. J Shoulder Elbow Surg/ American Shoulder and Elbow Surgeons [et al]. 2017;26(10):1844–53.
64. Rice RS, Sperling JW, Miletti J, Schleck C, Cofield RH. Augmented glenoid component for bone deficiency in shoulder arthroplasty. Clin Orthop Relat Res. 2008;466(3):579–83.
65. Cil A, Sperling JW, Cofield RH. Nonstandard glenoid components for bone deficiencies in shoulder arthroplasty. J Shoulder Elbow Surg/ American Shoulder and Elbow Surgeons [et al]. 2014;23(7):e149–57.
66. Stephens SP, Spencer EE, Wirth MA. Radiographic results of augmented all-polyethylene glenoids in the presence of posterior glenoid bone loss during total shoulder arthroplasty. J Shoulder Elbow Surg/ American Shoulder and Elbow Surgeons [et al]. 2017;26(5):798–803.
67. Favorito PJ, Freed RJ, Passanise AM, Brown MJ. Total shoulder arthroplasty for glenohumeral arthritis associated with posterior glenoid bone loss: results of an all-polyethylene, posteriorly augmented glenoid component. J Shoulder Elbow Surg/American Shoulder and Elbow Surgeons [et al]. 2016;25(10):1681–9.
68. Wright TW, Grey SG, Roche CP, Wright L, Flurin PH, Zuckerman JD. Preliminary results of a posterior augmented glenoid compared to an all polyethylene standard glenoid in anatomic total shoulder arthroplasty. Bull Hosp Jt Dis (2013). 2015;73(Suppl 1):S79–85.

Severe Glenoid Erosion (B2, B3, C, E2, E3) Treated with RSA

5

Francesco Ascione and Howard D. Routman

Introduction

Severe glenoid erosion or deficiency is a challenge in shoulder arthroplasty that is frequently encountered in patients with arthritis and is more commonly an indication for the surgeon to perform reverse shoulder arthroplasty (RSA) instead of total shoulder arthroplasty (TSA). Severe glenoid bone loss can occur in many situations, including osteoarthritis, rheumatoid arthritis, rotator cuff tear arthropathy, fractures, chronic instability, congenital deformities, tumors, and revision arthroplasty.

Acquired glenoid bone defects may necessitate altering surgical technique to make implantation of the baseplate possible and ultimately achieve a successful glenoid in RSA. Standard surgical techniques can be modified to accommodate acquired osseous defects of the glenoid. The current options in RSA to address glenoid-sided bone loss include complete or partial correction of deformity by reaming, the use of either allograft or autograft, the use of augmented glenoid components, or a combination of the above. The importance of adequate preoperative imaging with 3D CT scanning cannot be overemphasized as severe glenoid deformity when encountered at the time of surgery is frequently difficult to visually assess in an accurate manner. In addition, preoperative imaging allows the surgeon to visualize the deformity with great detail and may allow the surgeon to utilize software to simulate the proposed surgery on a computer, understand the limits of the current bone stock, manufacture guides using 3D printing techniques that can be used at the time of surgery, and even prepare a surgical plan that can be executed at the time of surgery using intraoperative navigation systems.

Neer et al. [50] described the combination of severe rotator cuff tearing and an arthritic condition of the glenohumeral joint known as *classic cuff tear arthropathy*. The mechanical factors associated with massive rotator cuff tears lead to unbalanced muscle forces, and an accelerated process of further cuff destruction and arthropathy, with a combination of superior and posterior erosion of the glenoid as the most common pattern of bone loss.

In osteoarthritis of the shoulder, a different set of circumstances affects the expected pattern of glenoid erosion. This disease process is generally considered to be protective of the rotator cuff, and the compressive effects of the surrounding

F. Ascione
Orthopedic Department, Campolongo Hospital, Salerno, Italy

Orthopedic and Traumatolgy Division, Madonna del Buon Consiglio Fatebenefratelli Hospital, Naples, Italy

H. D. Routman (✉)
The Palm Beach Shoulder Service at Atlantis Orthopaedics, Palm Beach Gardens, FL, USA
e-mail: h.routman@atlantisortho.com

R. Z. Tashjian (ed.), *Complex and Revision Shoulder Arthroplasty*,
https://doi.org/10.1007/978-3-030-02756-8_5

musculature combined with stronger internal than external rotators can lead to predictable patterns of glenoid bone loss. As osteoarthritis advances, it can result in progressive posterior glenoid bone loss, erosive changes with retroversion of the glenoid, loss of normal glenoid vault anatomy, and posterior subluxation of the humeral head.

The understanding of the frequency and severity of glenoid morphologic alterations in patients undergoing RSA is improving, as recent technologies have allowed a better assessment of the glenoid [9, 39, 40]. In RSA, glenoid bone erosion is encountered frequently in patients with rotator cuff tear arthropathy, which is the primary indication for RSA. Acquired glenoid bone defects are present in nearly 39% of this patient population [15, 17, 39]. Whereas bone deficiency may occur in any location on the glenoid, it most commonly occurs on the posterior (18%) and superior (9%) portions of all patients undergoing RSA and includes global erosions in 6% and anterior erosions in 4% of patients [17, 39].

Classifications of the Glenoid in Glenohumeral Osteoarthritis and Rotator Cuff Arthropathy

Osteoarthritis is the most common indication for TSA and frequently results in glenoid bone loss (Fig. 5.1). Walch et al. [66] classified such glenoid defects as follows: *A1*, minor concentric erosion; *A2*, concentric and centrally major erosion (centered humeral head, resultant strengths equally distributed against the surface of the glenoid); *B1*, posteriorly subluxated (no bony erosion, asymmetric distributed loads); *B2*, posteriorly eroded and subluxated (excessive retroversion, posterior cupula with an unusual biconcave aspect of the glenoid); and *C*, retroverted (more than 25°, dysplastic origin, well-centered or slightly posteriorly subluxated head). Recently, Bercik et al. [4] proposed several revisions to the original classification. They added *B3* and *D* glenoids and a more precise definition of the A2 glenoid, which demonstrated improved interobserver and intraobserver reliability. The *B3*

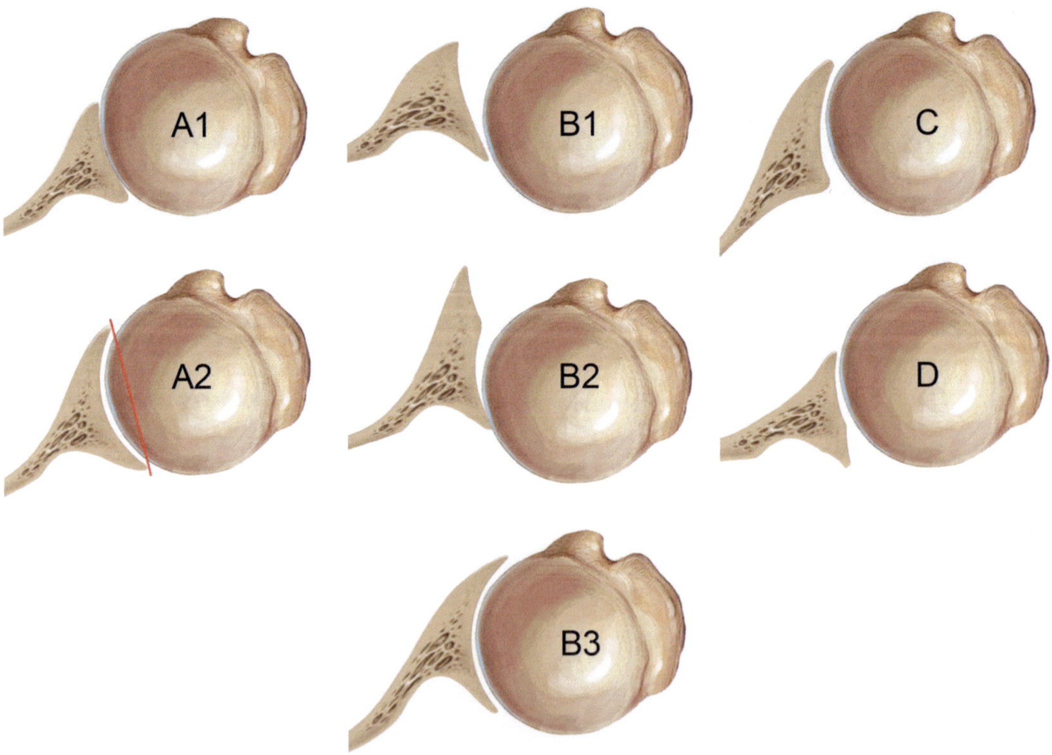

Fig. 5.1 The Walch classification (new)

glenoid was defined as a monoconcave and posteriorly worn glenoid with at least 15° of retroversion or at least 70% posterior humeral head subluxation or both. They defined the *D* glenoid as one with any level of glenoid anteversion or with humeral head subluxation of less than 40% and *A2* as "cupula" glenoids in which a line drawn from the anterior to posterior rims of the native glenoid transects the humeral head. This more precise definition of the *A2* glenoid better differentiated it from the A1.

Favard et al. [15] created a classification scheme to describe glenoid wear in patients with rotator cuff arthropathy. The five grades included *E0*, the head of the humerus migrated upward without erosion of the glenoid; *E1*, concentric glenoid wear; *E2*, superior wear; *E3*, superior and inferior glenoid erosion; and *E4*, glenoid erosion predominantly in the inferior pole (Fig. 5.2).

Lévigne and Franceschi [43] proposed a classification system of stages to describe glenoid wear due to rheumatoid arthritis, a less common indication for reverse shoulder arthroplasty. The stages are as follows: *Stage 1*, intact or minimally deformed subchondral bone; *Stage 2*, wear reaches the foot of the coracoid; and *Stage 3*, wear goes beyond the foot of the coracoid.

Visotsky et al. [65] proposed a biomechanical classification of cuff tear arthropathy and relative glenoid degree and direction of bone erosion called the *Seebauer classification*. Four distinct groups were formed based on the biomechanics, clinical outcomes of arthroplasty, the degree of superior migration from the center of rotation, and the amount of instability of the center of rotation.

Glenoid Defects in Glenohumeral Arthritis

Glenoid version changes that occur in the arthritic shoulder frequently can be associated with abnormal subluxation of the humeral head

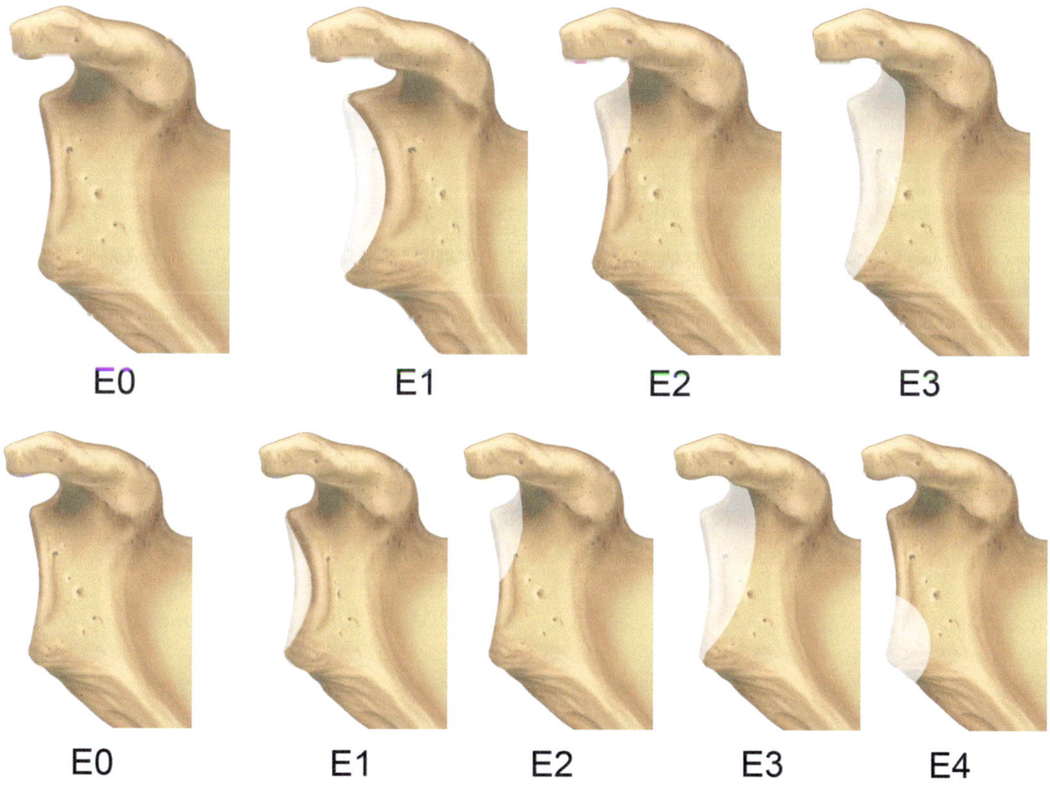

Fig. 5.2 The Favard classification

relative to the glenoid. Decision-making in shoulder arthroplasty needs to account for this, particularly in OA with posterior subluxation, or early failure of the glenoid component can occur. A posterior subluxation (index >65%) has been reported to contribute to early glenoid loosening in TSA [20].

Static posterior subluxation present preoperatively can recur despite glenoid version reorientation at the time of surgery. The amount of this translation is proportional to the degree of glenoid retroversion. This is true regardless of whether increased retroversion is due to posterior glenoid bone loss or increased retroversion is due to dysplasia. The B2 subtype, or biconcave glenoid, is characterized by a normal anterior glenoid (paleoglenoid) that represents the native glenoid fossa and varying amounts of posterior bone loss [49]. The humeral head translates posteriorly to articulate with the new posterior concavity (neoglenoid). The anterior-posterior dimension and depth of this concavity are highly variable (the intermediate glenoid). In the classic B2 glenoid, the anterior 50% of the native glenoid fossa is preserved. Alternatively, some shoulders have less than 10% of the native anterior glenoid remaining, making the surgical treatment of this glenoid subtype challenging [5, 20, 33]. When minimal anterior glenoid remains, the biconcavity is less pronounced, and the glenoid appears to have more uniform retroversion. The humeral head also appears to be more centered. In some cases, this morphology resembles a C glenoid. The wide variation in pathologic conditions among B2 glenoids makes it difficult to compare the treatment methods or outcome of any one specific surgical procedure in the overall management of the B2 glenoid.

The vault model can be used to differentiate a B2 glenoid with these characteristics from a C glenoid with congenital retroversion [60]. Researchers have shown it has a highly consistent and conserved three-dimensional (3D) shape across individuals and can be used to estimate native glenoid version and inclination in both non-pathologic and pathologic shoulders [19, 60]. A pathologic glenoid with acquired bone loss, such as a B2 glenoid, will have a vault version measurement within the range of normal, whereas a pathologic glenoid with developmental or congenital retroversion, such as a C glenoid, will have a vault version measurement that shows increased retroversion. Determining the premorbid glenoid version has important surgical implications. High retroversion in the pathologic B2 glenoid should be corrected during arthroplasty. This may not be the case in the pathologic C glenoid, in which high retroversion is typical of normal premorbid anatomy.

The B3 glenoid may form via one of two mechanisms. The B2 glenoid may convert into a B3 glenoid as increased erosion completely destroys the paleoglenoid. Alternatively, persistent posterior subluxation may preferentially erode the posterior glenoid, leading to significant retroversion without an interval biconcave period. The development of anterior osteophytes also contributes to the retroverted appearance of the B3 glenoid in either situation. The limit of 15° or more of retroversion was set to define the B3 glenoid because researchers have shown that eccentric reaming in glenoids with that amount of retroversion does not allow for proper implantation of an anatomic glenoid without perforating the glenoid walls [11, 21, 53].

Diagnosis and Assessment of the Severely Eroded Glenoid

For a normal glenoid, plain radiographs, including anteroposterior (Grashey) and axillary views, may be sufficient, and the evaluation of the glenoid should start with or without two-dimensional (2D) computed tomography (CT) scans. Frankle et al. [17] reported no significant differences among radiographic images, 2D CT-scan techniques, and 3D CT-scan techniques for differentiating between normal and abnormal glenoid morphology. During RSA surgical planning, using radiographs and CT scans is helpful to further assess the version and posterior subluxation. For the abnormal glenoid, the 2D techniques became insufficient to further differentiate subclasses of abnormal glenoid deformity. The 3D models have been shown to be more accurate for identifying the localized erosions and guiding surgical decision-making. If the abnormality becomes obvious, 3D CT reconstruction models should be considered to further define the location and severity of erosion and to help to guide placement of the central fixation of the baseplate into adequate bone for initial fixation [60]. Researchers have reported that 2D CT scans portray glenoid version less reliably than 3D reconstructions that analyze the scapula as a free body [4, 9, 40]. These 3D reconstructions provide corrected axial 2D images that are strictly in the scapular plane regardless of patient orientation, allowing for more accurate assessments of version and subluxation. In the future, 3D reconstructions will probably become the standard of care because their benefits are not only academic but may lead to better clinical results [34].

The glenoid vault model is a 3D virtual tool that can be used to determine premorbid glenoid anatomy. The vault model has been shown to accurately predict premorbid glenoid version, inclination, and joint-line position [19, 60]. It can also help the surgeon identify the extent and location of bone loss in the B2 glenoid. The surgeon can use this information to place the glenoid component in the location and orientation that best restores native glenoid version and inclination. This information also can help the surgeon select the optimal implant to restore native glenoid anatomy while avoiding peg perforation [31, 60].

TSA Versus RSA for the Severely Eroded Glenoid

In primary, non-constrained shoulder arthroplasty, glenoid bone erosion has been shown to negatively affect outcomes, regardless of technique [25, 30, 33, 44, 47, 67, 68]. Researchers have reported failure rates of up to ten times that of primary arthroplasty without glenoid bone loss [5, 10, 20, 28, 33, 47, 62]. Moreover, resurfacing the moderately to severely deficient glenoid using structural bone grafting is technically difficult and characterized by a relatively high rate of complications as well [28, 51]. Iannotti and Norris [33] found that patients with posterior subluxation of the humeral head and posterior glenoid erosion had lower final American Shoulder and Elbow Surgeons (ASES) scores, increased pain, and decreased active external rotation after TSA or hemiarthroplasty than other patients in their study.

Glenoid component loosening is the most common cause of failure of anatomic shoulder replacement and revision surgery [5, 14, 16, 18, 25, 30, 46, 47, 62]. Researchers have shown a correlation with glenoid loosening and eccentric loading of the humeral head secondary to posterior glenoid wear, retroversion, and posterior humeral subluxation. According to Ho et al. [29], glenoid retroversion of greater than 15° can increase the odds of developing osteolysis around the central glenoid peg in TSA. Placing the glenoid in 15° of retroversion significantly decreases glenohumeral contact area, increases contact pressure, and decreases inferior and posterior glenohumeral forces, resulting in eccentric loading of the glenoid component and possibly leading to wear and loosening [61].

Some patients have combinations of acquired central and posterior bone loss. These deformities do not fit into any one Walch classification category and present as the most challenging cases for standard shoulder arthroplasty. Walch et al. ([67], *J Shoulder Elbow Surg*) reported 94 anatomic TSAs in patients with a biconcave glenoid and demonstrated acceptable objective and subjective results but an unacceptably high rate of complications: loosening (20.6%), posterior instability (5.5%), and revision (16.3%) at the 6-year follow-up. When preoperative glenoid retroversion was greater than 27°, the risk of loosening or instability after anatomic TSA was 44%, demonstrating the preoperative version was the strongest predictor of glenoid loosening and recurrent posterior humeral head subluxation in patients treated with anatomic TSA and a standard glenoid component. Similarly, 60% of the postoperative dislocations occurred when preoperative subluxation of the humeral head was greater than 80%. In another study, Walch et al. ([68], *J Bone Joint Surg Am*) studied loosening patterns of keeled glenoid components after TSA for primary osteoarthritis and noted an increased rate of posterior tilting and loosening of the glenoid component in patients with preoperative static posterior subluxation.

RSA is now being utilized as a primary treatment alternative for the posterior-superior-eroded glenoid in osteoarthritis as a result of the high rate of failure of posterior bone grafting and the inability to durably correct posterior instability of the humeral head during anatomic arthroplasty. One of the greatest advantages of RSA for large glenoid deficiencies is that it allows reconstruction of the glenoid with large structural grafts that can be fixed to the native bone with baseplate screws and an extended peg, screw, or cage traversing the graft into native bone. This theoretically allows a high rate of graft union regardless of whether the graft is an autograft or allograft. Compared with anatomic TSA, the RSA presents a favorable environment for glenoid graft incorporation. Immediate graft fixation and compression are obtained by the combination of the long-peg baseplate and screws in the native scapula, and compression forces (after 30° of abduction) are favorable to graft healing and incorporation.

The semi-constrained design of an RSA implant may provide a solution to the static posterior instability of the humeral head in some patients with glenohumeral arthritis. Several factors inherent in the RSA design increase the constraint of the shoulder relative to that of an anatomic TSA and make stability and proper soft tissue tension attainable making RSA a viable option. In addition, when attempting to achieve glenoid component stability, the rigid screw fixation of the glenoid baseplate used for RSA may be advantageous compared with the cemented polyethylene glenoid component typically used for anatomic TSA. Finally, the greater surface contact area between the glenosphere and humeral polyethylene cup in conjunction with the reversal of the articulation neutralizes the destabilizing force of the deltoid.

RSA Utilized for Glenoid Bone Loss

Reverse shoulder arthroplasty, for some surgeons, has become the treatment of choice in severe glenoid defects, with or without glenoid bone grafting, regardless of the preoperative status of the cuff. Mizuno et al. [49] reported good results with RSA in patients with a B2 glenoid and osteoarthritis with an intact rotator cuff. They included 27 patients with a mean preoperative retroversion of 32° and mean humeral head subluxation of 87%. Seventeen patients had RSA without bone graft, and ten had a bone graft to address posterior glenoid bone loss. Bone grafting was performed when glenoid version could not be corrected to less than 10° with asymmetric reaming or when bone loss resulted in an unsupported baseplate of greater than 20%. At a mean follow-up of 54 months, patients had improved functional outcomes without recurrence of posterior instability. They also observed no correlation between initial glenoid retroversion or posterior subluxation and the postoperative clinical outcomes. Reverse shoulder arthroplasty for bone loss is a particularly attractive choice for older and less active patients. Managing this pathologic condition in younger or more active patients remains difficult.

Klein et al. [39] compared outcomes of RSA in patients with and without glenoid bone loss. Of the 56 patients considered to have abnormal glenoids due to bone loss, 22 required a bone graft (21 autograft humeral heads, 1 allograft femoral head). No differences were observed in clinical outcomes at the 2-year follow-up between normal and abnormal glenoids; patients with acquired glenoid bone defects may accommodate bone loss and, therefore, have clinical outcomes comparable to those in patients with normal glenoid morphology. They reported no evidence of graft failure on postoperative radiographs regardless of the level and location of bone loss. Despite the challenges presented by bone loss, clinical results in all outcomes measured were not statistically or clinically different from those achieved by the group with normal glenoid morphology.

The challenge with RSA and glenoid bone loss lies with obtaining predictable and sustainable glenoid component fixation and restoring the joint line to optimize soft tissue tensioning [64]. In the setting of acquired glenoid bone defects, initial fixation of the baseplate is of paramount importance to the surgeon's ability to successfully implant a glenoid component. Surgical techniques in glenoid component fixation should attempt to maximize fixation by using the best centerline and bone stock available and maximizing the length of peripheral screws, even when bone loss is present. For posterior, global, and anterior erosions, the surgical centerline for baseplate implantation is shorter, resulting in a lack of bone stock for fixation. If fixation of the glenoid component is questionable, an alternative direction of glenoid component placement should be considered. The additional *alternative scapular centerline* along the scapular spine is an alternative axis for glenoid component fixation [17] and is defined as the point that originated in the center of the glenoid aligned with the scapular spine, not perpendicular to the native glenoid surface. The goal is to implant the baseplate within 10° of neutral version in relation to the native glenoid which is typically anteverted while utilizing the alternative scapular centerline. In the coronal plane, the baseplate should be neutral or slightly inferiorly tilted relative to the floor of the supraspinatus fossa (i.e., the central fixation parallel to the line of the supraspinatus fossa). It is not typically used in a normal glenoid because this requires implanting the component at an anteverted angle relative to the glenoid surface; however, Frankle et al. [17] reported no higher rate of dislocations, and the fixation provides sufficient bone for central devices. A similar observation was made with regard to peripheral screw placement. Caution should be employed if not utilizing a lateralized glenosphere system, as was done in the Frankle et al. series, as a medialized Grammont style sphere with an alternate centerline baseplate may lead to impingement and subsequent instability.

Adverse consequences can also occur from implanting an RSA in patients with severely eroded glenoids if bone loss is not corrected. Excessive medialization of the baseplate can lead to inferomedial and anteroposterior impingement, causing scapular notching that results in bone erosion, and polyethylene wear, as well as limitation of external and internal rotation and decrease of deltoid wrapping also potentially leading to instability (Fig. 5.3). Not correcting superior glenoid bone loss (i.e., Favard types E2 and E3) can lead to superior tilt and failure of the baseplate, increased scapular impingement, instability, inferior scapular notching, and medial polyethylene wear [27, 41]. Biomechanically, superior tilt increases destabilizing shear forces and decreases the stabilizing compressive forces experienced by the RSA glenoid component during deltoid contraction, potentially leading to early loosening [23, 24]. In osteoarthritis with severe retroversion and biconcavity (i.e., Walch type B2 glenoid) or excessive hypoplastic glenoid retroversion (type C glenoid), not correcting posterior bone loss can lead to retroversion of the baseplate, reduced external rotation, posterior scapular notching, and posteromedial polyethylene wear [42, 45].

Technical Options and Results for Treating Eroded Glenoids

Numerous investigators have suggested strategies for addressing glenoid bone loss in RSA [1, 7, 13, 17, 39, 49, 52, 56]. However, few researchers have examined the clinical results [7, 51]. Techniques that preserve subchondral glenoid bone and minimize glenoid reaming are now being used, and they may be superior and provide long-term fixation. Surgical solutions addressing the glenoid in RSA have been adapted from primary shoulder arthroplasty and include asymmetric reaming, bone grafting, combined asymmetric reaming and bone grafting, and augmented baseplate components.

Large structural grafts from the humeral head or iliac crest have been used to reconstruct posterior, superior, and anterior defects. Screws used for baseplate fixation can be used to secure the graft. More recently, extended-length fixation baseplates have been used to assist fixation to the native scapula beyond the structural graft. Advantages of this technique include maintaining proper joint lateralization and preserving glenoid bone stock. Disadvantages include the technical difficulty, fixation failure, and graft resorption that could secondarily lead to component loosening.

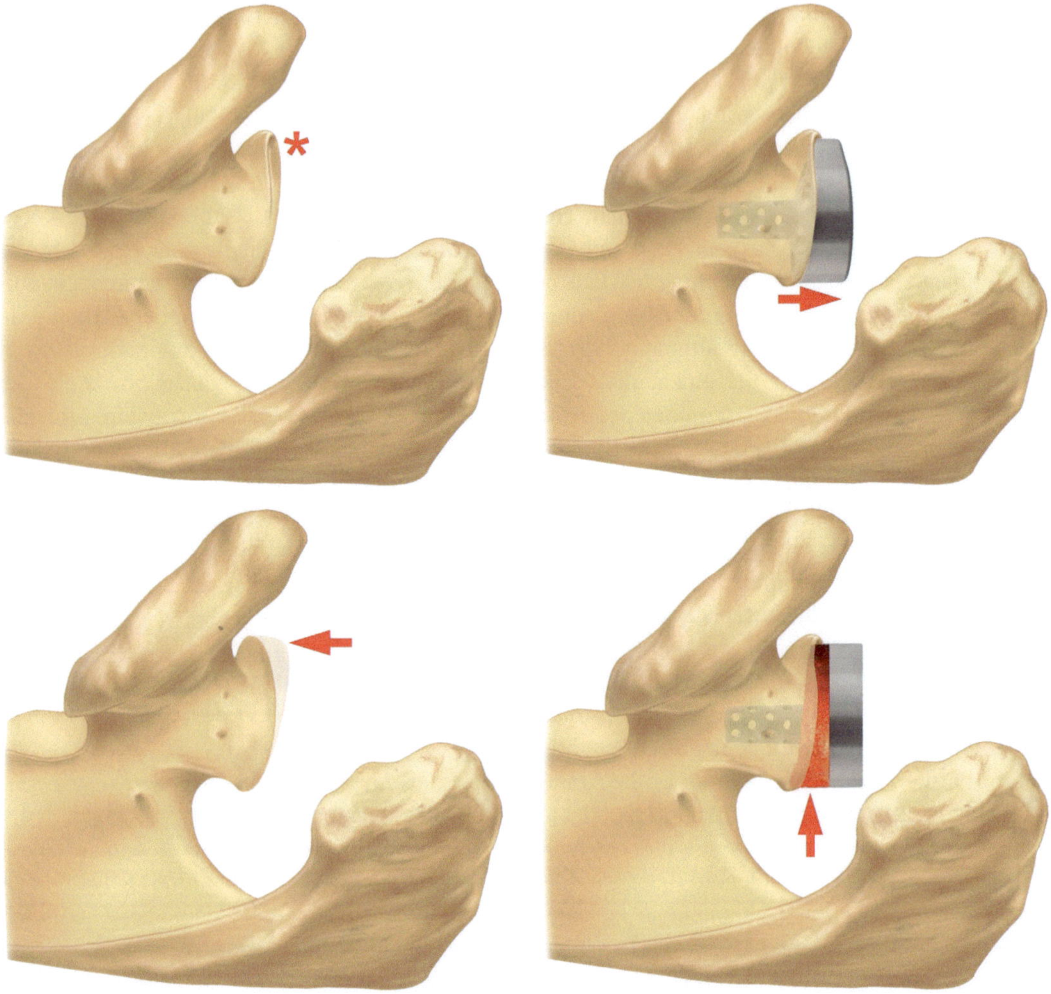

Fig. 5.3 Loss of wrap and instability

Norris et al. [52] reported a technique for managing glenoid bone loss using the reverse prosthesis and bulk tricortical autologous iliac crest bone graft. The authors describe preparing the baseplate directly on the iliac crest and then removing it from the crest with the graft attached. The same authors also describe a technique to manage severe posterior bone loss in patients with intact rotator cuff osteoarthritis using a humeral head graft [26]. This technique involves "shaping" the humeral head autograft to match the neoglenoid retroversion with the goal of correcting retroversion and restoring glenoid bone. Results in patients with B2, B3, and C glenoids were comparable to those observed for TSA in patients with glenohumeral arthritis and A1, A2, and B1 glenoids and similar to results reported by Mizuno et al., demonstrating no episodes of instability or subluxation when RSA is performed for B2 glenoids, lending further support to the idea that the semi-constrained design of RSA prevents and protects from this mode of failure often seen with treatment using anatomic shoulder replacement.

Neyton et al. [51] reviewed the cases of nine patients with a Grammont-type RSA who underwent glenoid bone grafting for severe bone loss. At a minimum 2-year follow-up, no incidence of radiographic loosening had occurred, pain relief was good, postoperative functional scores were low (mean Constant score = 53 points), and six patients had radiographic evidence of inferior scapular notching.

Boileau et al. [6] described a similar harvesting technique using a humeral head autograft as Norris et al. [52] described from the iliac crest to achieve bony lateralization of the center of rotation in RSA (BIO-RSA) . They used a 7- to 10-mm graft and extended central fixation on the baseplate to achieve central fixation in the native scapula. Screws through the baseplate achieved fixation, as well. They achieved a 98% incorporation rate, with no loosening or revisions 28 months postoperatively, and reported a 19% notching rate for 42 patients, recommending implanting the baseplate in a lower position.

Boileau et al. [7] reported results of an angled BIO-RSA technique for eroded glenoids. The technique was used to not only lateralize but also correct version and inclination associated with severe glenoid erosion. The humeral head autograft may be symmetrical (BIO-RSA) or asymmetrical (angled BIO-RSA), depending on the presence, amount, and orientation of glenoid deficiency. Purpose-designed instrumentation is used to harvest the graft from the humeral head so that it is trapezoidal to match the glenoid bone defect. Potential advantages of this technique include flexibility to reconstruct multiplanar deformity (i.e., to correct baseplate version and inclination), restoration of glenoid bone stock, and the ability to lateralize the center of rotation. Glenoid loosening occurred in three (5%) patients in the first 6 months after the operation and was revised with iliac crest bone graft. One failure occurred secondary to a technical mistake: persistent superior inclination. Radiographs and CT images demonstrated union between the cancellous bone graft and the surface of the native glenoid in 94% (51 of 54) of the patients. At final follow-up, 13 (25%) patients had grade 1 to 3 scapular notching, and no patients had grade 4 inferior scapular notching. The correction of glenoid orientation was significant in both inclination and version measured using the multiplanar mode in the scapular plane. In the patients with combined vertical and horizontal glenoid bone loss, the angled BIO-RSA technique allowed simultaneous correction of both the posterior and superior defects, which is one of the main advantages of using a cancellous bone graft. Other advantages of the angled BIO-RSA technique include minimal donor-site morbidity compared with structural iliac crest graft [8, 28, 37, 52, 54], no potential for disease transmission compared with allograft [31], and no additional cost compared with allograft or augmented baseplate [22, 35, 56]; however, it cannot be used for revision of a previous arthroplasty, when necrosis is present, or when the humeral head is absent. In addition, the use of humeral head autograft for baseplate fixation is dependent on humeral head bone quality, which can be variably porotic in the patient population in which RSA is typically performed.

Jones et al. [36] recently reported on allograft bone grafting in the setting of RSA. They demonstrated a higher rate of structural graft incorporation in RSA for autografts than allografts (86% complete or partial incorporation for autografts versus 66% for allografts) in a series that included revision cases. The graft was fully incorporated in 51.7% of the cohort, partially incorporated in 29.3%, and not incorporated in 19.5%, and it was considered to have radiographically loose baseplates determined by lucency around the screws or a change in the position of the baseplate over time in 13.6%. How much graft incorporation is necessary for stability of the implant is unknown, and using radiographs to assess how much graft remains is difficult. Some of the unincorporated graft could certainly be providing stability and could explain why, although a significant amount of resorption of some grafts appears to occur, very few patients had clinical symptoms and needed revision surgery.

Melis et al. [48] examined 37 anatomic TSAs requiring revisions to RSA; of these, 29 required a bone graft consisting of a structural iliac crest or cancellous autograft, and 3 allografts were used. At the mean follow-up of 47 months, 76% of the grafts were incorporated. A postoperative complication rate of 30% with a 22% repeat revision rate was reported. Recurrent glenoid loosening occurred in three of these patients and was considered to be related to using a short peg in the baseplate that did not extend past the graft into the native bone. Reimplantation with a long central fixation baseplate was performed in two patients. The authors did not differentiate between the results of patients with allografts and with autografts.

Bateman and Donald [3] reported using a hybrid grafting technique consisting of an allograft femoral neck packed with cancellous autograft in five patients (five cases). They used extended central fixation in all cases and reported no loosening or implant failures at the minimum 12-month follow-up. All grafts incorporated as early as 6 months. Bone grafting remains a frequently recommended technique for addressing severe glenoid wear with RSA. Indications for bone grafting and the best technique remain to be defined.

Despite these efforts, substantial glenoid bone loss present at the time of either primary or revision TSA has been associated with inferior outcomes [10, 12, 17, 28, 33, 51, 55]. Using bone grafting is generally associated with a high percentage of radiolucency, glenoid component failure, graft failures, and instability [2, 54, 59, 63].

In comparison to bone grafting, augmented baseplates have been considered less flexible because the degree of correction that the augmented baseplate can achieve is based on the geometry of the manufactured implant. Some augmented baseplates can allow for correction of deformity in multiple planes, and newer designs of off-the-shelf augmented baseplates do allow for more difficult correction. In addition, patient-specific augmented baseplates have been custom-fabricated and used to correct complex multiplanar deformity associated with severe bone loss, although the process to build such an implant is more complicated and expensive. In addition, it does not offer the possibility to reconstruct the glenoid bone stock.

Augmented glenoid components in RSA are commercially available, have been biomechanically studied, are favored because of the relative ease of insertion compared to more complex grafting techniques, do not require incorporation of a structural graft for success, and the designs continue to evolve [22, 32, 38, 56, 58]. Limited clinical data is available on augmented components in RSA currently although they may be a viable alternative to asymmetric reaming, bone grafting, or combined asymmetric reaming and bone grafting in the setting of moderate to severe glenoid erosion. They are typically inserted using an off-axis reaming technique relative to the plane of the deformity that preserves cortical bone and maintains a greater implant-to-bone contact area, potentially improving long-term glenoid fixation. Eliminating a structural graft using the augmented baseplate also eliminates concern for resorption of the graft or nonunion of the graft with subsequent baseplate loosening. A posterior augmented baseplate also can preserve anterior bone, correct version, and restore the native joint line.

Roche et al. [56, 69] compared fixation of standard and superior augmented glenoid baseplates. A superior glenoid defect was created and was corrected with either eccentric reaming with implantation of a standard glenoid baseplate or off-axis reaming with implantation of a superior augment glenoid baseplate. No differences in baseplate displacement were observed before or after cyclic loading between groups.

Authors Preferred Surgical Indications and Technique for Severely Eroded B2, B3, C, E2, and E3 Glenoids

The author's current technique for management of glenoid deformity relies heavily on adequate preoperative imaging using a 3D CT in all cases where deformity is suspected. E0 and E1 deformity is treated with standard glenoid preparation with minimal reaming and no use of bone graft. E2 and E3 glenoids are treated with minimal reaming and either a 10° superior or a combined posterior-superior augment that corrects 8° of posterior and 10° of superior deformity. The surgical goal is to preserve the patient's native bone stock and ream as little as possible. E3 glenoid deformity that medializes the joint line to the level of the coracoid is treated with autograft reconstruction using the convexity of the patient's native humeral head as the ideal graft. While correction to neutral glenoid version is the ultimate goal, 10–15° of residual glenoid component retroversion or anteversion is not considered catastrophic and acceptable in our hands as long as intraoperatively the surgeon can confirm that there is no scapular or coracoid contact with range of motion of the humerus via palpation. Superior inclination should be avoided, but up to 15° of inferior inclination can be accepted if the only other option is to ream away good cortical bone. B2 glenoid management is broken down into shallow B2 and deep (medialized) B2 glenoid deformities. Our first and preferred option is to lightly ream eccentrically and correct the deformity to a degree and use an off-the-shelf augmented product, targeting 60% back-side contact on good-quality bone as an acceptable amount, and correction of the deformity to within 10–15° (ideally within 10°) of neutral. This is usually achievable in patients with shallow B2 deformity with preserved paleoglenoids, and with the use of preoperative planning software and intraoperative navigation, both the final version and back-side contact can be confidently planned and intraoperatively confirmed. This is the most common deformity type seen and the most common reconstructive technique required in our hands. If the B2 deformity is too deep and this reaming will result in severe destruction of the bone and adequate back-side contact is a concern (based on preoperative planning), humeral head autograft is considered, if it is available. If the autologous humeral head is not available, femoral head allograft has been more reliably obtainable at our institution and is therefore our allograft of choice. Initial reaming to create a smooth prepared surface and initial fixation are contemplated using K-wires off-axis. Gentle reaming of the graft/glenoid construct is then done to allow for good bone implant contact. Primary fixation of the graft is usually achieved with the extended central fixation of the implant into the native scapula, and multiple screws are used for compression into the native scapula and stability of the construct. C-type glenoids are fortunately rare and need to be handled with extreme care as there can be very little and poor-quality bone to work with. Preoperative planning is essential in these cases, and they frequently require a combination of grafting and augmented components or custom-made glenoids.

Revision arthroplasty with cavitary defects can be managed with aggressive cancellous allograft impaction grafting into the vault and longer central and peripheral fixation with compression of the graft. Non-contained defects in younger patients are managed with autograft iliac crest, and in older patients, allograft femoral head is utilized, always obtaining fixation in the native glenoid with the central fixation and usually using more than the normal amount of screws on the baseplate.

Full glenoid exposure is necessary to be able to visualize and palpate the glenoid neck to assess the "zero axis." More recently, the use of intraoperative navigation has allowed for a much more simplified, no-K-wire-based approach that has provided intraoperative feedback of drill and reamer orientation and a precise reconstruction. For virtually every case, using preoperative planning is critical to understanding the deformity pattern, and using software to simulate your final reconstruction provides a high level of confidence going into the operating room. It is rare to have to troubleshoot the glenoid intraoperatively if a good preoperative plan is in place using software.

Rehabilitation

Boileau et al. [7] reported very little difference between rehabilitation protocols used for the graft augmented RSA and standard RSA. Patients were discharged 1 or 2 days after surgery. During the first 4–6 weeks, they wore a sling with or without an abduction pillow. Self-directed rehabilitation started immediately and included five 5-minute sessions each day of pendulum, elbow, wrist, and hand exercises performed without the sling. Patients were also allowed to remove the sling for hygiene. They were encouraged to immediately use the hand for activities of daily living, such as eating, drinking, holding a newspaper or a book, typewriting, and dressing. However, no active lifting was allowed. After 4–6 weeks, sling use was discontinued, formal rehabilitation with a physiotherapist started, physical therapy consisting of gradual range of motion and progressive strengthening exercises was initiated, and progression of activities as tolerated was allowed. Aquatherapy in a swimming pool was recommended. Heavy lifting was prohibited until 12 weeks after surgery to ensure solid bony union of the graft was obtained. Return to all types of activities, including gardening or leisure sports, was permitted after 3–6 months.

Conversely, Romano et al. [57] used a more cautious rehabilitation protocol for this "high-care" category of patients who were treated with eccentric reaming, bone graft, or augmented baseplates and reported satisfactory clinical and radiological results. The required duration of immobilization and the need for a structured therapy program after RSA remains a topic of debate, with some surgeons minimizing or eliminating both of these postoperative treatments and others continuing to apply a formal protocol. Our current protocol for grafted and non-grafted cases is the same, with a 3-week window of sling immobilization without swathe. During this time, we instruct patients that shoulder extension should be avoided and that ideally the position of the arm should be so that they can easily see their elbow (avoiding extension behind the body). Patients are encouraged to perform gentle pendulum exercises when the regional anesthetic has worn off for 5 min, five times a day, as well as simple active hand and elbow ROM (elbow flexion, extension, pronation, supination, and fisting). Patients are encouraged to remove the sling for simple seated activities such as eating, holding a book, and brushing their teeth during this first 3-week window. After 3 weeks, the sling is removed, and patients are encouraged to use the arm more freely but to avoid lifting anything heavier than a cup of coffee for the first 2 months. After 2 months, activity is gradually increased with a restriction on the most vigorous parts of golf and tennis (golf bunker shots and overhead tennis shots) until 5 months. Occupational and physical therapists are utilized during the first week after surgery to confirm that the patient is performing the pendulum program correctly, and after this first week, for most patients there is no supervised program used at our center.

Conclusions

Severe glenoid erosion includes a broad spectrum of pathologic conditions and is a frequent problem encountered by shoulder surgeons performing arthroplasty, with many proposed techniques to manage this condition. Varying amounts of bone loss produce distinctly different types of deformity. Meticulous preoperative planning is important to determine the best surgical approach. In cases of complex or extreme bone loss, RSA offers a reliable solution that is particularly attractive for older and less active patients, and its use is supported by the demonstration of unreliable results using TSA in the same group of patients. Familiarity with the full spectrum of treatment options will allow the surgeon to make the best decision for patients when these patterns of deformity are encountered. This procedure remains technically demanding regardless of the technique performed to accommodate bone loss.

References

1. Allred JJ, Flores-Hernandez C, Hoenecke HR Jr, D'Lima DD. Posterior augmented glenoid implants require less bone removal and generate lower stresses: a finite element analysis. J Shoulder Elb Surg. 2016;25:823–30. https://doi.org/10.1016/j.jse.2015.10.003.
2. Ascione F, Bugelli G, Domos P, Neyton L, Godeneche A, Bercik MJ, Walch G. Reverse shoulder arthroplasty with a new convertible short stem: preliminary 2- to 4-year follow-up results. J Shoulder Elb Arthropl. 2017; https://doi.org/10.1177/2471549217746272.
3. Bateman E, Donald S. Reconstruction of massive uncontained glenoid defects using a combined autograft-allograft construct with reverse shoulder arthroplasty: preliminary results. J Shoulder Elb Surg. 2012;21:925–34. https://doi.org/10.1016/j.jse.2011.07.009.
4. Bercik MJ, Kruse K 2nd, Yalizis M, Gauci MO, Chaoui J, Walch G. A modification to the Walch classification of the glenoid in primary glenohumeral osteoarthritis using three-dimensional imaging. J Shoulder Elb Surg. 2016;25:1601–6. https://doi.org/10.1016/j.jse.2016.03.010.

5. Boileau P, Avidor C, Krishnan SG, Walch G, Kempf JF, Molé D. Cemented polyethylene versus uncemented metal-backed glenoid components in total shoulder arthroplasty: a prospective, double-blind, randomized study. J Shoulder Elb Surg. 2002;11:351–9. https://doi.org/10.1067/mse.2002.125807.
6. Boileau P, Moineau G, Roussanne Y, O'Shea K. Bony increased-offset reversed shoulder arthroplasty: minimizing scapular impingement while maximizing glenoid fixation. Clin Orthop Relat Res. 2011;469:2558–67. https://doi.org/10.1007/s11999-011-1775-4.
7. Boileau P, Morin-Salvo N, Gauci MO, Seeto BL, Chalmers PN, Holzer N, et al. Angled BIO-RSA (bony-increased offset-reverse shoulder arthroplasty): a solution for the management of glenoid bone loss and erosion. J Shoulder Elb Surg. 2017;26(12):2133–42. https://doi.org/10.1016/j.jse.2017.05.024.
8. Boone DW. Complications of iliac crest graft and bone grafting alternatives in foot and ankle surgery. Foot Ankle Clin. 2003;8:1–14. https://doi.org/10.1016/S1083-7515(02)00128-6.
9. Budge MD, Lewis GS, Schaefer E, Coquia S, Flemming DJ, Armstrong AD. Comparison of standard two-dimensional and three-dimensional corrected glenoid version measurements. J Shoulder Elb Surg. 2011;20:577–83. https://doi.org/10.1016/j.jse.2010.11.003.
10. Cheung EV, Sperling JW, Cofield RH. Reimplantation of a glenoid component following component removal and allogenic bone-grafting. J Bone Joint Surg Am. 2007;89:1777–83. https://doi.org/10.2106/JBJS.F.00711.
11. Clavert P, Millett PJ, Warner JJ. Glenoid resurfacing: what are the limits to asymmetric reaming for posterior erosion? J Shoulder Elb Surg. 2007;16:843–8. https://doi.org/10.1016/j.jse.2007.03.015.
12. Cofield RH, Edgerton BC. Total shoulder arthroplasty. complications and revision surgery. Instr Course Lect. 1990;39:449–62.
13. Denard PJ, Walch G. Current concepts in the surgical management of primary glenohumeral arthritis with a biconcave glenoid. J Shoulder Elb Surg. 2013;22:1589–98. https://doi.org/10.1016/j.jse.2013.06.017.
14. Deshmukh AV, Koris M, Zurakowski D, Thornhill TS. Total shoulder arthroplasty: long-term survivorship, functional outcome, and quality of life. J Shoulder Elb Surg. 2005;14:471–9. https://doi.org/10.1016/j.jse.2005.02.009.
15. Favard L, Lautmann S, Sirveaux F, Oudet D, Kerjean Y, Huguet D. Hemiarthroplasty versus reverse arthroplasty in the treatment of osteoarthritis with massive rotator cuff tear. In: Walch G, Boileau P, Molé D, editors. 2000 shoulder prostheses: two to ten year follow-up. Montpellier: Sauramps Médical; 2001. p. 261–8.
16. Fox TJ, Cil A, Sperling JW, Sanchez-Sotelo J, Schleck CD, Cofield RH. Survival of the glenoid component in shoulder arthroplasty. J Shoulder Elb Surg. 2009;18:859–63. https://doi.org/10.1016/j.jse.2008.11.020.
17. Frankle MA, Teramoto A, Luo ZP, Levy JC, Pupello D. Glenoid morphology in reverse shoulder arthroplasty: classification and surgical implications. J Shoulder Elb Surg. 2009;18:874–85. https://doi.org/10.1016/j.jse.2009.02.013.
18. Franta AK, Lenters TR, Mounce D, Neradilek B, Matsen FA 3rd. The complex characteristics of 282 unsatisfactory shoulder arthroplasties. J Shoulder Elb Surg. 2007;16:555–62. https://doi.org/10.1016/j.jse.2006.11.004.
19. Ganapathi A, McCarron JA, Chen X, Iannotti JP. Predicting normal glenoid version from the pathologic scapula: a comparison of 4 methods in 2- and 3-dimensional models. J Shoulder Elb Surg. 2011;20:234–44. https://doi.org/10.1016/j.jse.2010.05.024.
20. Gerber C, Costouros JG, Sukthankar A, Fucentese SF. Static posterior humeral head subluxation and total shoulder arthroplasty. J Shoulder Elb Surg. 2009;18:505–10. https://doi.org/10.1016/j.jse.2009.03.003.
21. Gillespie R, Lyons R, Lazarus M. Eccentric reaming in total shoulder arthroplasty: a cadaveric study. Orthopedics. 2009;31:21. https://doi.org/10.3928/01477447-20090101-07.
22. Gilot GJ. Addressing glenoid erosion in reverse total shoulder arthroplasty. Bull Hosp Jt Dis (2013). 2013;71(Suppl 2):S51–3.
23. Gutiérrez S, Greiwe RM, Frankle MA, Siegal S, Lee WE 3rd. Biomechanical comparison of component position and hardware failure in the reverse shoulder prosthesis. J Shoulder Elb Surg. 2007;16(3 Suppl):S9–12. https://doi.org/10.1016/j.jse.2005.11.008.
24. Gutiérrez S, Walker M, Willis M, Pupello DR, Frankle MA. Effects of tilt and glenosphere eccentricity on baseplate/bone interface forces in a computational model, validated by a mechanical model, of reverse shoulder arthroplasty. J Shoulder Elb Surg. 2011;20:732–9. https://doi.org/10.1016/j.jse.2010.10.035.
25. Habermeyer P, Magosch P, Lichtenberg S. Recentering the humeral head for glenoid deficiency in total shoulder arthroplasty. Clin Orthop Relat Res. 2007;457:124–32. https://doi.org/10.1097/BLO.0b013e31802ff03c.
26. Harmsen S, Casagrande D, Norris T. "Shaped" humeral head autograft reverse shoulder arthroplasty: treatment for primary glenohumeral osteoarthritis with significant posterior glenoid bone loss (B2, B3, and C type). Orthopade. 2017;46(12):1045–54. https://doi.org/10.1007/s00132-017-3497-0.
27. Hettrich CM, Permeswaran VN, Goetz JE, Anderson DD. Mechanical tradeoffs associated with glenosphere lateralization in reverse shoulder arthroplasty. J Shoulder Elb Surg. 2015;24:1774–81. https://doi.org/10.1016/j.jse.2015.06.011.

28. Hill JM, Norris TR. Long-term results of total shoulder arthroplasty following bone-grafting of the glenoid. J Bone Joint Surg Am. 2001;83:877–83. https://doi.org/10.2106/00004623-200106000-00009.
29. Ho JC, Sabesan VJ, Iannotti JP. Glenoid component retroversion is associated with osteolysis. J Bone Joint Surg Am. 2013;95:e82. https://doi.org/10.2106/JBJS.L.00336.
30. Hsu JE, Ricchetti ET, Huffman GR, Iannotti JP, Glaser DL. Addressing glenoid bone deficiency and asymmetric posterior erosion in shoulder arthroplasty. J Shoulder Elb Surg. 2013;22:1298–308. https://doi.org/10.1016/j.jse.2013.04.014.
31. Iannotti JP, Frangiamore SJ. Fate of large structural allograft for treatment of severe uncontained glenoid bone deficiency. J Shoulder Elb Surg. 2012;21:765–71. https://doi.org/10.1016/j.jse.2011.08.069.
32. Iannotti JP, Lappin KE, Klotz CL, Reber EW, Swope SW. Liftoff resistance of augmented glenoid components during cyclic fatigue loading in the posterior-superior direction. J Shoulder Elb Surg. 2013;22:1530–6. https://doi.org/10.1016/j.jse.2013.01.018.
33. Iannotti JP, Norris TR. Influence of preoperative factors on outcome of shoulder arthroplasty for glenohumeral arthritis. J Bone Joint Surg Am. 2003;85:251–8. https://doi.org/10.2106/00004623-200302000-00011.
34. Iannotti JP, Weiner S, Rodriguez E, Subhas N, Patterson TE, Jun BJ, et al. Three-dimensional imaging and templating improve glenoid implant positioning. J Bone Joint Surg Am. 2015;97:651–8. https://doi.org/10.2106/JBJS.N.00493.
35. Jones RB, Wright TW, Roche CP. Bone grafting the glenoid versus use of augmented glenoid baseplates with reverse shoulder arthroplasty. Bull Hosp Jt Dis (2013). 2015;73(Suppl 1):S129–35.
36. Jones RB, Wright TW, Zuckerman JD. Reverse total shoulder arthroplasty with structural bone grafting of large glenoid defects. J Shoulder Elb Surg. 2016;25:1425–32. https://doi.org/10.1016/j.jse.2016.01.016.
37. Kelly JD 2nd, Zhao JX, Hobgood ER, Norris TR. Clinical results of revision shoulder arthroplasty using the reverse prosthesis. J Shoulder Elb Surg. 2012;21:1516–25. https://doi.org/10.1016/j.jse.2011.11.021.
38. Kirane YM, Lewis GS, Sharkey NA, Armstrong AD. Mechanical characteristics of a novel posterior-step prosthesis for biconcave glenoid defects. J Shoulder Elb Surg. 2012;21:105–15. https://doi.org/10.1016/j.jse.2010.12.008.
39. Klein SM, Dunning P, Mulieri P, Pupello D, Downes K, Frankle MA. Effects of acquired glenoid bone defects on surgical technique and clinical outcomes in reverse shoulder arthroplasty. J Bone Joint Surg Am. 2010;92:1144–54. https://doi.org/10.2106/JBJS.I.00778.
40. Kwon YW, Powell KA, Yum JK, Brems JJ, Iannotti JP. Use of three-dimensional computed tomography for the analysis of the glenoid anatomy. J Shoulder Elb Surg. 2005;14:85–90. https://doi.org/10.1016/j.jse.2004.04.011.
41. Laver L, Garrigues GE. Avoiding superior tilt in reverse shoulder arthroplasty: a review of the literature and technical recommendations. J Shoulder Elb Surg. 2014;23:1582–90. https://doi.org/10.1016/j.jse.2014.06.029.
42. Lévigne C, Boileau P, Favard L, Garaud P, Molé D, Sirveaux F, et al. Scapular notching in reverse shoulder arthroplasty. J Shoulder Elb Surg. 2008;17:925–35. https://doi.org/10.1016/j.jse.2008.02.010.
43. Lévigne C, Franceschi JP. Rheumatoid arthritis of the shoulder: radiographic presentation and results of arthroplasty. In: Walch G, Boileau P, editors. Shoulder arthroplasty. Berlin: Springer-Verlag; 1999. p. 221–30.
44. Levine WN, Djurasovic M, Glasson JM, Pollock RG, Flatow EL, Bigliani LU. Hemiarthroplasty for glenohumeral osteoarthritis: results correlated to degree of glenoid wear. J Shoulder Elb Surg. 1997;6:449–54. https://doi.org/10.1016/S1058-2746(97)70052-1.
45. Li X, Knutson Z, Choi D, Lobatto D, Lipman J, Craig EV, et al. Effects of glenosphere positioning on impingement-free internal and external rotation after reverse total shoulder arthroplasty. J Shoulder Elb Surg. 2013;22:807–13. https://doi.org/10.1016/j.jse.2012.07.013.
46. Matsen FA 3rd, Clinton J, Lynch J, Bertelsen A, Richardson ML. Glenoid component failure in total shoulder arthroplasty. J Bone Joint Surg Am. 2008;90:885–96. https://doi.org/10.2106/JBJS.G.01263.
47. Matsen FA 3rd, Warme WJ, Jackins SE. Can the ream and run procedure improve glenohumeral relationships and function for shoulders with the arthritic triad? Clin Orthop Relat Res. 2015;473:2088–96. https://doi.org/10.1007/s11999-014-4095-7.
48. Melis B, Bonnevialle N, Neyton L, Lévigne C, Favard L, Walch G, et al. Glenoid loosening and failure in anatomical total shoulder arthroplasty: is revision with a reverse shoulder arthroplasty a reliable option? J Shoulder Elb Surg. 2012;21:342–9. https://doi.org/10.1016/j.jse.2011.05.021.
49. Mizuno N, Denard PJ, Raiss P, Walch G. Reverse total shoulder arthroplasty for primary glenohumeral osteoarthritis in patients with a biconcave glenoid. J Bone Joint Surg Am. 2013;95:1297–304. https://doi.org/10.2106/JBJS.L.00820.
50. Neer CS 2nd, Craig EV, Fukuda H. Cuff-tear arthropathy. J Bone Joint Surg Am. 1983;65:1232–44. https://doi.org/10.2106/00004623-198365090-00003.
51. Neyton L, Boileau P, Nové-Josserand L, Edwards TB, Walch G. Glenoid bone grafting with reverse design prosthesis. J Shoulder Elb Surg. 2007;16(3 Suppl):S71–8. https://doi.org/10.1016/j.jse.2006.02.002.
52. Norris TR, Kelly JD 2nd, Humphrey CS. Management of glenoid bone defects in revision shoulder arthroplasty: a new application of the reverse total shoulder

prosthesis. Tech Shoulder Elb Surg. 2007;8:37–46. https://doi.org/10.1097/BTE.0b013e318030d3b7.
53. Nowak DD, Bahu MJ, Gardner TR, Dyrszka MD, Levine WN, Bigliani LU, et al. Simulation of surgical glenoid resurfacing using three-dimensional computed tomography of the arthritic glenohumeral joint: the amount of glenoid retroversion that can be corrected. J Shoulder Elb Surg. 2009;18:680–8. https://doi.org/10.1016/j.jse.2009.03.019.
54. Phipatanakul WP, Norris TR. Treatment of glenoid loosening and bone loss due to osteolysis with glenoid bone grafting. J Shoulder Elb Surg. 2006;15:84–7. https://doi.org/10.1016/j.jse.2005.06.004.
55. Rice RS, Sperling JW, Miletti J, Schleck C, Cofield RH. Augmented glenoid component for bone deficiency in shoulder arthroplasty. Clin Orthop Relat Res. 2008;466:579–83. https://doi.org/10.1007/s11999-007-0104-4
56. Roche CP, Stroud NJ, Martin BL, Steiler CA, Flurin PH, Wright TW, et al. Achieving fixation in glenoids with superior wear using reverse shoulder arthroplasty. J Shoulder Elb Surg. 2013;22:1695–701. https://doi.org/10.1016/j.jse.2013.03.008.
57. Romano AM, Oliva F, Nastrucci G, Casillo P, Di Giunta A, Susanna M, et al. Reverse shoulder arthroplasty patient personalized rehabilitation protocol: preliminary results according to prognostic groups. Muscle Ligaments Tendons J. 2017;7:263–70. https://doi.org/10.11138/mltj/2017.7.2.263.
58. Sabesan V, Callanan M, Sharma V, Iannotti JP. Correction of acquired glenoid bone loss in osteoarthritis with a standard versus an augmented glenoid component. J Shoulder Elb Surg. 2014;23:964–73. https://doi.org/10.1016/j.jse.2013.09.019.
59. Sears BW, Johnston PS, Ramsey ML, Williams GR. Glenoid bone loss in primary total shoulder arthroplasty: evaluation and management. J Am Acad Orthop Surg. 2012;20(9):604–13. https://doi.org/10.5435/JAAOS-20-09-604.
60. Scalise JJ, Bryan J, Polster J, Brems JJ, Iannotti JP. Quantitative analysis of glenoid bone loss in osteoarthritis using three-dimensional computed tomography scans. J Shoulder Elb Surg. 2008;17:328–35. https://doi.org/10.1016/j.jse.2007.07.013.
61. Shapiro TA, McGarry MH, Gupta R, Lee YS, Lee TQ. Biomechanical effects of glenoid retroversion in total shoulder arthroplasty. J Shoulder Elb Surg. 2007;16(3 Suppl):S90–5. https://doi.org/10.1016/j.jse.2006.07.010.
62. Singh JA, Sperling JW, Cofield RH. Revision surgery following total shoulder arthroplasty: analysis of 2588 shoulders over three decades (1976 to 2008). J Bone Joint Surg Br. 2011;93:1513–7. https://doi.org/10.1302/0301-620X.93B11.26938.
63. Stephens SP, Paisley KC, Jeng J, Dutta AK, Wirth MA. Shoulder arthroplasty in the presence of posterior glenoid bone loss. J Bone Joint Surg Am. 2015;97(3):251–9. https://doi.org/10.2106/JBJS.N.00566.
64. Valenti P, Sauzières P, Katz D, Kalouche I, Kilinc AS. Do less medialized reverse shoulder prostheses increase motion and reduce notching? Clin Orthop Relat Res. 2011;469:2550–7. https://doi.org/10.1007/s11999-011-1844-8.
65. Visotsky JL, Basamania C, Seebauer L, Rockwood CA, Jensen KL. Cuff tear arthropathy: pathogenesis, classification, and algorithm for treatment. J Bone Joint Surg Am. 2004;86(Suppl 2):35–40. https://doi.org/10.2106/00004623-200412002-00007.
66. Walch G, Badet R, Boulahia A, Khoury A. Morphologic study of the glenoid in primary glenohumeral osteoarthritis. J Arthroplast. 1999;14:756–60. https://doi.org/10.1016/S0883-5403(99)90232-2.
67. Walch G, Moraga C, Young A, Castellanos-Rosas J. Results of anatomic nonconstrained prosthesis in primary osteoarthritis with biconcave glenoid. J Shoulder Elb Surg. 2012;21:1526–33. https://doi.org/10.1016/j.jse.2011.11.030.
68. Walch G, Young AA, Boileau P, Loew M, Gazielly D, Molé D. Patterns of loosening of polyethylene keeled glenoid components after shoulder arthroplasty for primary osteoarthritis: results of a multicenter study with more than five years of follow-up. J Bone Joint Surg Am. 2012;94:145–50. https://doi.org/10.2106/JBJS.J.00699.
69. Wright TW, Roche CP, Wright L, Flurin PH, Crosby LA, Zuckerman JD. Reverse shoulder arthroplasty augments for glenoid wear: comparison of posterior augments to superior augments. Bull Hosp Jt Dis (2013). 2015;73(Suppl 1):124–8.

Treatment of Post-traumatic Sequelae with Shoulder Arthroplasty

6

Christopher Chuinard

Treatment of Post-traumatic Sequelae with Shoulder Arthroplasty

The approach to treating proximal humerus fracture sequelae involves understanding how patient complaints relate to the pathoanatomy. Lifestyle limitations that result from pain and loss of function and lifestyle demands define the treatment strategy. The incidence of proximal humerus fractures accounts for approximately 5–8% of all fractures, with over 80% treated non-operatively [1–3]. However, operative treatment rates have increased with the advent of newer technologies like locked platting and reverse shoulder arthroplasty [4, 5]. Furthermore, with the increase in extreme sports and predominance of snowboarding over skiing, higher-energy fractures are becoming more frequent in the younger population, and fragility fractures may increase with the aging population in the USA. As a result, the sequelae of proximal humerus fractures are increasing.

Osteoporosis, diabetes, smoking, and other comorbidities influence the rates of healing of proximal humeral fractures, and patients with these conditions are at a high risk for treatment failure or avascular necrosis with humeral bone collapse [2]. Metaphyseal comminution and surgical neck translation of greater than 30% are some of the anatomic factors that influence the rate of nonunion which has been reported to be between 1.1% and 10% [3].

An in-depth understanding of the pathoanatomy is essential to select the optimal treatment, and algorithms based upon clinical outcomes can assist the physician. When evaluating a malunion, the mechanism that created the injury may have influence over the deficit the injury creates. Was it simply a failure of conservative management? Did the patient do well for a period of time and only become symptomatic many years later? If the malunion followed surgical treatment, are implant factors or other technical considerations responsible for the current deformity? How do the scapular dynamics contribute to the patient's function? Furthermore, did neurovascular injury, patient compliance, or other host factors play a role?

The status of the humeral head and tuberosities must be carefully evaluated. Ideally, if the head has collapsed but the tuberosities are in a relatively good position, success can be achieved by accepting the deformity and implanting a new joint surface, facilitated by implants that do not require diaphyseal fixation (Fig. 6.1). But what if a tuberosity osteotomy must be performed or another deformity must be corrected to implant an anatomic prosthesis (Fig. 6.2a, b)? The status of the greater and lesser tuberosities and their corresponding rotator cuff muscles is of paramount importance to shoulder function; if there

C. Chuinard (✉)
Great Lakes Orthopaedic Center,
Traverse City, MI, USA

R. Z. Tashjian (ed.), *Complex and Revision Shoulder Arthroplasty*,
https://doi.org/10.1007/978-3-030-02756-8_6

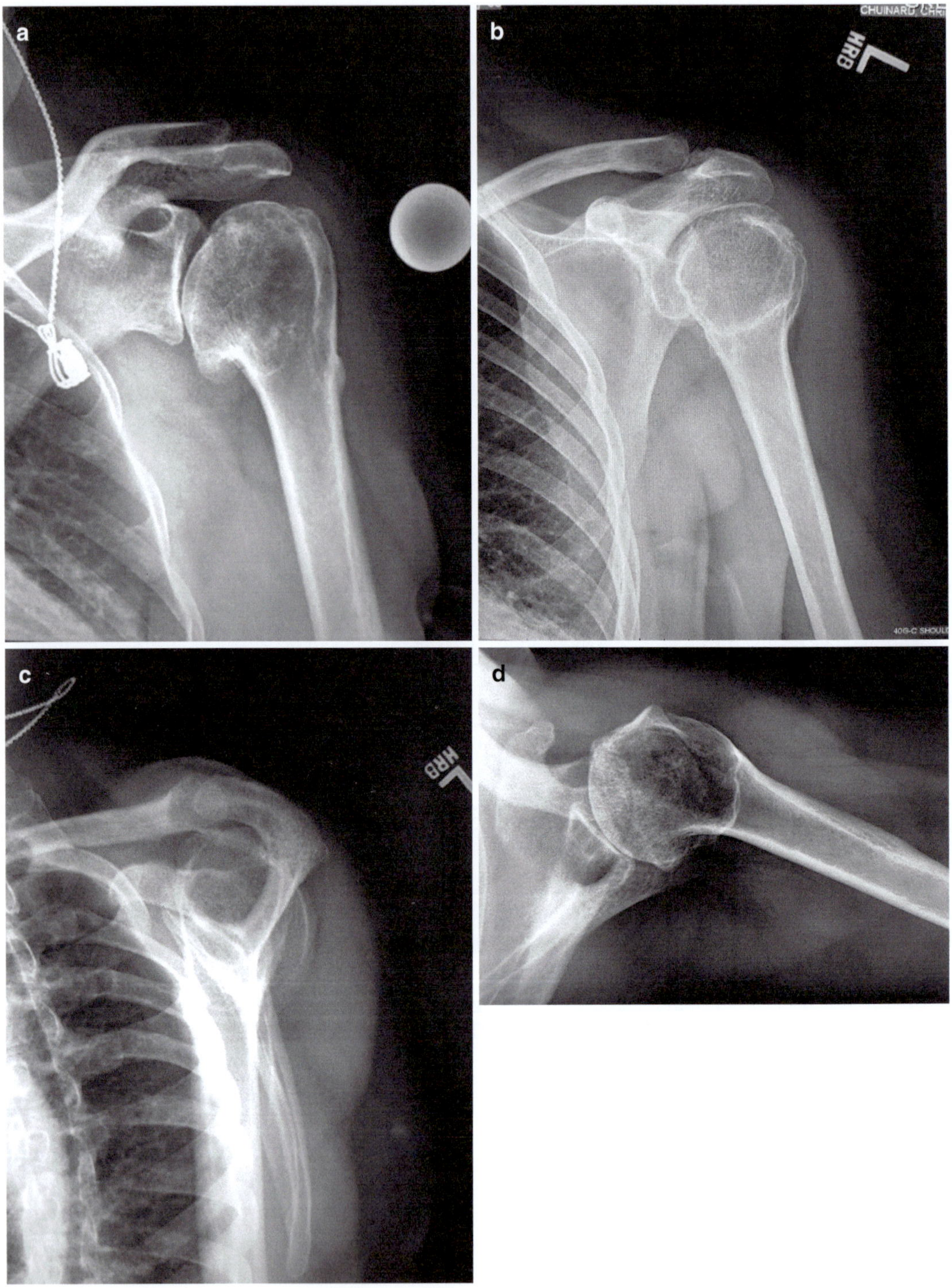

Fig. 6.1 The x-rays demonstrate a type 1 fracture (**a**–**d**) sequela which resulted from a valgus impacted fracture. The tuberosities are in a good position; therefore this can be managed with a stemless total shoulder implant (**e**–**h**)

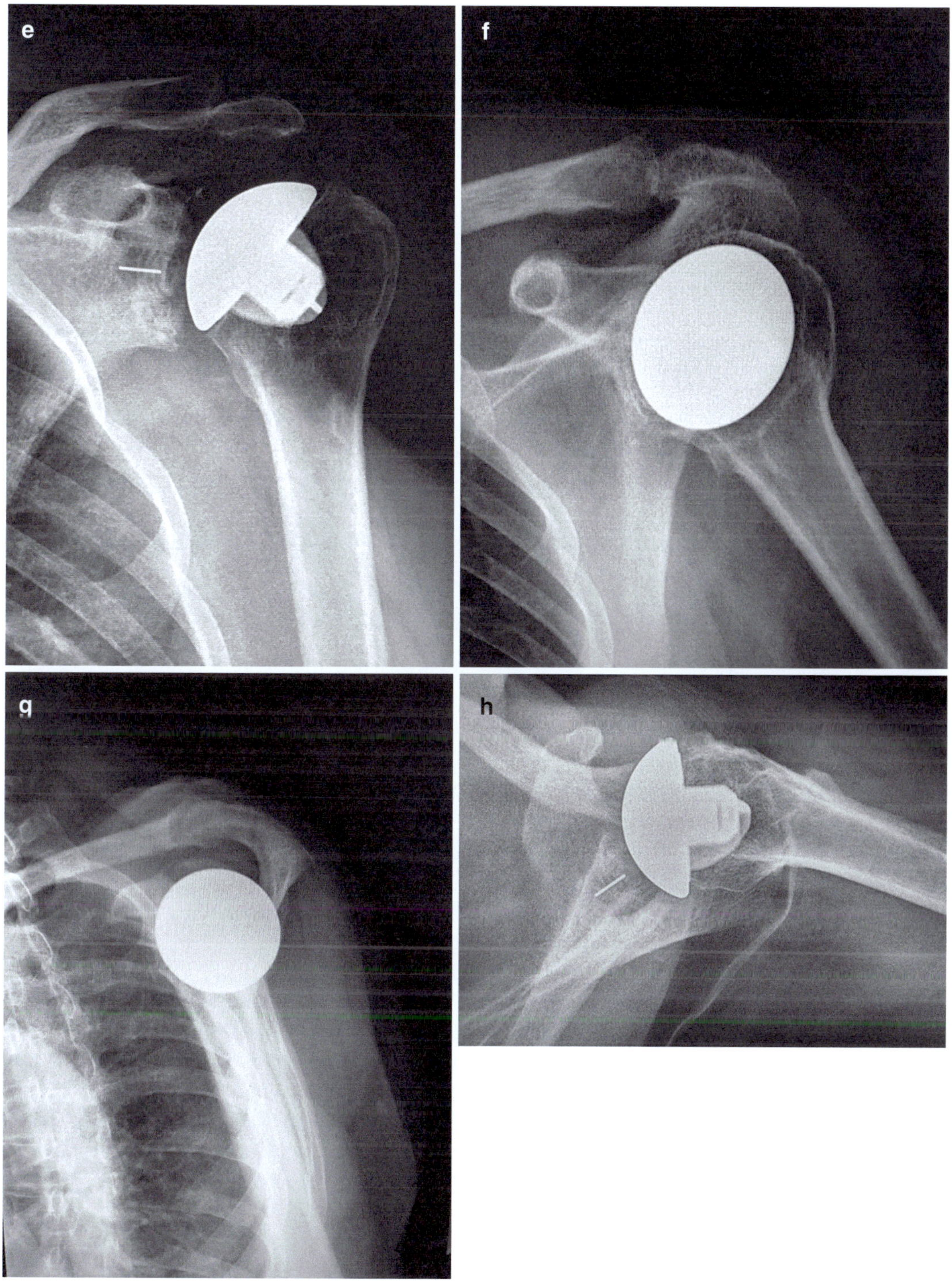

Fig. 6.1 (continued)

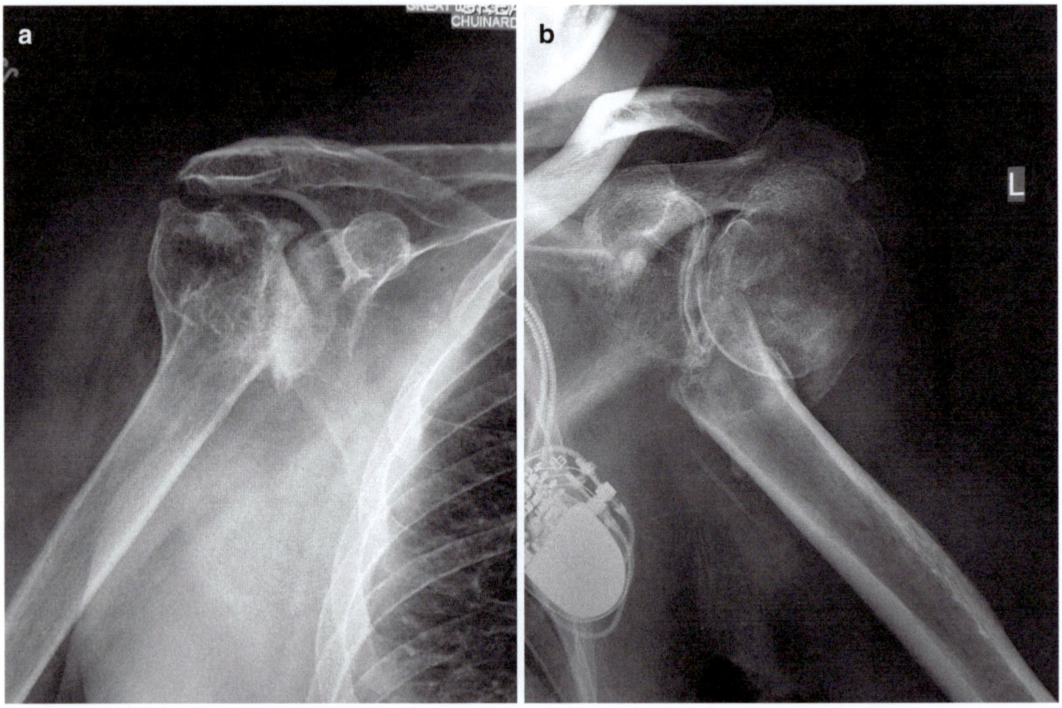

Fig. 6.2 (**a**) Demonstrates a malunion that would be a challenging anatomic reconstruction without a tuberosity osteotomy; (**b**) demonstrates a malunion with heterotopic ossification and malrotation. Both would be considered type 4 sequela as neither would do well with an anatomic replacement or osteotomy

is any doubt about the health of the cuff or the relative position of the tuberosities, the treatment may need to vary accordingly (Fig. 6.3a, b).

Nonunions of the proximal humerus require the same considered approach (Fig. 6.4). What factors led to the nonunion? Are host factors to be blamed? Is it failure of non-operative management? Was the surgical treatment appropriate? Was there excessive motion at the implant or inadequate immobilization? If pain is the main issue, is the hardware prominent? And in cases of either malunion or nonunion, was there an infection work-up performed to rule out other concomitant problems?

Surgical malunions or hardware failure may require staged operations. For patients with previous shoulder surgery, there must be a high index of suspicion for occult infection/colonization. Asymmetric blushing (Fig. 6.5a, b) on the skin adjacent to surgical incisions and chronic axillary nodes are frequent cutaneous manifestations of a subclinical infection. Traditional infection markers like sedimentation rate, CRP, and elevated WBC are rarely elevated, but pain is a frequent symptom. *Propionibacterium acnes* (*P. acnes*), *Staphylococcus*, and *Streptococcus* species are normal flora in high density around the neck and shoulder girdle. Moreover, these facultative anaerobes create a biofilm that adheres to foreign material and blocks the host defenses. Consequently, it is crucial to remove as much implant and suture burden as possible at the time of any revision operation or to stage any significant revision. Sutures and anchors should be removed and cultures obtained.

Some patients may decompensate after doing well for many years; the treating physician should obtain the injury films and all treatment records if possible. A careful neurovascular examination is imperative to rule out associated plexus or axillary nerve/vessel injuries, especially if there was a dislocation or displacement of the fracture fragments medial to the conjoined tendon. An EMG and vascular study may be necessary as injuries to the axillary nerve and brachial plexus are common, even with low-energy trauma, and axillary artery injuries

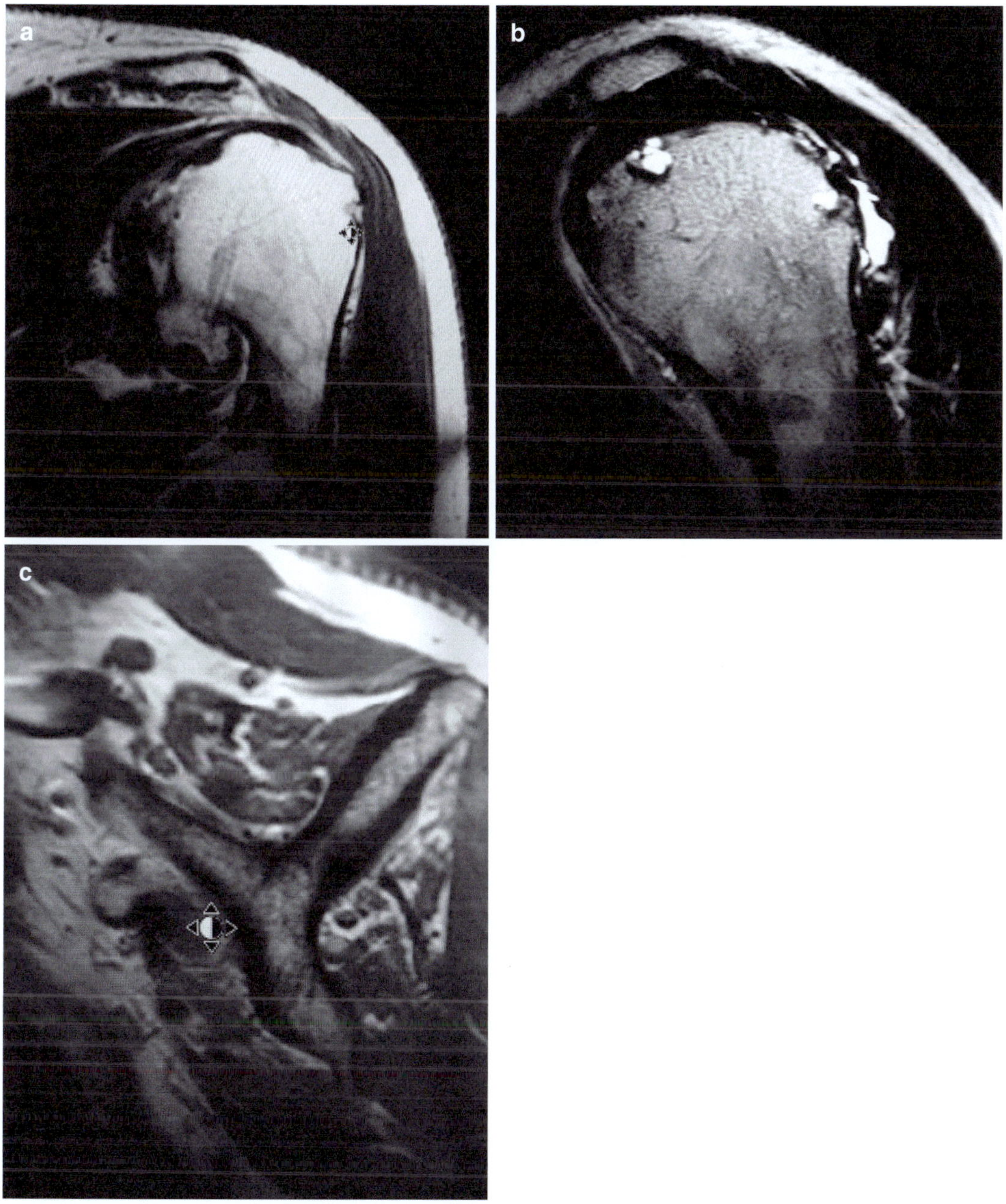

Fig. 6.3 (**a**) Coronal and (**b**) sagittal images demonstrating significant post-traumatic arthropathy with only minimal angular deformity. For a younger patient, anatomic arthroplasty may be appropriate, but for the elderly patient, reverse shoulder arthroplasty may be the treatment of choice due to the attenuated rotator cuff. (**c**) Sagittal image demonstrates atrophy and fatty infiltration of the supraspinatus and infraspinatus

are easily overlooked (Fig. 6.6). Rotational deformities of the proximal humerus or greater tuberosity can lead to suprascapular nerve entrapment, resulting in pain and weakness. Ultimately, the physician must understand the patient's goals: is it pain relief, improvement in function, or both? And what is realistic for both the patient and the surgeon?

Location of the scar and choice of surgical approach may have resulted in deltoid dehiscence or devascularization; nerve injury may be

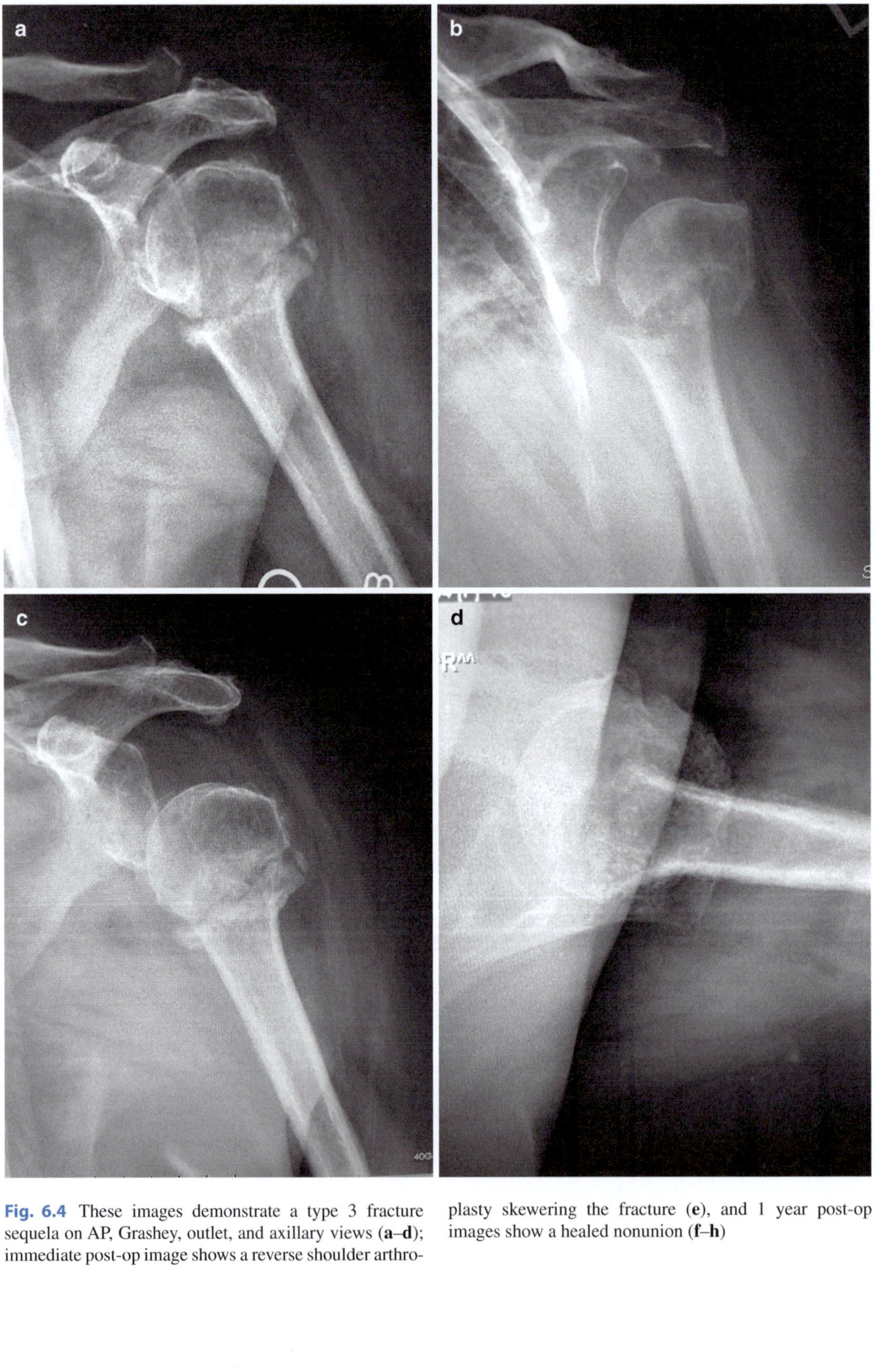

Fig. 6.4 These images demonstrate a type 3 fracture sequela on AP, Grashey, outlet, and axillary views (**a–d**); immediate post-op image shows a reverse shoulder arthroplasty skewering the fracture (**e**), and 1 year post-op images show a healed nonunion (**f–h**)

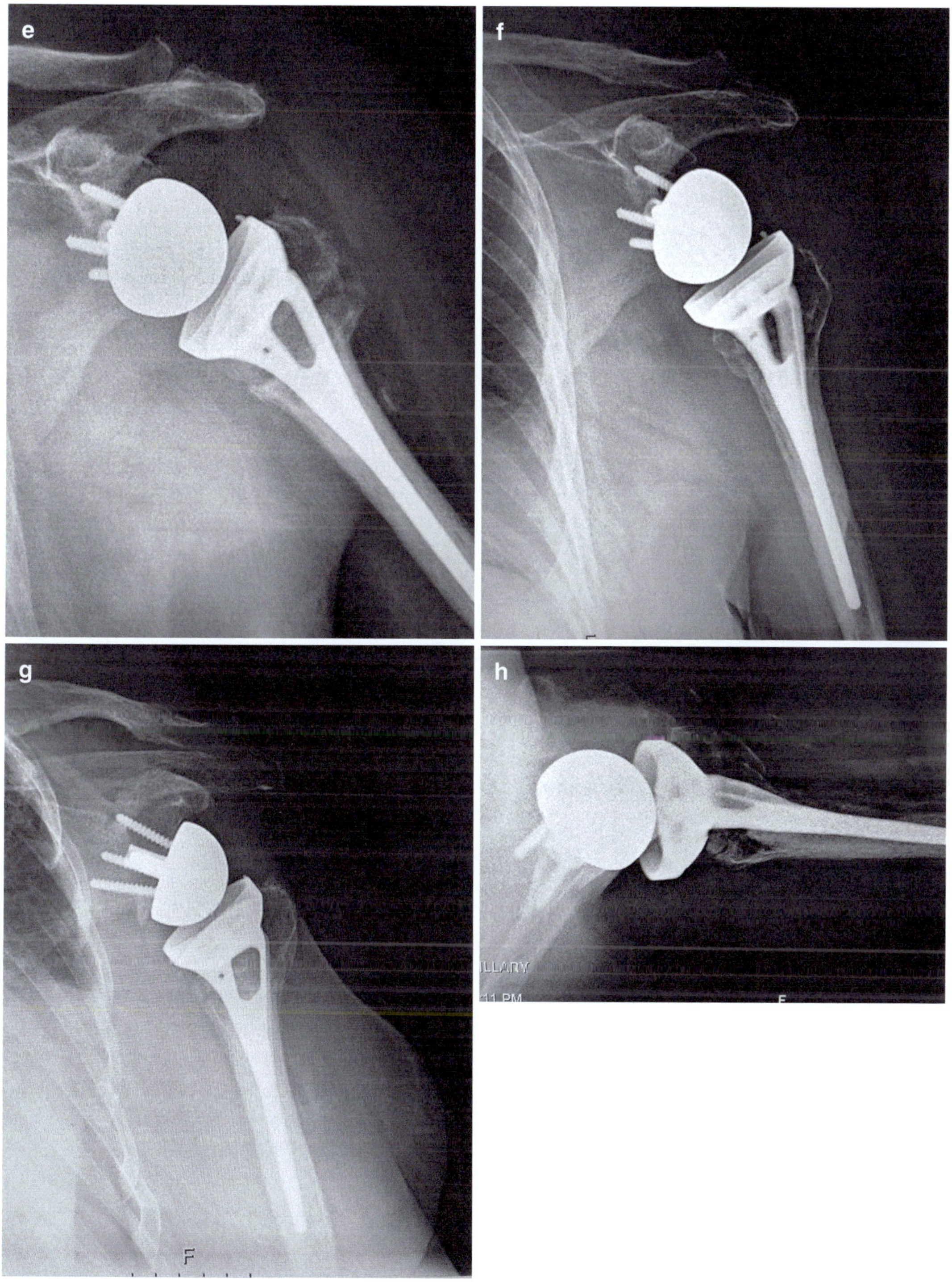

Fig. 6.4 (continued)

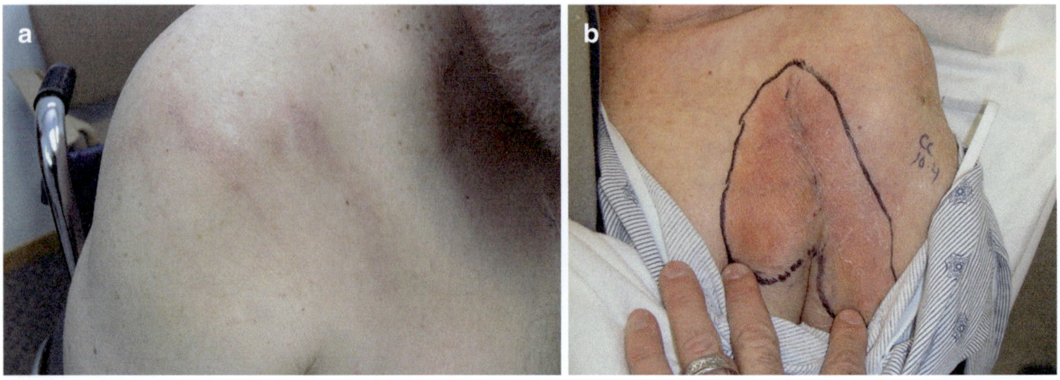

Fig. 6.5 (**a**) Subtle cutaneous streaking that can be indicative of an indolent *P. acnes* infection; (**b**) not so subtle redness consistent with infection

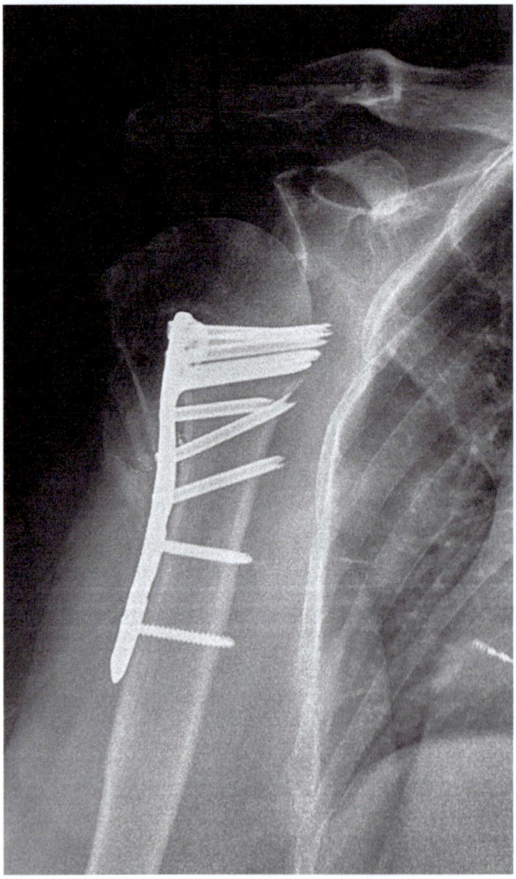

Fig. 6.6 An elderly woman suffered a proximal humerus fracture with an unrecognized brachial plexus injury. This Grashey image demonstrates ptosis of the shoulder, loss of humeral reduction, and hardware malposition with screw protrusion

suggested by overall shoulder asymmetry. Alcoholism, diabetes, smoking, obesity, or osteoporosis may have been factors in the initial trauma as well as the outcome of the treatment [1–5]. Less common factors like metal allergy or infection may have contributed to failure of the previous operative treatment (Fig. 6.7).

A classification scheme to categorize the fracture sequelae and guide the treatment is useful because these patients are often younger and more active than patients treated for osteoarthritis; intracapsular injuries may have different consequences than extracapsular injuries. Furthermore, with increased life expectancy and increased utilization of locking plates, physicians will be caring for older patients with greater hardware complications [1, 11–14]. While no classification supplants good clinical judgment, it can provide a foundation for critical decisions [1, 11–15]. However, small case series with ill-defined, heterogeneous pathology have made it challenging to standardize treatment [6–12, 16–51]. Therefore, simply describing the injury as a "nonunion" or a "malunion" is not enough: How old is the patient, and what are the comorbidities? What does the rotator cuff look like with advanced imaging? What is the status of the greater tuberosity? The viability of the greater tuberosity is of great importance and may dictate the treatment options [1, 2, 12, 34].

The complexity and variation of the anatomy of proximal humeral fracture sequelae have made

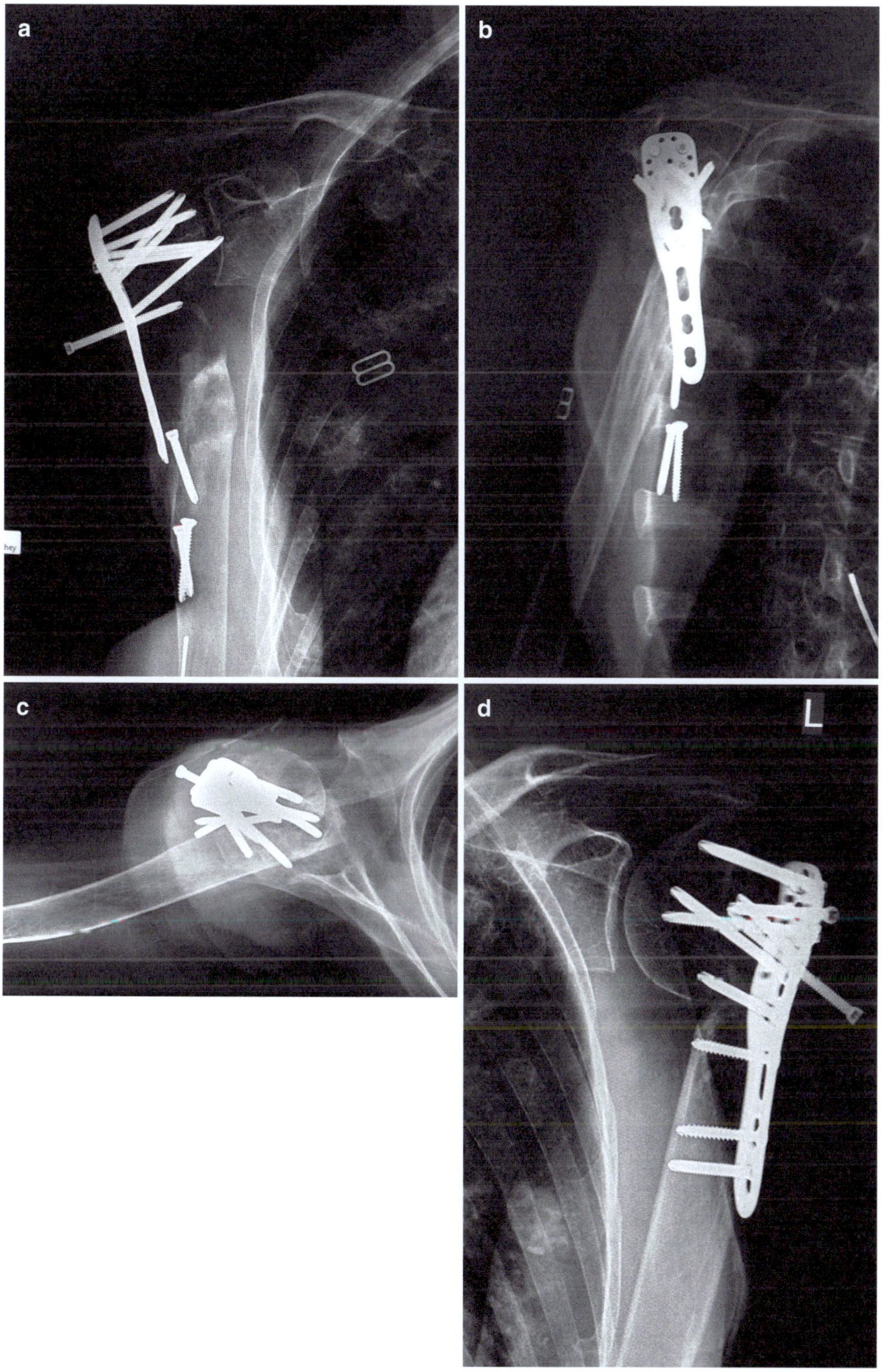

Fig. 6.7 A 60-year-old female patient referred primary for pain. She smokes two packs per day and has a nickel allergy, and operative cultures demonstrated *P. acnes* infection which contributed to her nonunion on the right side (**a–c**) and a malunion on the left (**d**); she was treated with arthroscopic hardware removal and 8 weeks of oral antibiotics. Her pain resolved and she has not sought further treatment (currently 3 years post-op (**e**, **f**))

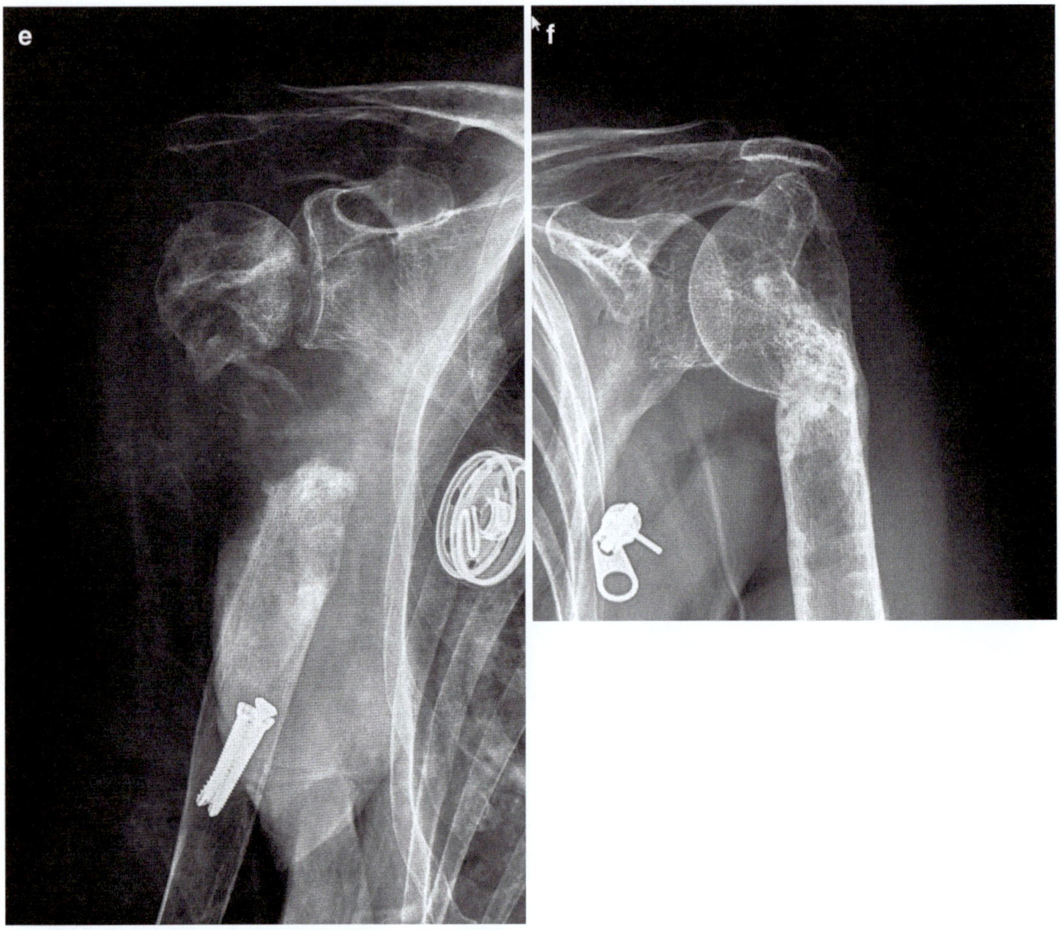

Fig. 6.7 (continued)

shoulder arthroplasty an unpredictable option; moreover few studies demonstrate excellent clinical outcomes for the non-arthroplasty treatment [6–9, 19–35, 37, 38]. The ideal sequelae classification should help the surgeon choose an appropriate surgical option based upon simple radiographic data, providing both the surgeon and the patient with some expectation of outcome; the system advocated here was borne out of a systematic retrospective review of treatment of sequelae with diligent follow-up and relies upon radiographs only and no advanced imaging (Fig. 6.8) [13, 14].

While an MRI or CT scan may be required to help the surgeon understand the distorted anatomy or evaluate the trophicity of the rotator cuff, with a standard series of x-rays (a Grashey, an anteroposterior, an axillary, and an outlet lateral x-ray), the surgeon evaluates the gross appearance and location of the humeral head, tuberosities, and humeral shaft. If the patient has had previous surgery, what kind of hardware remains, and how should it be removed or left behind: plate, screws, and arthroplasty? Is there hardware penetration into the joint [19, 21]? What does the location of the tuberosity indicate, i.e., anatomic, nonunion with retraction, or malunion to the shaft of the humerus or glenoid? Superior tuberosity displacement can limit abduction either mechanically blocking motion or by limiting the mechanical advantage of the rotator cuff; posterior tuberosity displacement can block external rotation and weaken the external rotators. Is this the result of a missed dislocation, and what are the current deformities? Is there a surgical neck nonunion or significant malunion or deformity of the fragments? The suprascapular nerve could be entrapped by a malunion, causing pain. Is there

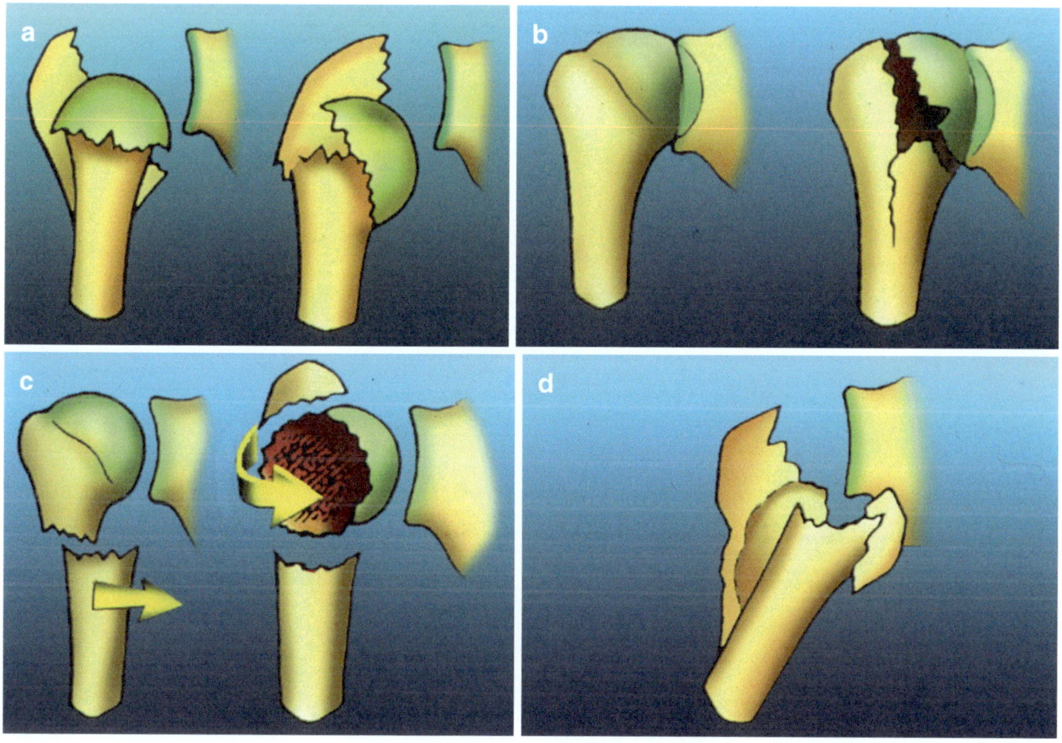

Fig. 6.8 Fracture sequela classification system. (**a**) Type 1 sequela: valgus impacted or varus fracture with cephalic collapse or necrosis; intracapsular/impacted injury. (**b**) Type 2: a chronic missed dislocation; intracapsular/impacted injury. (**c**) Type 3: surgical neck non-union with an intact or healed greater tuberosity; extracapsular/disimpacted injury. (**d**) Type 4 fracture sequela: severe tuberosity malunion or non-union, massive hardware failure, or failure of a previous prosthesis for fracture; extracapsular/disimpacted injury

cephalic collapse or avascular necrosis (AVN)? If so, does the articular surface remain spherical?

What follows is an approach to classifying and treating fracture sequelae based upon five types (Fig. 6.8). As with any classification system, it represents only a guideline, and all treatment must be individualized to the patient. Type 1 sequela is characterized by AVN or cephalic collapse on the plain radiographs; the greater tuberosity must be healed to the humerus in a near anatomic height and orientation. This pattern results from valgus impacted or varus fractures with cephalic collapse (Fig. 6.1a–d). Arthroscopic capsular releases may be an option for young patients who present with stiffness but minimal to moderate arthritis, provided that the humeral head remains spherical and the glenoid is not biconcave. Arthroplasty with either a "stemless" or a modular, adaptable prosthesis is the more reliable solution for those patients that have more significant arthropathy or associated glenoid changes, provided the prosthesis can be implanted without further damage to the greater tuberosity (Fig. 6.1). Tauber and Resch recommended that if there were greater than 1 cm of posterior displacement of the tuberosity, and the patient were young without significant risk factors (smoking, diabetes, etc.), a corrective oblique osteotomy with a large surface area and periosteal sleeve may be successfully performed with cerclage fixation, as they found that better tuberosity alignment resulted in better function and pain relief (Fig. 6.9a–c) [34, 35]. Specific fracture stems that enhance tuberosity fixation and allow for bone grafting may improve results; however (Fig. 6.9d), Cofield's series demonstrated a 20% complication rate and significantly worse range of motion if a tuberosity osteotomy was performed [37, 38].

Short metaphyseal filling implants may be preferable to resurfacing or stemless ones for patients with significant AVN (Fig. 6.10a–d),

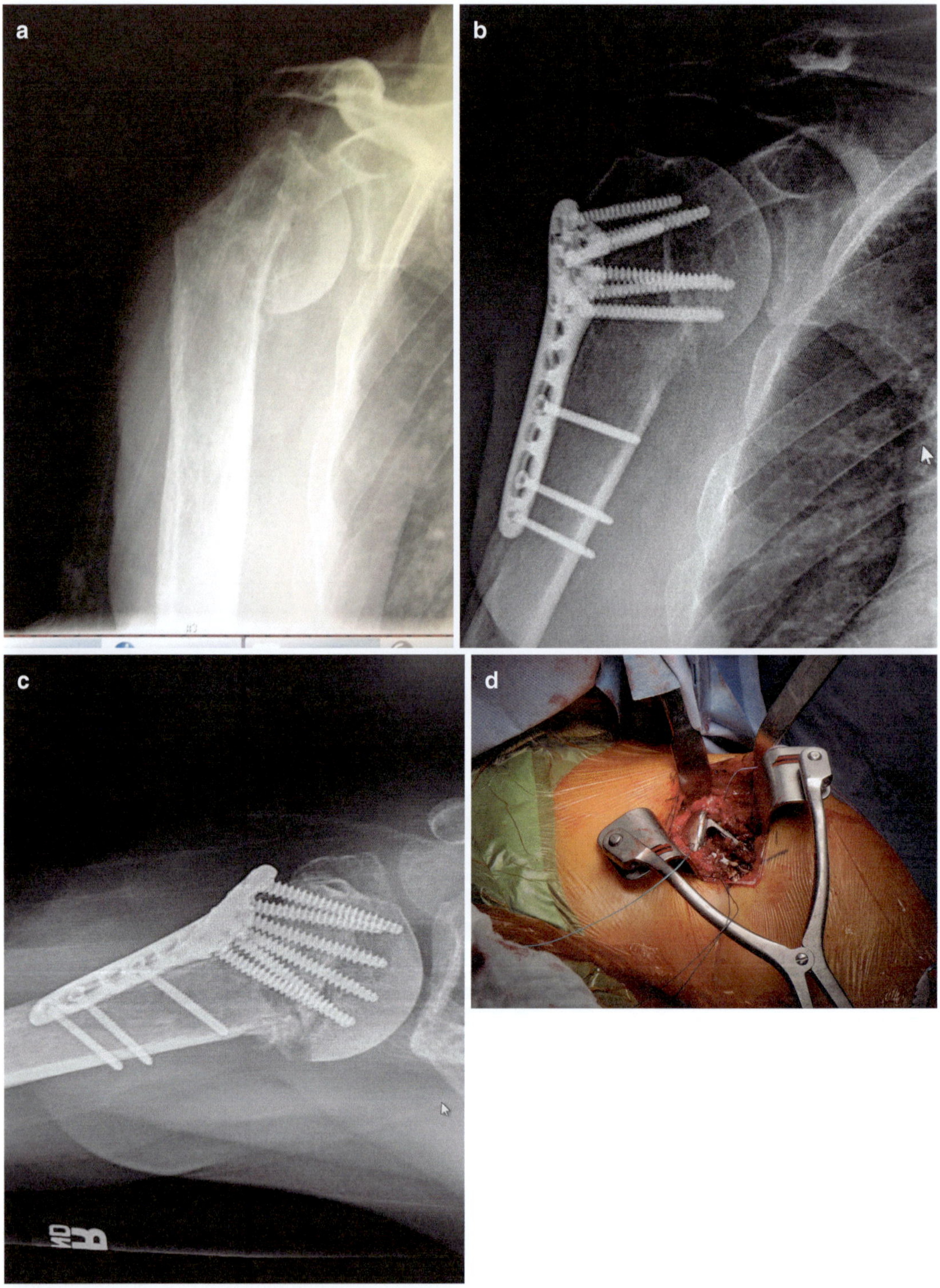

Fig. 6.9 A 50-year-old manual laborer underwent a derotational osteotomy with locking plate fixation for a proximal humeral malunion 1 year after his injury. Pre-op (**a**) and post-op (**b**, **c**). Case courtesy of Jesse McCarron. (**d**) A younger patient treated with a fracture-specific stem that provides for enhanced tuberosity fixation. (**e**) Demonstrates the intraoperative photograph of tuberosity osteotomy, reconstruction, and bone grafting; (**f**) is one year follow up showing a healed tuberosity

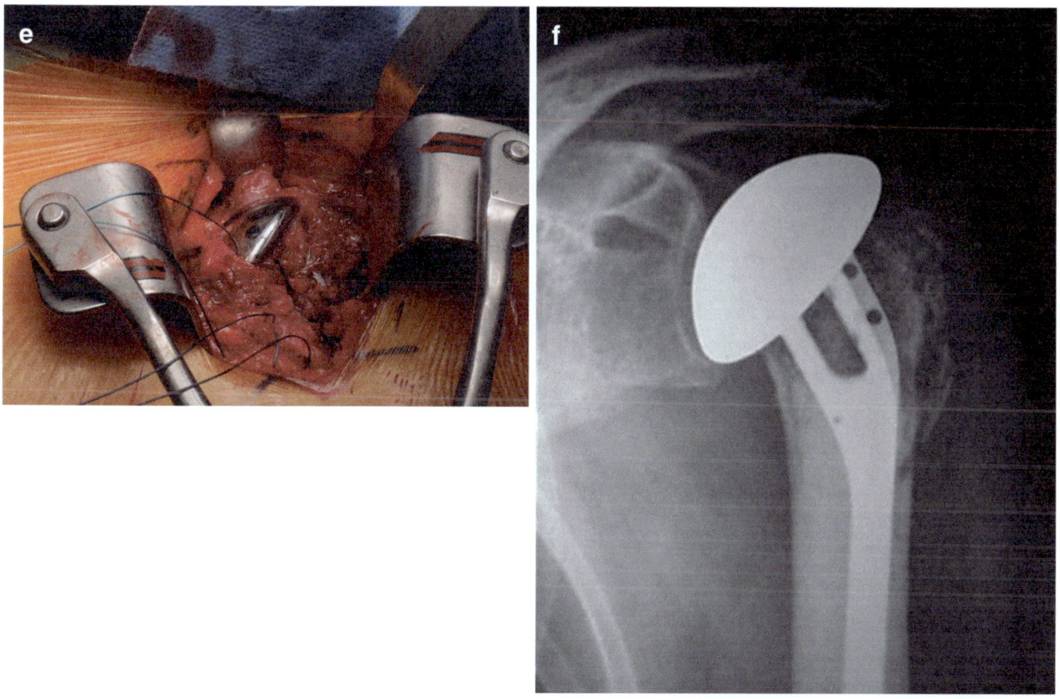

Fig. 6.9 (continued)

as there may be little cancellous bone left for purchase; moreover, the underlying necrotic bone could serve as a source of chronic pain if it is not adequately removed or decompressed (Fig. 6.10e–h) [1].

If the greater tuberosity is in a normal relationship with the acromion, then place the prosthesis so that the head is in a normal or anatomic position; small cemented stems can provide an extra degree of freedom, allowing the surgeon to "float" the implant in the correct position. The prosthesis must be inserted with minimal insult to the surrounding soft tissues because rotator cuff integrity influences outcome (minimal fatty infiltration and an acromial-humeral distance of >7 mm) [14, 23, 28, 30, 39].

Type 2 sequela results from a chronic missed dislocation (Fig. 6.8b). Good to excellent results can be achieved with a standard prosthesis for most cases of a chronic posterior dislocation [12, 13, 16, 17, 19, 26, 33, 45]. However, resurfacing may be inadequate due to changes on the glenoid; therefore soft tissue plication or alteration of stem version may be necessary to prevent recurrent prosthetic dislocation. If very large components are required to address a patulous, redundant soft tissue envelope, if the patient is elderly, or there is glenoid bone loss, a reverse shoulder arthroplasty (RSA) potentially with glenoid bone grafting will lead to more reliable outcomes (Fig. 6.11). Moreover, the constraint of RSA is the preferred option for chronic anterior dislocations.

A type 3 sequela, surgical neck nonunion, most often results from an initial failure to treat the patient operatively (Fig. 6.4). If the x rays show an intact greater tuberosity or one that is healed to the proximal fragment, and an arthropathy is not present, the nonunion should be addressed with non-prosthetic options if the proximal fragment is well vascularized. Bone peg autograft (Fig. 6.12a) or fibular or ulnar strut allograft (Fig. 6.12b) with plate fixation is a reasonable treatment option, whereby the head is impacted onto the graft and compressed with a locking plate or blade plate [11, 13, 36]. Prosthetic options should be considered if there is cephalic necrosis or minimal proximal osseous structure;

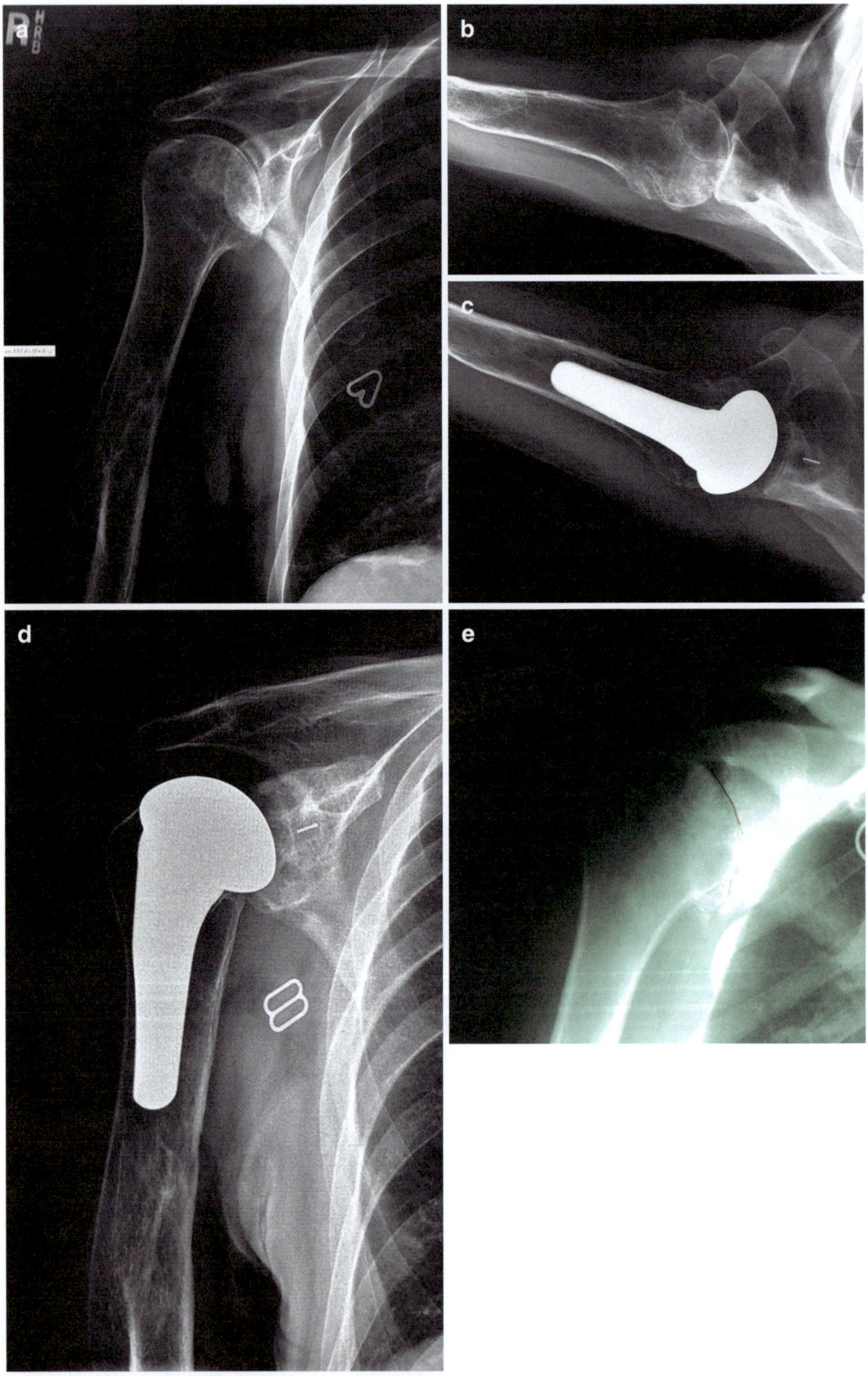

Fig. 6.10 Type 1 sequela with AVN of the head and an older shaft fracture (**a**, **b**); placement of a modular prosthesis (**c**, **d**); post-traumatic AVN (**e**, **f**) that was inadequately treated as diseased bone remained behind (**g**, **h**)

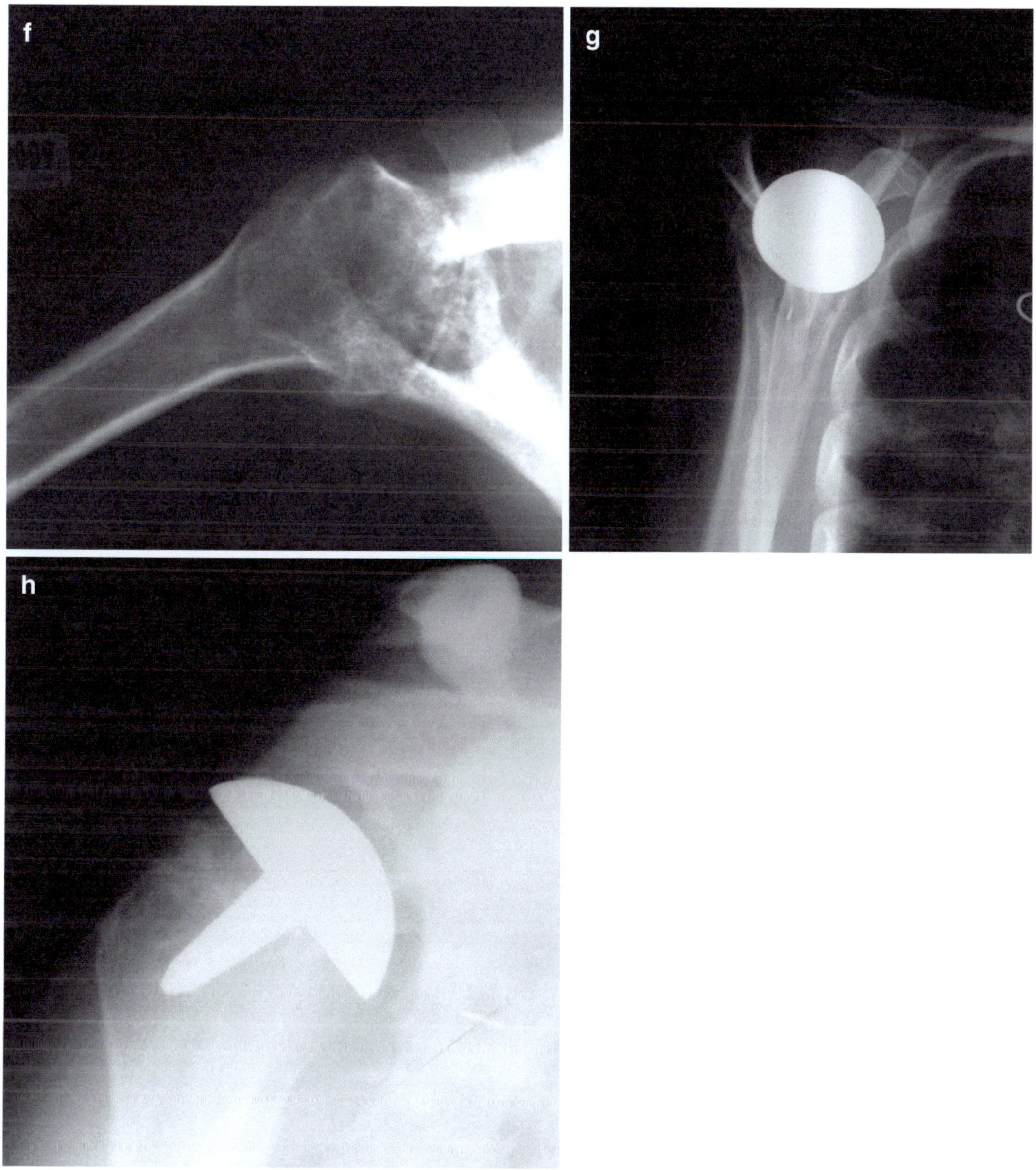

Fig. 6.10 (continued)

in which case the head can be "shish-ka-bobed" by a low-profile anatomic fracture stem, for a young patient, or by a reverse prosthesis for an elderly one (Fig. 6.4) [1, 14, 43, 49]. Occult infection or inadequate hardware may lead to failure of operative treatment; if so, revision fixation with bone grafting may be appropriate, but the surgeon should assume that there is an infection until proven otherwise. Similarly in these revision cases, the proximal bone is often compromised requiring arthroplasty as the solution.

Severe tuberosity malunion or nonunion, massive hardware failure, or failure of a previous prosthesis for fracture is the hallmark of a type 4 sequela (Fig. 6.13). Very often, non-prosthetic management is unrealistic because of accompanying soft tissue contractures or loss of rotator cuff function due to tuberosity complications.

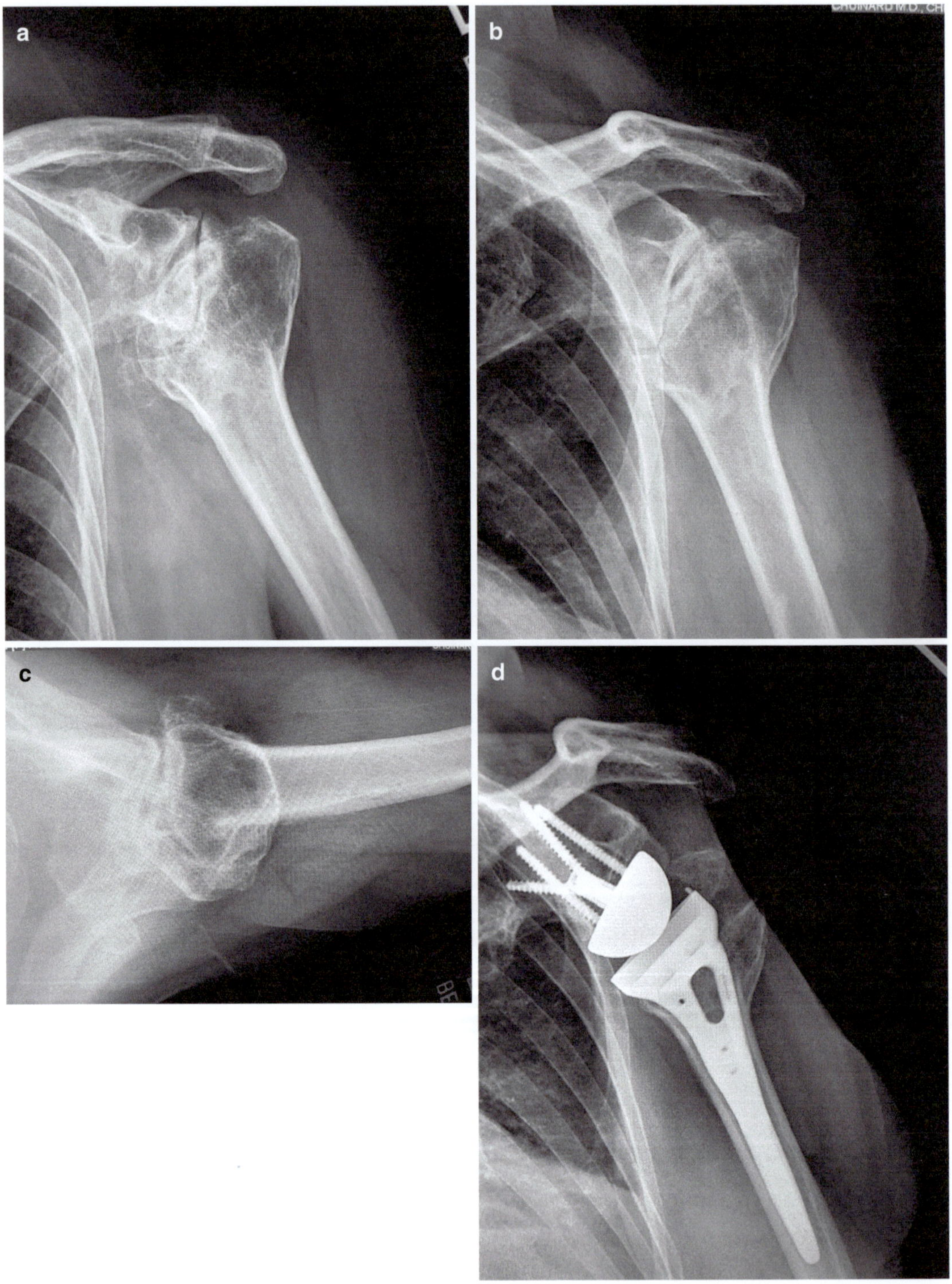

Fig. 6.11 Type 2 sequela with locked posterior dislocation (**a**–**c**); an older patient was treated with semi-constrained arthroplasty with good results (**d**–**f**)

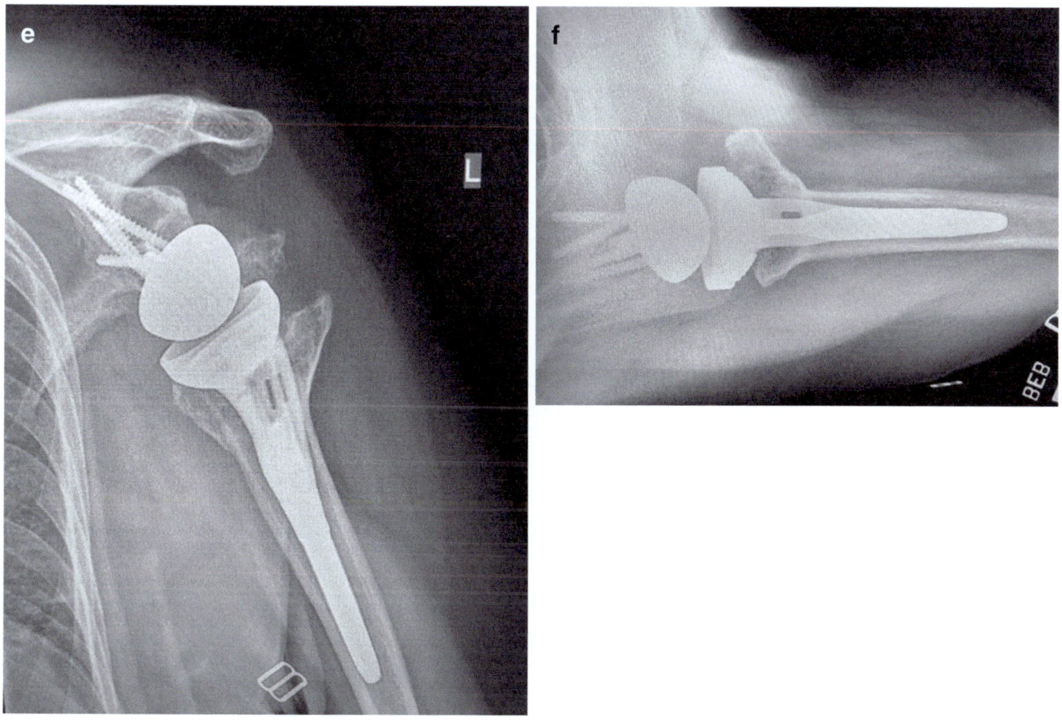

Fig. 6.11 (continued)

The x-rays may show that the tuberosities are healed to the posterior aspect of the head or are resorbed; hardware may be loose, eroding into the glenoid, or demonstrating implant failure. Anatomic reconstruction should be reserved for the very young and may require specialized implants or a staged approach. Complication rates are highest for conversion of a previous hemiarthroplasty with tuberosity failure to a reverse arthroplasty or resection [47–49]. Reverse shoulder arthroplasty may be the only option, and concomitant latissimus dorsi and teres major transfer may be necessary to restore external rotation [23, 29, 47, 48].

Extreme caution must be observed with conversion of a failed hemiarthroplasty to a reverse due to high complication rates, especially instability (Fig. 6.14). Because the contracted soft tissues (especially posteriorly and inferiorly) act as a fulcrum to dislocate the reverse when the arm is brought into extension (as exemplified by the heterotopic ossification seen in images Fig. 6.14c and d), the approach requires extensive soft tissue mobilization and may require constrained implants. Furthermore, it is incumbent upon the surgeon to obtain scaled radiographs of the contralateral limb to estimate appropriate humeral length intraoperatively. Neurovascular structures that are encased in scar are at heightened risk for injury; intraoperative nerve monitoring, coracoid osteotomy, and preoperative angiography may all be useful adjuncts to enhance the safety of the operation. And while "convertible" prostheses may enable retention of the humeral stem, this option may be obviated by improper placement at the index procedure, and the surgeon should be prepared to explant the stem at the time of the revision.

The focus of the treatment of type 4 fracture sequela should be pain relief, as functional gains may be limited, especially with prosthetic revision, and the physician must emphasize this as part of the discussion of the realistic goals and expected outcomes of intervention. If possible, modular, adaptable implants that enable the surgeon to adapt to the patient's anatomy may pro-

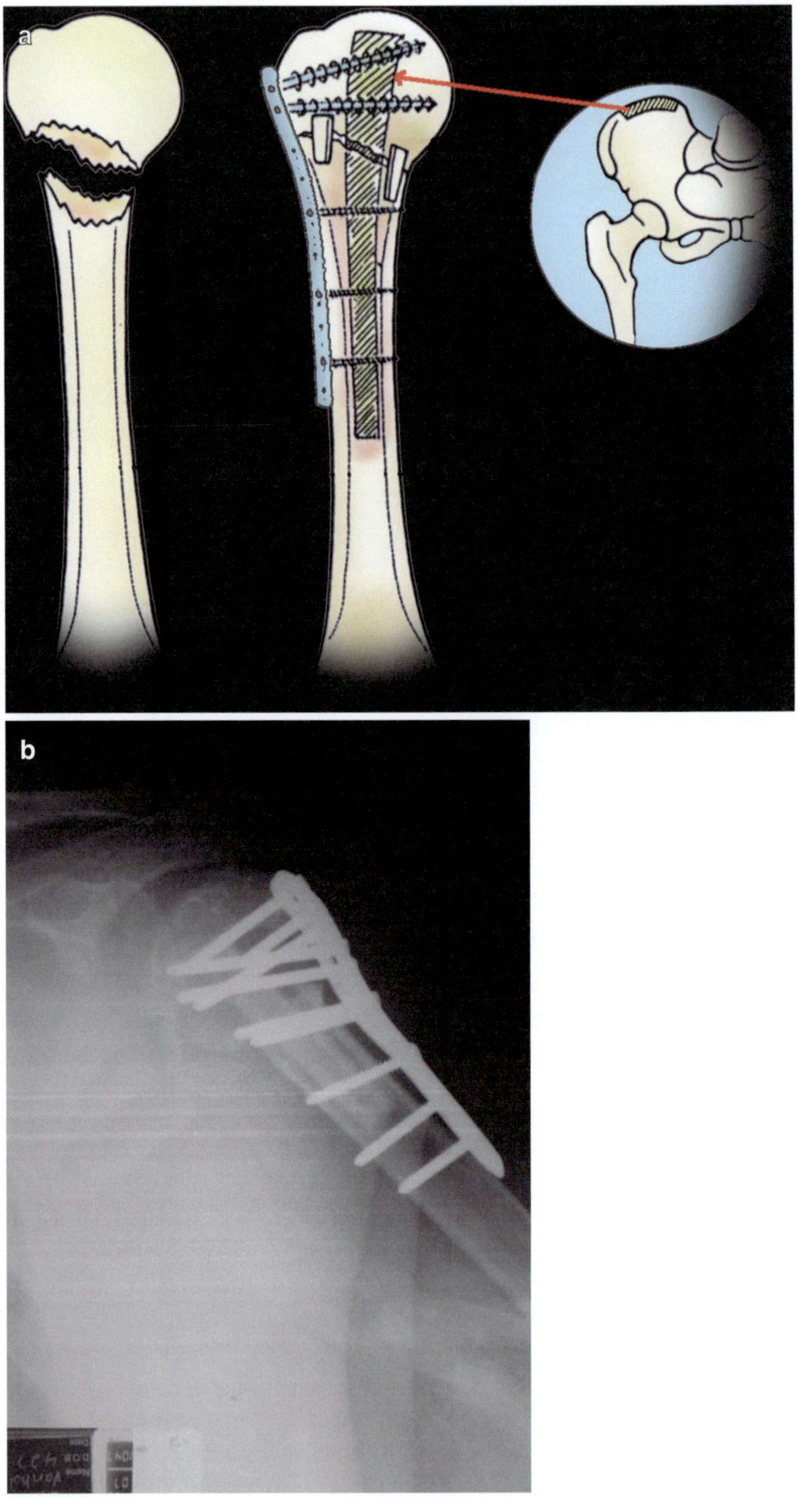

Fig. 6.12 Schematic of bone peg autograft for the treatment of type 3 sequela (**a**); patient treated with fibular strut allograft (**b**)

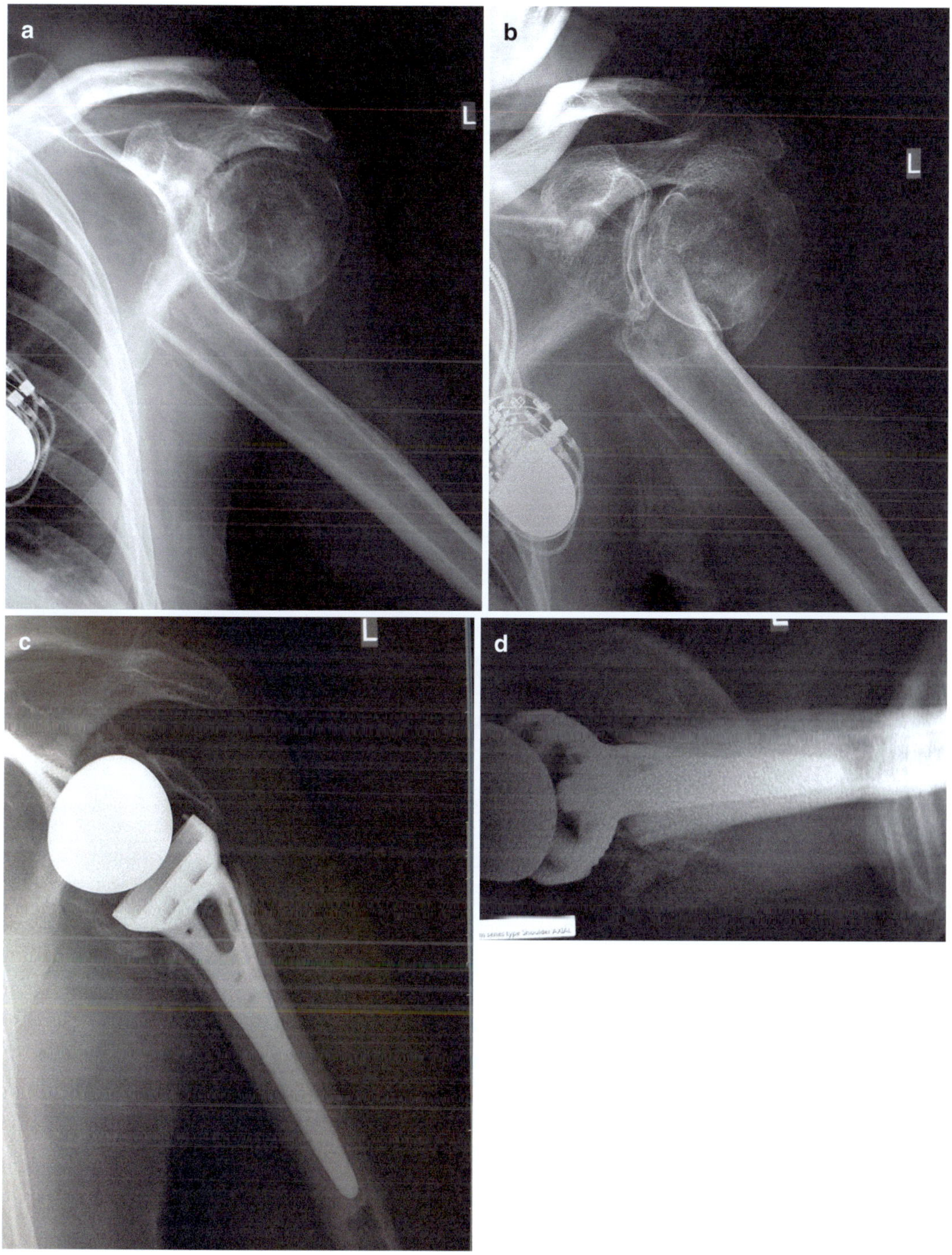

Fig. 6.13 Type 4 sequela with combined nonunion and malunion treated with RSA (**a**–**d**); type 4 treated with conversion to RSA (**e**–**h**)

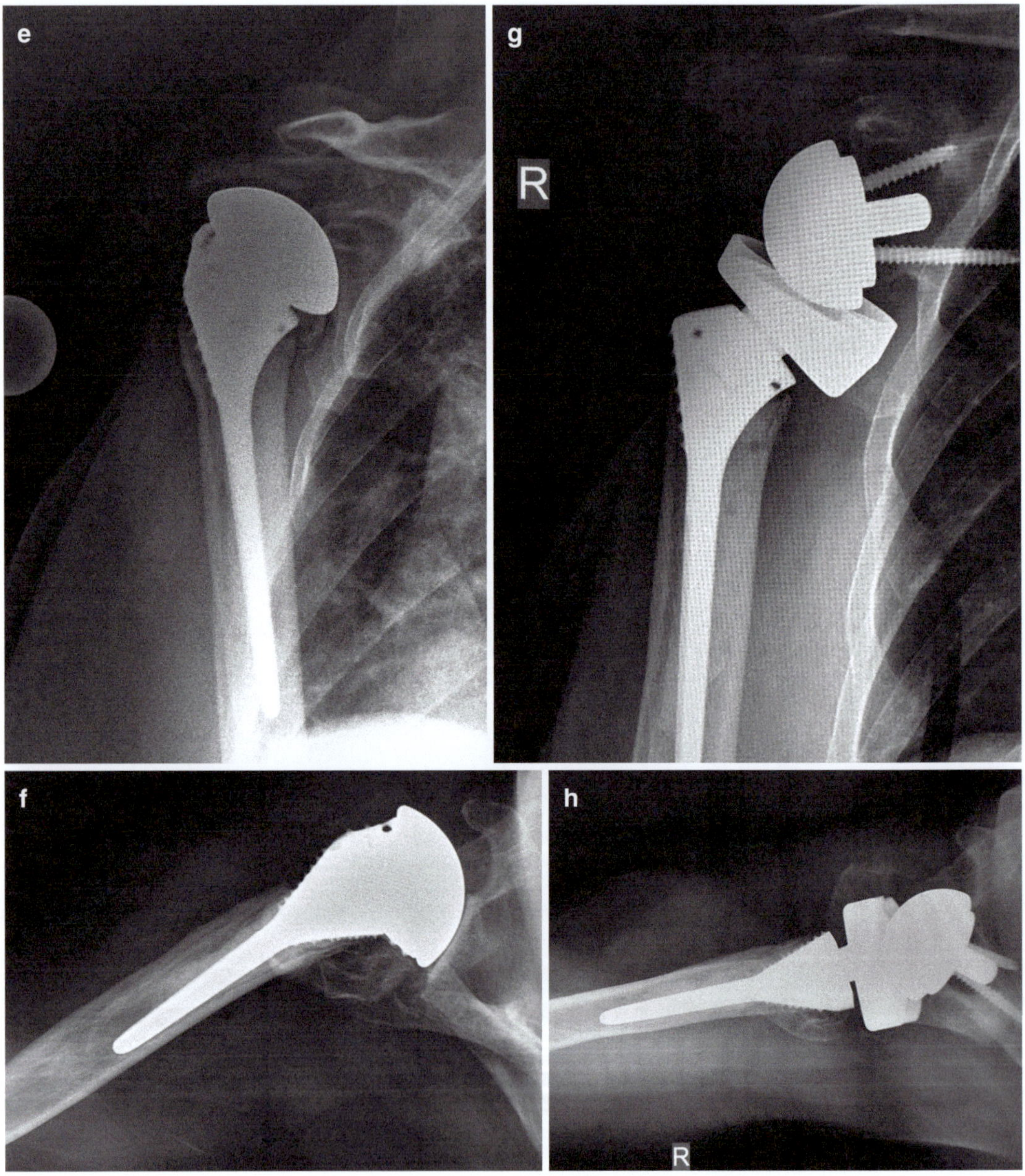

Fig. 6.13 (continued)

vide good results with minimal surgical trauma (Fig. 6.15). Furthermore, staged operations may be necessary to reduce complications related to occult infection. Open or arthroscopic capsular release with biopsies to remove suture and hardware and obtain cultures with empiric antibiotic treatment may be the preferred approach to decrease the risk of chronic infection after arthroplasty is performed. For some patients, this initial stage may provide enough relief to delay definitive treatment.

If the cultures are positive but the hardware and sutures were effectively removed at the time of the arthroscopy, antibiotic treatment should be continued in conjunction with input from infectious disease. Depending on the patient's symptoms, a second stage could be delayed indefinitely. However, it may be necessary to

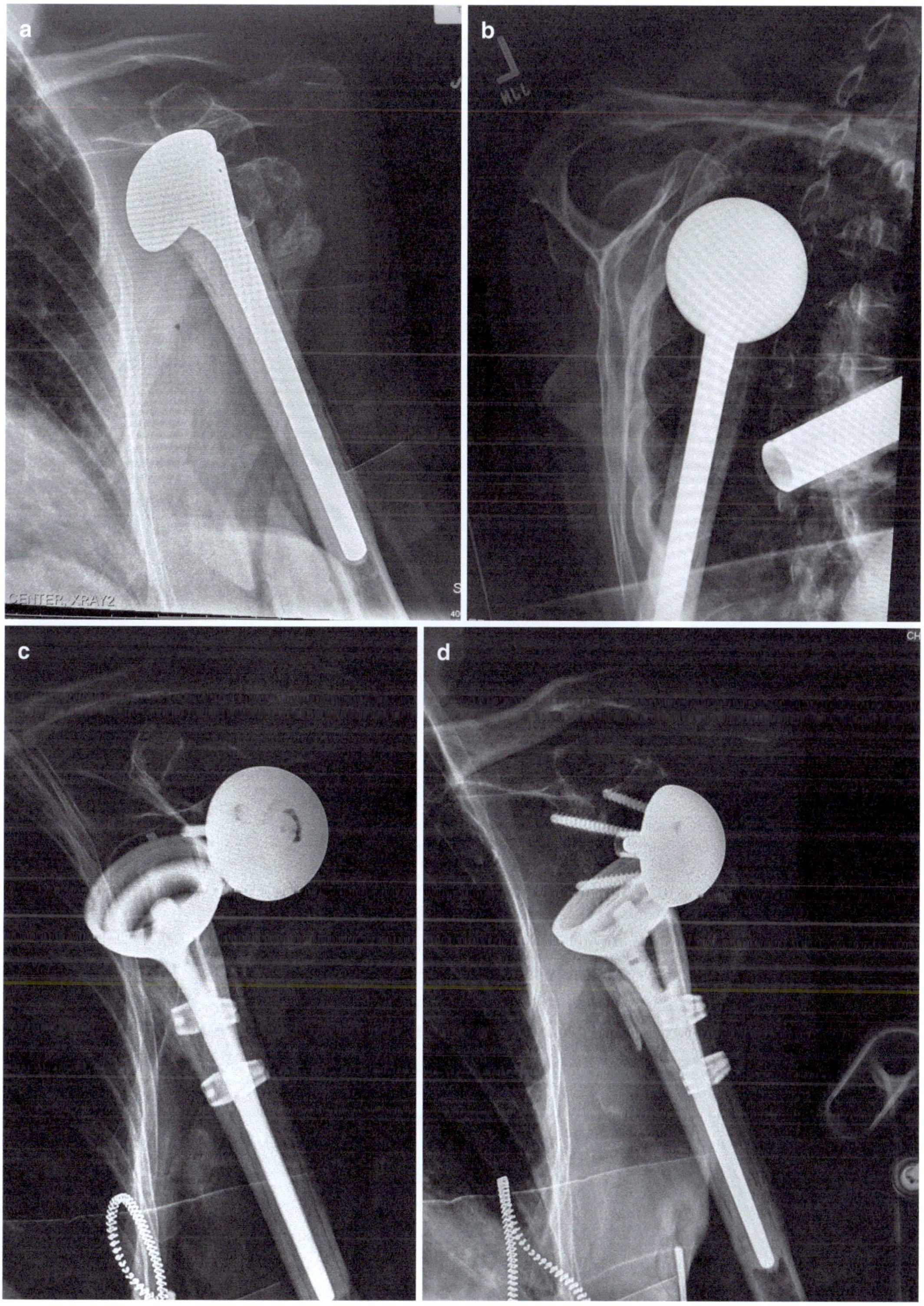

Fig. 6.14 An elderly patient was treated with a hemiarthroplasty for a four-part proximal humerus fracture and presented with a dislocation (**a**, **b**); revision to a reverse was complicated by a dislocation because the posterior soft tissues were inadequately released (**c**, **d**); subsequent revision included extensive soft tissue resection and placement of a constrained liner (**e**, **f**)

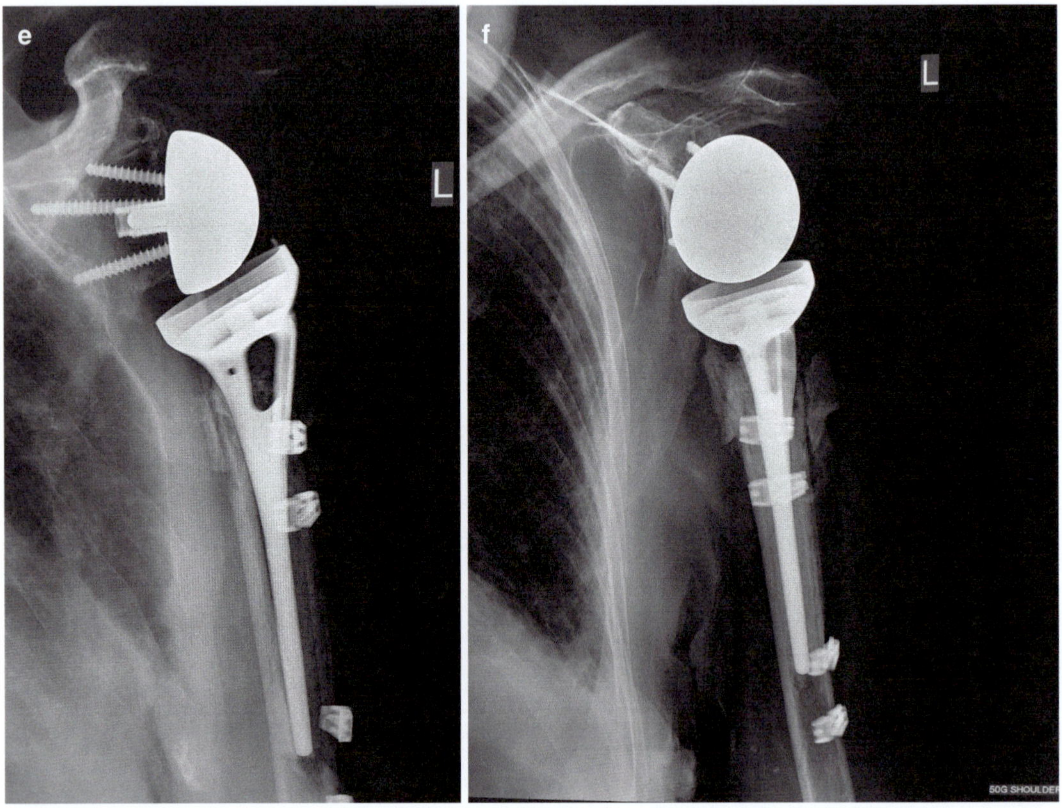

Fig. 6.14 (continued)

consider application of a cement spacer prior to revision arthroplasty if the cultures are positive and hardware remains, as is typically the case with a hemiarthroplasty.

Lastly, type 5 fracture sequelae are isolated GT nonunions or malunions (Fig. 6.16). Posterior tuberosity displacement can block external rotation; superior tuberosity displacement can limit abduction either mechanically or by limiting the mechanical advantage of the rotator cuff (Fig. 6.16c). Treatment, again, must be individualized to the patient. Younger patients may benefit from osteotomy and repair of the fragment; smaller fractures may be treated arthroscopically; larger ones may benefit from direct lateral approaches. In cases where loss of external rotation is a major complaint, muscle transfers like a L'Episcopo or lower trapezius transfer may be indicated. Elderly patients, however, may require a reverse shoulder arthroplasty with or without accompanying arthritis (Fig. 6.16d–h).

As the incidence of proximal humerus fractures increases, so too will the prevalence of proximal humeral fracture sequelae across a broad age range. By focusing on realistic goals and symptomatic management, a treatment plan can be guided by the following: (1) if there was previous surgery, (2) if there was hardware placed, (3) the extent of proximal humeral anatomy distortion, (4) the tuberosity-diaphysis continuity, and (5) the necessity for a greater tuberosity osteotomy. An unconstrained total shoulder replacement can yield predictable functional results, provided that there is tuberosity-diaphysis continuity and minimal proximal deformity (types 1 and 2 fracture sequelae); chronic dislocations likely require semi-constrained implants. The surgeon should adapt both the technique and the prosthesis to accommodate the distorted anatomy, not the other way around. By maximizing the head offset to cover the tuberosity,

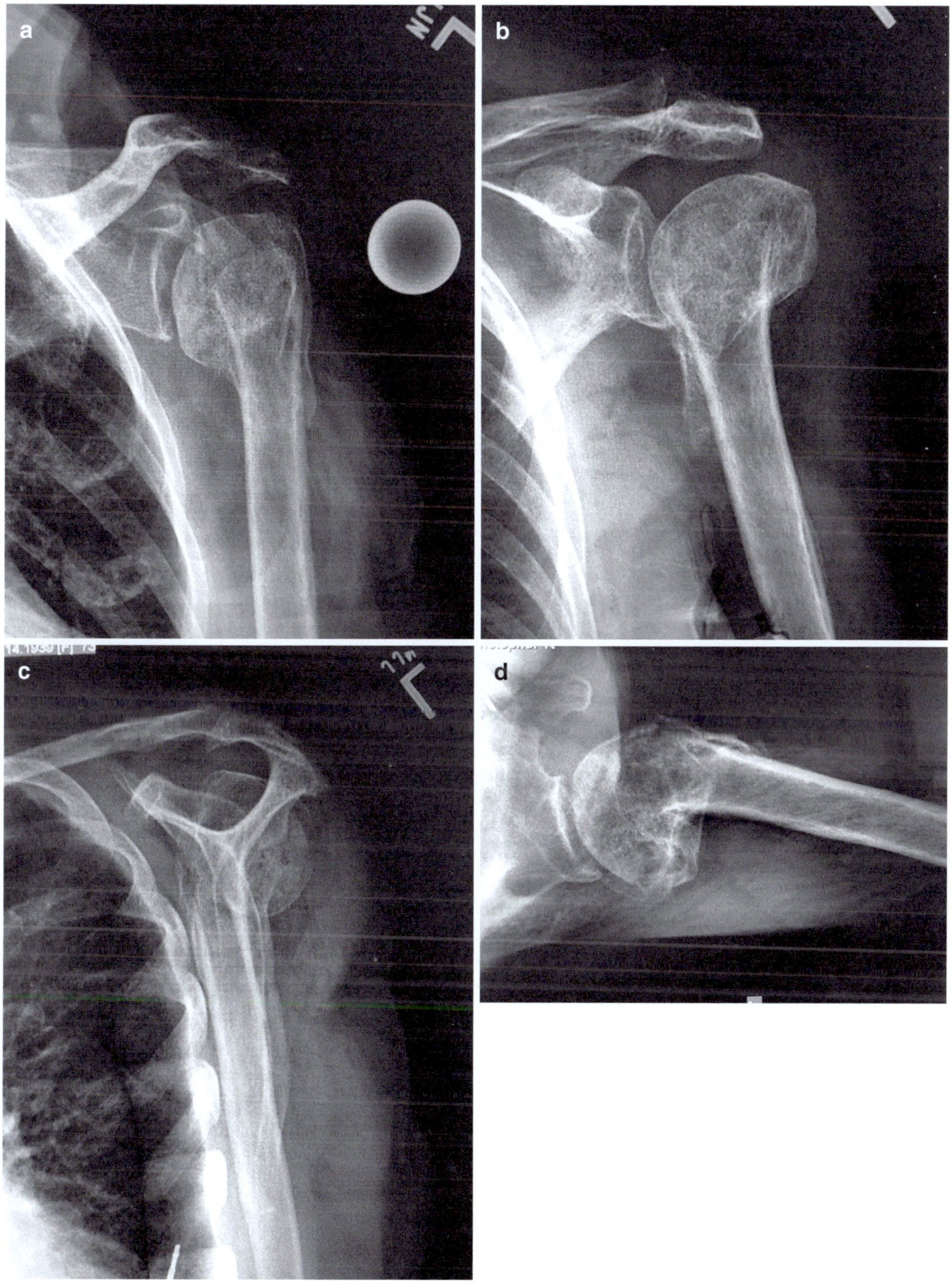

Fig. 6.15 A 75-year-old woman who did well with non-operative treatment for 3 years, but she presented with a type 4 fracture sequela as the pain began to affect her (**a**–**d**); reverse shoulder arthroplasty with a modular, adaptable prosthesis was used for the reconstruction, allowing the implant to sit in the proximal defect (**e**–**h**)

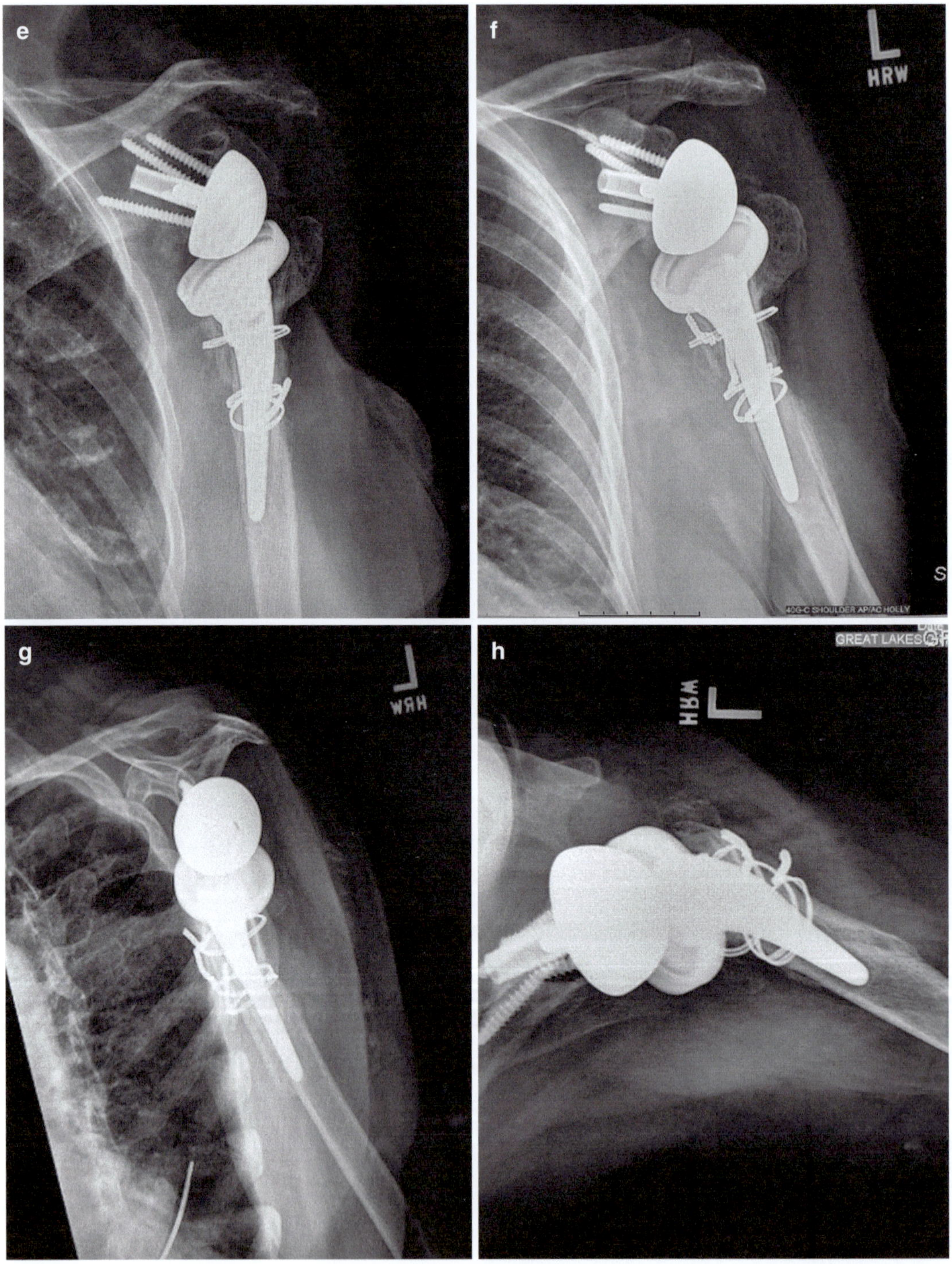

Fig. 6.15 (continued)

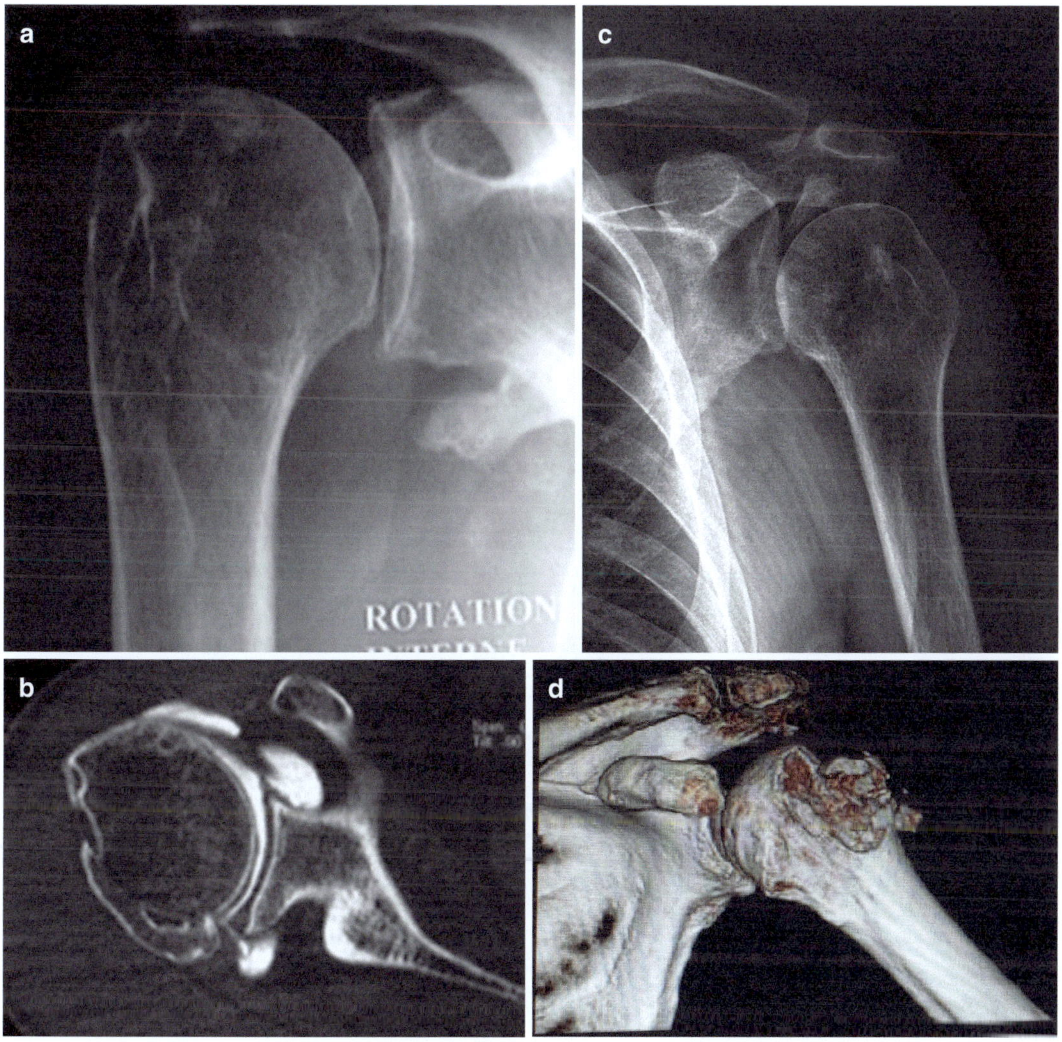

Fig. 6.16 (**a**) A Grashey x-ray demonstrating a type 5 fracture sequela; (**b**) CT scan showing a posterior malunion of the greater tuberosity; (**c**) an AP x-ray showing a greater tuberosity nonunion that can mechanically block motion as well as indicate the loss of the attachment of the external rotators; (**d–h**) CT scan and x-rays demonstrating a greater tuberosity nonunion that was treated with reverse shoulder arthroplasty

little to no head cut may be required if the prosthesis can be passed directly through the head fragment. The stem can be cemented in a valgus or lateralized position. Don't hesitate to use c-arm and a curette to "sound" the humeral canal prior to broaching or reaming. Elderly patients, those with extreme stiffness or rotator cuff deficiency, may benefit from RSA for type 1 sequelae, but they should be advised that while their pain relief will be good, their functional outcomes, especially with respect to external rotation, will likely pale compared to arthroplasty in a non-sequela patient [52].

For the type 2 sequela, a total shoulder will provide better pain relief than attempts at reduction and stabilization if the dislocation is over 10 months old. For a posterior dislocation, the stem should be placed in low to neutral retroversion and the patient placed in a neutral or external rotation brace for at least 6 weeks to minimize the risk of recurrent posterior instability [16, 17,

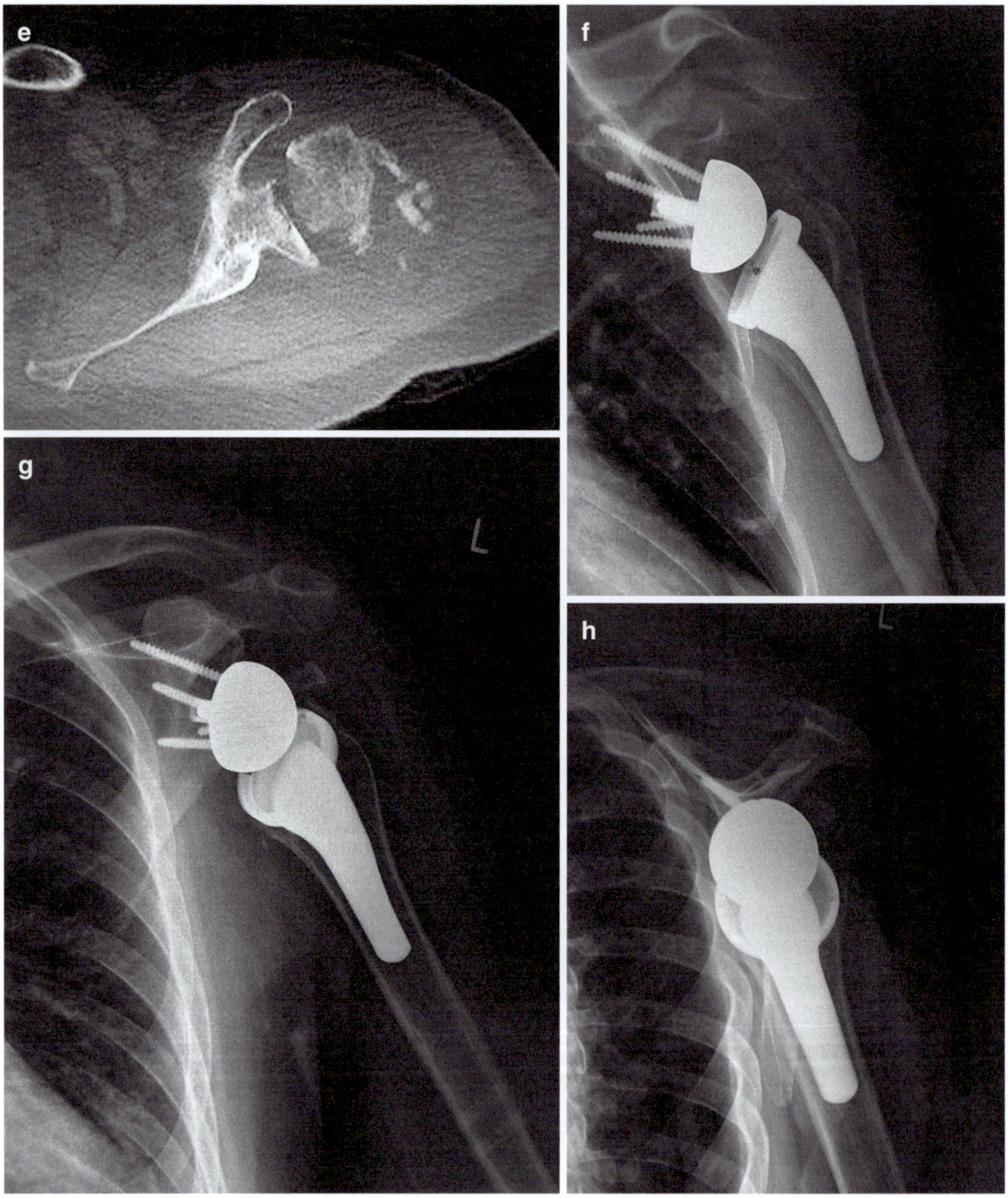

Fig. 6.16 (continued)

26, 33, 45]. Elderly patients are likely best treated with a RSA to avoid instability.

Intramedullary peg bone graft with iliac crest autograft or strut allograft and osteosynthesis to focus on enhancing the biology is recommended for type 3 fracture sequelae (surgical neck non-union) because displaced, non-impacted, extra-capsular fractures occur in this watershed area. Recent data suggests that bone grafting may not be necessary to achieve good results in terms of union and functional outcomes with locking plate fixation [53]. If there is a tuberosity-diaphysis discontinuity (type 3 fracture sequelae) and/or a severe distortion of the anatomy (type 4 fracture sequelae), anatomic or unconstrained shoulder replacement with a greater tuberosity osteotomy yields poor functional results. A type 3 fracture sequela is a *relative* contraindication to a non-constrained shoulder prosthesis [1, 6, 11, 12, 18, 24, 27, 39, 40, 42, 46]. However, a "low-profile" anatomic fracture prosthesis that allows bone grafting or RSA may be indicated if there is osteoarthritis or AVN of the proximal segment or simply in an elderly patient with a low chance for healing of the nonunited fracture if it is fixated [47, 49]. The placement of copious bone graft between the epiphysis and the diaphysis may improve osteosynthesis, although a reverse arthroplasty may be necessary for elderly patients [8, 14]. Loss or fracture of the tuberosities can lead to higher rates of instability if reverse shoulder arthroplasty is chosen [54].

In type 4 fracture sequelae (severe tuberosity malunion or nonunion or major surgery), reverse shoulder arthroplasty reliably restores forward flexion and abduction and provides better pain relief than non-constrained options because of the severe distortion of the anatomy but may require a staged approach [14, 23, 25, 32, 47].

Utilization of a RSA may have a lower complication rate for type 4 (10%) when compared to RSA for type 3 sequelae (40%) [54–57]. A proximal humeral allograft-reverse shoulder composite, as described by Levy and Frankle, should be considered in cases of severe proximal humeral bone loss; furthermore, Sanchez-Sotelo has reported excellent survivability with a low complication rate (15%) [48, 58]. For the patient with loss of both deltoid and rotator cuff function or severe brachial plexus damage, a shoulder fusion might be the only available option [35, 59]. Type 5 sequelae should be managed based upon the viability of the remaining bone and rotator cuff as determined by an MRI or CT scan. Osteotomy and repair may be considered for younger patients, while reverse shoulder arthroplasty is likely the most predictable treatment in the elderly. Regardless of the treatment chosen, patients must be aware that operative intervention for a proximal humerus fracture carries a higher risk for the development of a complication; therefore surgeons and patients must be realistic about the expectations of treatment.

References

1. Chuinard C, Boileau P, Walch G. Evaluation and prosthetic management of proximal humeral malunions. In: Iannotti JP, Williams GR, editors. Disorders of the shoulder: reconstruction. Philadelphia: Lippincott Williams and Wilkins; 2014.
2. Jost B, Spross C, Grehn H, Gerber C. Locking plate fixation of fractures of the proximal humerus: analysis of complications, revision strategies and outcome. J Shoulder Elb Surg. 2013;22:542–9.
3. Cadet ER, Yin B, Schulz B, Ahmad CS, Rosenwasser MP. Proximal humerus and humeral shaft nonunions. J Am Acad Orthop Surg. 2013;21:538–47.
4. Kim SH, Szabo RM, Marder RA. Epidemiology of humerus fractures in the United States: nationwide emergency department sample, 2008. Arthritis Care Res. 2012;64:407–14.
5. Bell JE, Leung BC, Spratt KF, Koval KJ, Weinstein JD, Goodman DC, Tosteson AN. Trends and variation in incidence, surgical treatment, and repeat surgery of proximal humeral fractures in the elderly. J Bone Joint Surg Am. 2011;93(2):121–31.
6. Antuna SA, Sperling JW, Sanchez-Sotelo J, Cofield RH. Shoulder arthroplasty for proximal humeral nonunions. J Shoulder Elb Surg. 2002;11:114–21.
7. Antuna SA, Sperling JW, Sanchez-Sotelo J, Cofield RH. Shoulder arthroplasty for proximal humeral malunions: Long-term results. J Shoulder Elb Surg. 2002;11:122–9.
8. Antuna SA, Sperling JW. Prosthetic replacement for nonunions of proximal humeral fractures. In: Cofield R, Sperling J, editors. Revision and complex shoulder arthroplasty. Philadelphia: Lippincott, Williams and Wilkins; 2010. p. 259–65.
9. Beredjiklian PK, Iannotti JP, Norris TR, Williams GR. Operative treatment of malunion a fracture of the proximal aspect of the humerus. J Bone Joint Surg. 1998;80A:1484–97.
10. Boileau P, Walch G. The three-dimensional geometry of the proximal humerus: implications for surgical technique and prosthetic design. J Bone Joint Surg. 1997;79B:857–65.
11. Boileau P, Walch G, Trojani C, Sinnerton R, Romeo AA, Veneau B. Sequelae of fractures of the proximal humerus : surgical classification and limits of shoulder arthroplasty. In: Walch G, Boileau P, editors. Shoulder arthroplasty. Berlin: Springer-Verlag; 1999. p. 349–58.
12. Boileau P, Trojani C, Walch G, Krishnan S, Romeo A, Sinnerton R. Shoulder arthroplasty for the treatment of the sequelae of fractures of the proximal humerus. J Shoulder Elb Surg. 2001;10:299–308.
13. Boileau P, Chuinard C, LeHuec JC, Walch G, Trojani C. Proximal humerus fracture sequelae: Impact of a new radiographic classification on arthroplasty. Clin Ortho Rel Res. 2006;442:121–30.
14. Chuinard C. Fracture sequelae revisited. In: Boileau P, editor. Shoulder concepts. Montpillier: Sauramps Medical; 2008. p. 179–91.

15. Constant CR, Murley AHG. A clinical method of functional assessment of the shoulder. Clin Orthop Relat Res. 1987;214:160–4.
16. Flatow EL, Neer CS II. Chronic anterior dislocation of the shoulder. J Shoulder Elb Surg. 1993;2(1): 2–10.
17. Hawkins RJ, Neer CS II. Locked posterior dislocation of the shoulder. J Bone Joint Surg. 1987;69A: 9–18.
18. Healy WL, Jupiter JB, Kristiansen TK, White RR. Nonunion of the proximal humerus. In: Post M, Morrey BF, Hawkins RJ, editors. Surgery of the shoulder. St. Louis: Mosby-Year Book; 1990. p. 59.
19. Huten D, Duparc J. L'arthroplastie prothétique dans les traumatismes complexes récents et anciens de l'épaule. Rev Chir Orthop. 1986;72:517–29.
20. Iannotti JP, Sidor ML. Malunions of the proximal humerus. In: Warner JP, Iannotti JP, Gerber C, editors. Complex and revision problems in shoulder surgery. Philadelphia: Lippincott-Raven Publishers; 1997. p. 245–64.
21. Keene JS, Huizenga RE, Engber WD, Rogers SC. Proximal humeral fractures: a correlation of residual deformity with long term function. Orthopedics. 1983;6:173.
22. Kyle RF, Conner TN. Post-traumatic avascular necrosis of the humeral head in displaced proximal humeral fractures. J Trauma. 1981;21:788–91.
23. Lollino N, Paladini P, Campi F, Merolla G, Rossi P, Porcellini G. Reverse shoulder prosthesis as revision surgery after fractures of the proximal humerus, treated initially by internal fixation or hemiarthroplasty. Musculoskelet Surg. 2009;93:S35–9.
24. Neer CS II. Nonunion of the surgical neck of the humerus. Orthop Trans. 1983;3:389.
25. Norris TR, Turner JA, Bovill D. Nonunion of the upper humerus: an analysis of the etiology and treatment in 28 cases. In: Post M, Morrey BF, Hawkins RJ, editors. Surgery of the shoulder. St. Louis: Mosby-Year Book; 1990. p. 63.
26. Pritchett JW. Prosthetic replacement for chronic unreduced dislocations of the shoulder. Clin Orthop Relat Res. 1987;216:89–93.
27. Dines DM, Klarren RF, Altcheck DW, Moeckel B. Posttraumatic changes of the proximal humerus: Malunion, nonunion, and osteonecrosis. Treatment with modular hemiarthroplasty or total shoulder arthroplasty. J Shoulder Elb Surg. 1993;2(1):11–21.
28. Mansat P, Guity M, Bellumore Y, Mansat M. Shoulder arthroplasty for late sequelae of proximal humeral fractures. J Shoulder Elb Surg. 2004;13:305–12.
29. Martin T, Iannotti J. Reverse total shoulder arthroplasty for acute fractures and failed management after proximal humeral fractures. Orthop Clin N Am. 2008;39:451–7.
30. Moineau G, Boileau P. Post-traumatic cephalic collapse and necrosis (Type-1 fracture sequelae): results of a nonconstrained anatomical prosthesis. In: Boileau P, editor. Shoulder concepts 2008. Montpillier: Sauramps Medical; 2008. p. 193–208.
31. Neer CS II. Old trauma in glenohumeral arthroplasty. In: Shoulder reconstruction. 3rd ed. Philadelphia: Saunders; 1990. p. 222–34.
32. Norris TR, Turner JA. Late prosthetic shoulder arthroplasty for displaced proximal humerus fractures. J Shoulder Elb Surg. 1995;4:271–80.
33. Rowe CR, Zarins B. Chronic unreduced dislocations of the shoulder. J Bone Joint Surg. 1982;64A:494–505.
34. Tauber M, Karpik S, Matis N, Schwartz M, Resch H. Shoulder arthroplasty for traumatic avascular necrosis. Predictors of outcome. Clin Orthop Relat Res. 2007;465:208–14.
35. Tauber M, Resch H. Prosthetic arthroplasty for delayed complications of proximal humerus fractures. In: Cofield R, Sperling J, editors. Revision and complex shoulder arthroplasty. Philadelphia: Lippincott, Williams and Wilkins; 2010. p. 250–8.
36. Walch G, Badet R, Nove-Josserand L, Levigne C. Nonunions of the surgical neck of the humerus: surgical treatment with an intramedullary bone peg, internal fixation and cancellous bone grafting. J Shoulder Elb Surg. 1996;5:161–8.
37. Cofield RH. Shoulder replacement: prognosis related to diagnosis. In: Kôlbel R, Helbig B, Blauth W, editors. Shoulder replacement. Berlin: Springer; 1987. p. 157–61.
38. Cofield R. Nonconstrained arthroplasty of the shoulder for severe malunions. In: Boileau P, editor. Shoulder concepts. Montpillier: Sauramps Medical; 2008. p. 259–63.
39. Cheung E, Sperling J. Management of proximal humeral nonunions and malunions. Orthop Clin N Am. 2008;39:475–82.
40. Duralde XA, Flatow EL, Pollock RG, Nicholson GP, Self EB, Bigliani LU. Operative treatment of nonunions of the surgical neck of the humerus. J Shoulder Elb Surg. 1996;5(3):169–80.
41. Frich LH, Sjoberg JO, Sneppen O. Shoulder arthroplasty in complex acute and chronic proximal humerus fractures. Orthopaedics. 1991;14:949–54.
42. Ritzman T, Iannotti J. Malunions, nonunions, and other complications of proximal humerus fractures. In: Iannotti J, Williams G, editors. Disorders of the shoulder, diagnosis and management. Philadelphia: Lippincott, Williams and Wilkins; 2007. p. 907–42.
43. Razemon JP, Baux S. Les séquelles des fractures de l'extrémité supérieure de l'humérus. Rev Chir Orthop. 1969;55:479–90.
44. Waiter JM, Flatow E. Posttraumatic arthritis. Ortho Clin North Am. 2000;31:63–76.
45. Walch G, Boileau P, Martin B, Dejour H. Unreduced posterior dislocations and fracture-dislocations of the shoulder. A review of 30 cases. J Orthop Surg. 1990;4:93–5.
46. Scheck M. Surgical treatment of nonunions of the surgical neck of the humerus. Clin Orthop Relat Res. 1982;167:255–9.
47. Stechel A, Fuhrmann U, Irlenbusch L, Rott O, Irlenbusch U. Reversed shoulder arthroplasty in cuff tear arthritis, fracture sequelae, and revision arthro-

plasty. Outcome in 59 patients followed for 2–7 years. Acta Orthop. 2010;81:367–72.
48. Levy J, Frankle M, Mighell M, Pupello D. The use of the reverse shoulder prosthesis for the treatment of failed hemiarthroplasty for proximal humeral fracture. J Bone Joint Surg. 2007;89A:292–300.
49. Neyton L, Garaud P, Boileau P. Results of reverse shoulder arthroplasty in proximal humerus fracture sequelae. In: Reverse shoulder arthroplasty. Montpellier: Sauramps Medical; 2006. p. 81–101.
50. Watson KC. Indications and considerations of shoulder replacement in post-traumatic conditions. In: Köbel R, Helbig B, Blauth W, editors. Shoulder replacement. Berlin: Springer; 1987. p. 129–33.
51. Lee CK, Hansen HR. Post-traumatic avascular necrosis of the humeral head in displaced proximal humeral fractures. J Trauma. 1981;21:788–91.
52. Raiss P, Alami G, Bruckner T, Magosch P, Habermeyer P, Boileau P, Walch G. Reverse shoulder arthroplasty for type 1 sequelae of a fracture of the proximal humerus. Bone Joint J. 2018;100-B:318–23.
53. Quadlbauer S, Hofmann GJ, Leixnering M, Rosenauer R4, Hausner T4, Reichetseder J. Open reduction and fixation with a locking plate without bone grafting is a reasonable and safe option for treating proximal humerus nonunion. Int Orthop. 2018;42:2199.
54. Raiss P, Edwards TB, da Silva MR, Bruckner T, Loew M, Walch G. Reverse shoulder arthroplasty for the treatment of nonunions of the surgical neck of the proximal part of the humerus (type-3 fracture sequelae). J Bone Joint Surg Am. 2014;96:2070–6.
55. Raiss P, Edwards TB, Collin P, Bruckner T, Zeifang F, Loew M, Boileau P, Walch G. Reverse shoulder arthroplasty for malunions of the proximal part of the humerus (Type-4 fracture sequelae). J Bone Joint Surg Am. 2016;98:893–9.
56. Schliemann B, Theisen C, Kösters C, Raschke MJ, Weimann A. Reverse total shoulder arthroplasty for type I fracture sequelae after internal fixation of proximal humerus fractures. Arch Orthop Trauma Surg. 2017;137:1677–83.
57. Grubhofer F, Wieser K, Meyer DC, Catanzaro S, Schürholz K, Gerber C. Reverse total shoulder arthroplasty for failed open reduction and internal fixation of fractures of the proximal humerus. J Shoulder Elb Surg. 2017;26:92–100.
58. Sanchez-Sotelo J, Wagner ER, Sim FH, Houdek MT. Allograft-prosthetic composite reconstruction for massive proximal humeral bone loss in reverse shoulder arthroplasty. J Bone Joint Surg Am. 2017;99:2069–76.
59. Wagner ER, McLaughlin R, Sarfani S, Cofield RH, Sperling JW, Sanchez-Sotelo J, Elhassan BT. Long-term outcomes of glenohumeral arthrodesis. J Bone Joint Surg Am. 2018;100:598–604.

Treatment of Deltoid Deficiency and Paralysis in Shoulder Arthroplasty

7

Julia Lee and Bassem Elhassan

Treatment of Deltoid Deficiency and Paralysis in Shoulder Arthroplasty

Deltoid deficiency and paralysis can be devastating to shoulder function. The deltoid is the powerhouse of the shoulder and provides over 50% of the abduction power for the shoulder in the scapular plane [1]. With improvements in shoulder arthroplasty technology, reconstruction of the deltoid in conjunction with arthroplasty is a viable option for restoration of shoulder function. The purpose of this chapter is to describe the epidemiology of deltoid deficiency, historical treatment options, current reconstructive options with arthroplasty, and their respective outcomes.

Epidemiology

The leading cause of deltoid paralysis is axillary nerve injury, either from a posttraumatic or iatrogenic etiology [2–5]. Deltoid paralysis or deficiency can also occur in the setting of a brachial plexus palsy, cervical disc pathology, peripheral compressive neuropathy, injury to the muscle belly, or infection [4, 6]. Loss of deltoid function can result in significant dysfunction as the deltoid provides abduction strength and stabilizes the glenohumeral joint [7]. In patients without a deltoid but with an intact rotator cuff, relatively good function can be maintained with minimal pain but easy fatigability [8]. However, in patients with osteoarthritis of the glenohumeral joint or with a concurrent massive rotator cuff tear, reconstruction of the deltoid in addition to shoulder arthroplasty may be the only option for pain relief and improved function (Fig. 7.1).

Historical Perspective

Traditionally, treatment for deltoid paralysis included glenohumeral arthrodesis which offered restoration of abduction but loss of passive glenohumeral motion and a high complication rate, including fractures, pseudarthrosis, and subsequent revision surgery [9, 10]. Due to the high complication rate and the permanence of the procedure, glenohumeral arthrodesis should be considered a salvage option. With improvements in shoulder arthroplasty, restoration of deltoid function in conjunction with a shoulder replacement may offer better function for patients with deltoid paralysis.

J. Lee · B. Elhassan (✉)
Mayo Clinic, Rochester, MN, USA
e-mail: elhassan.bassem@mayo.edu

R. Z. Tashjian (ed.), *Complex and Revision Shoulder Arthroplasty*,
https://doi.org/10.1007/978-3-030-02756-8_7

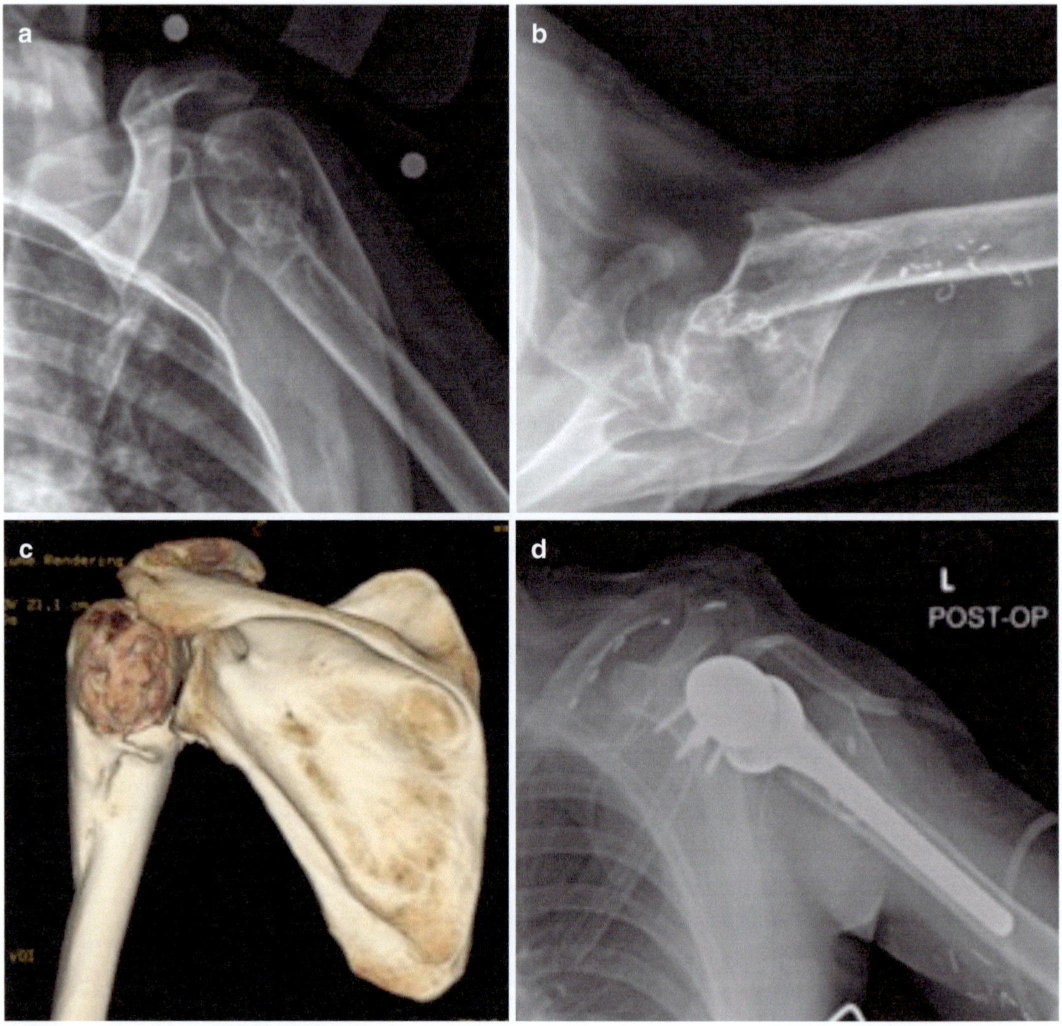

Fig. 7.1 Patient with proximal humerus malunion and deltoid palsy who was reconstructed with pedicled pectoralis major tendon and reverse shoulder arthroplasty. (**a**) Anteroposterior radiograph of the left shoulder showing proximal humerus malunion. (**b**) Axillary radiograph of the left shoulder showing proximal humerus malunion. (**c**) Three-dimensional reconstruction of proximal humerus malunion. (**d**) Postoperative radiograph of pedicled pectoralis major tendon transfer (note the cortical fixation device on the underside of the clavicle and acromion) and reverse shoulder arthroplasty

Current Options for Deltoid Deficiency

There are two techniques to reconstruct the deltoid: nerve reinnervation or tendon transfer. By reconstructing the deltoid or restoring its function, there are more options with shoulder arthroplasty.

Axillary Nerve Reinnervation for Deltoid Deficiency

For the injured axillary nerve, there are different ways to reinnervate depending on the injury. Primary repair of axillary nerve is an option if the defect length is not too great and the nerve can be reapproximated in a tension-free repair. If the distance is too far for primary repair, nerve grafting may be utilized.

Another option is nerve transfer. Witoonchart et al. published on a nerve transfer to the deltoid using the motor branch radial nerve [11, 12]. The nerve branch from the radial nerve innervating the long head of triceps is identified, mobilized, and transferred to the anterior branch of the axillary nerve. Proximity of this radial nerve branch to the axillary nerve may actually be shorter than some nerve grafts. Outcomes show improvements in shoulder range of motion with abduction >90° with M4 strength and improved DASH scores with no elbow extension weakness [12, 13].

Short-term results comparing nerve grafting to nerve transfers show that both groups improve deltoid function but still associate a disability to the affected shoulder [14]. The main advantage of the radial-to-axillary nerve transfer compared to interposition nerve grafting is the closer proximity of the donor nerve to the target muscle, which results in earlier reinnervation.

These nerve transfers, however, can have a long recovery with varied outcomes. Initial deltoid muscle function does not happen until 6–8 months following surgery with useful shoulder function recovering up to 1.5–2 years postoperatively [12, 13]. Nerve repairs, similarly, have varied results and must be conducted within a certain time frame after nerve injury. Recovery of deltoid muscle function must be confirmed prior to reverse shoulder arthroplasty.

Outcomes After Nerve Reinnervation and Shoulder Arthroplasty

Salazar et al. reported on one patient with rotator cuff deficiency and axillary nerve palsy who underwent a reverse shoulder arthroplasty after a radial-to-axillary nerve transfer [15]. After maximal restoration of deltoid function, the patient underwent reverse shoulder arthroplasty 18 months after the nerve transfer. Postoperative results after arthroplasty yielded significant improvements in range of motion as well as improved DASH and ASES scores.

Deltoid Reconstruction with Tendon Transfer

Muscle tendon transfers offer an alternative to nerve repair or transfers. Advantages of a tendon transfer include a shorter healing time without a time-sensitive window of treatment (Table 7.1). Postoperative immobilization for a tendon transfer can coincide with immobilization for shoulder arthroplasty, thus expediting the overall recovery process if arthroplasty and tendon transfer are done in a single-stage procedure. Tendon transfer options for deltoid reconstruction include a trapezius transfer, a pedicled pectoralis major transfer, or a pedicled latissimus dorsi transfer.

The trapezius tendon transfer was first described with the use of a fascia lata graft to extend the trapezius insertion to the deltoid tuberosity [9]. The use of the allograft resulted in gradual stretching, and the trapezius transfer was modified with the use of a bone block from the trapezius scapular spine insertion to attach to the humerus [16]. The procedure was later further modified by mobilizing the upper and middle trapezius tendons proximally; elevating the trapezius insertions along the lateral portion of the clavicle, the acromioclavicular joint, and the acromion; and transferring to the proximal humerus [9, 17]. This last modifica-

Table 7.1 Comparison of nerve restoration and tendon transfer for deltoid dysfunction or deficiency

	Nerve reinnervation	Tendon transfer
Indications	Nerve injury to axillary nerve	Nerve injury to axillary nerve Deltoid muscle injury or resection Brachial plexus palsy
Restoration of abduction	Yes	Yes
Time-sensitive	Yes	No
Single-stage procedure with RSA	No (must confirm restoration of deltoid function prior to RSA)	Yes (immobilization time for RSA similar to that of tendon transfer)

tion offered a more proximal release and a more distal transfer, providing better mechanical advantage for the deltoid.

Results of upper trapezius tendon transfer without RSA in the setting of brachial plexus injury show overall good results and high patient satisfaction [9, 16, 18]. Poor outcomes were associated with concurrent rotator cuff tears or baseline glenohumeral joint instability [16]. Average reported gain of motion was between 45° and 60° of abduction with resolution of preoperative glenohumeral subluxation and high patient satisfaction [18–20].

The second option for deltoid reconstruction with tendon transfer is a pedicled latissimus transfer [21–23]. The latissimus muscle is located at its insertion on the humerus and traced proximally to its origin on the thoracic and lumbar vertebrae. The neurovascular bundle is located on the underside of the muscle with numerous vascular tributaries to the muscle that need to be appropriately cauterized for hemostasis. The pedicle for the latissimus is relatively long, and muscle can be rotated on the pedicle to cover nearly the entire deltoid (Fig. 7.2).

Muramatsu et al. reported on a pedicled latissimus dorsi transfer without RSA for deltoid reconstruction in patients with musculoskeletal tumors requiring deltoid muscle excision. In these patients, the rotator cuff remained intact. All four patients had greater than 160° of shoulder abduction [22]. Itoh et al. reported abduction greater than 90° in their ten patients with latissimus dorsi transfer for deltoid pathology without RSA and noted the importance of the rotator cuff for good results [21].

The third option for deltoid reconstruction with tendon transfer is a pedicled pectoralis major transfer. Resch et al. described this procedure in 2008, where the clavicular origin and a portion of the sternal origin of the pectoralis muscle are elevated and the pectoralis flipped on its neurovascular pedicle, where the underside becomes the topside, and is reattached to the lateral clavicle and anterior acromion [24] (Fig. 7.3). The pectoralis insertion can also be elevated and distalized for better muscle tension. Resch et al. reported statistically significant improvements in shoulder abduction, shoulder forward elevation, and Constant scores. Smaller case series have also reported restoration of shoulder joint stability, deltoid muscle contour, abduction, and forward flexion with the pedicled deltoid flap [25, 26].

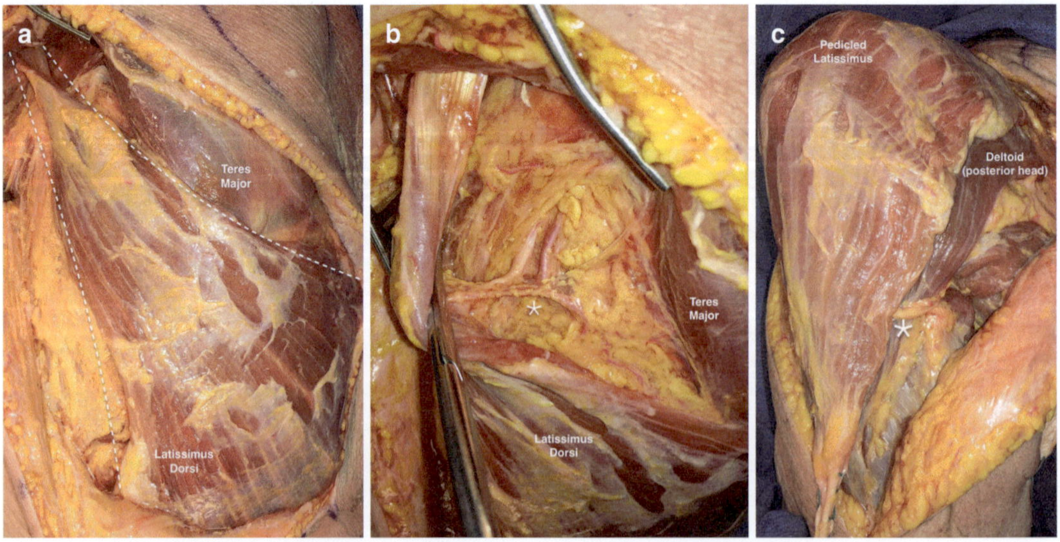

Fig. 7.2 Pedicled latissimus dorsi transfer for deltoid dysfunction. (**a**) Latissimus dorsi muscle with a broad muscular origin and narrow tendinous insertion at top left. (**b**) Neurovascular pedicle of latissimus dorsi (asterisk). (**c**) Latissimus dorsi muscle rotated over its pedicle (asterisk) to cover the entire deltoid

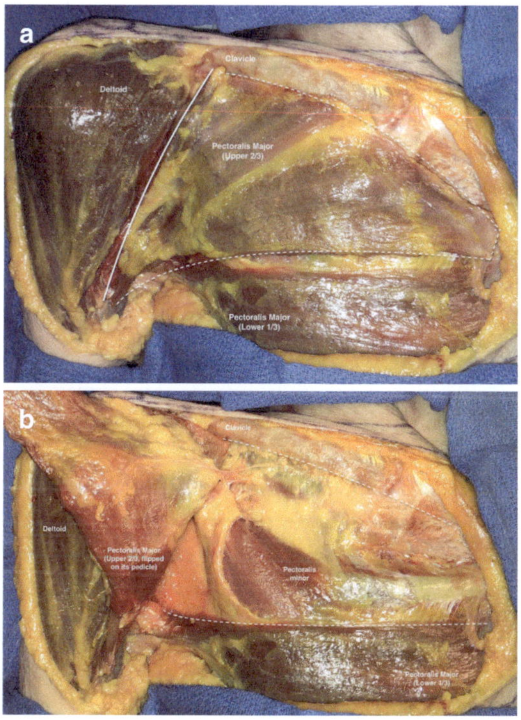

Fig. 7.3 Anatomy for pedicled pectoralis major transfer. (**a**) Anatomy of the anterior deltoid and pectoralis major. (**b**) Pectoralis major (upper 2/3) elevated to expose the neurovascular bundle on the underside of the muscle. Also shows the broad coverage of the deltoid offered by the pedicled pectoralis transfer

Outcomes After Tendon Transfer and Shoulder Arthroplasty

Elhassan et al. provided the initial report of 31 patients who underwent pedicled pectoralis major tendon in conjunction with reverse shoulder arthroplasty [27]. All patients had chronic deltoid paralysis due to axillary nerve injury with symptomatic glenohumeral arthritis and rotator cuff deficiency. With an average follow-up of 37 months, overall subjective shoulder value in patients improved from 7% to 53%, DASH scores improved from 54 to 33, forward elevation improved from 11° to 83° (range 50–110°, $p < 0.05$), and external rotation improved from 3° to 16° (range 5–30°, $p < 0.05$). Complications in this series included two acromion fractures, three seromas that resolved spontaneously, and two patients that had proximal partial detachment of the transfer, but the patients were overall satisfied and elected not to have further surgery.

Two case studies of a pedicled latissimus dorsi transfer for deltoid deficiency have also been reported, although only one of these cases had the transfer and arthroplasty procedures conducted in single-stage fashion rather than in a stepwise fashion [28, 29]. Goel et al. reported on one patient who underwent a concurrent reverse shoulder arthroplasty with latissimus dorsi pedicle flap. At 1 year after the procedure, the patient had restoration of shoulder range of motion with forward elevation to 135°, external rotation to 20°, and internal rotation to L2 with no evidence of latissimus dorsi muscle denervation on EMG and a well-seated implant on radiographs [29]. Dosari et al. reported on a RSA in a delayed fashion 5 months after a latissimus pedicled transfer with good restoration of shoulder range of motion and pain relief [28].

Authors' Preferred Treatment Strategy

The senior author's treatment algorithm includes clinical and electromyelogram confirmation of axillary nerve dysfunction correlating with MRI confirmation of deltoid muscle atrophy. On physical exam, at least the anterior and middle heads, with or without posterior head, of the deltoid are confirmed to be paralyzed. The dysfunction needs to have been present for a minimum of 18 months without nerve repair, nerve reconstruction intervention, or clinical improvement. If there was a nerve repair or reconstruction, proof of continued nerve dysfunction must be confirmed at 18 months after the nerve procedure. Additionally, the patient must have symptomatic glenohumeral arthritis with concurrent rotator cuff dysfunction.

For younger, more active patients, a glenohumeral arthrodesis may be appropriate. Or if nerve injury was within 6–8 months, nerve transfers to restore nerve function may be appropriate. However, as mentioned above, we have not performed a nerve transfer after reverse shoulder arthroplasty for deltoid paralysis because these patients almost always get referred after the 18-month time frame. If there is improvement in sequential EMG studies, it may be prudent to delay reconstruction until axillary nerve function has definitively plateaued. Again, shoulder arthroplasty with a pedicled pectoralis tendon should be considered a salvage procedure, especially in young, active individuals.

If this option is chosen, patients are counseled on postoperative functional and activity expectations with respect to a reverse shoulder arthroplasty in addition to the deformity from pectoralis transfer. If the patient cannot actively externally rotate past neutral, a tendon transfer for external rotation, either lower trapezius tendon or latissimus dorsi tendon, is done at the same time.

Authors' Preferred Pedicled Pectoralis Muscle Surgical Technique

The senior author's preferred technique was recently described [27]. The main reasons we favor the pedicled pectoralis transfer over the latissimus transfer are due to anatomy and synergistic function. The anatomy of shoulder girdle is such that the pectoralis lies adjacent to deltoid and the surgery can be done through the same anterior approach. The patient can be positioned in the beach chair during the pectoralis transfer versus the need for lateral positioning during the latissimus transfer. Anatomy of the pedicled pectoralis transfer requires minimal dissection of the neurovascular pedicle, which is in contrast to the latissimus transfer, where the muscle requires extensive dissection proximally to the level of the axillary vascular pedicle. Additionally, in terms of synergistic function, the upper part of the pectoralis major spontaneously contracts during shoulder flexion, especially if the forearm is positioned in pronation.

The surgical technique for pedicled pectoralis transfer with reverse shoulder arthroplasty is performed as follows. Briefly, the patient is placed either in a beach chair or modified lateral decubitus position. The incision is performed starting 2 cm distal and inferior to the sternoclavicular joint, extending from the sternum superiorly along the lower border of the clavicle toward the acromioclavicular joint and then distally toward the deltoid insertion via the deltopectoral interval. Full-thickness skin flaps are raised to expose pectoralis major muscle. The three parts of the muscle are identified: the clavicular head, the upper sternal head, and the lower part of the sternal head. Harvesting of the pectoralis major is based on its neurovascular bundles with the clavicular head and upper sternal head sharing a different neurovascular bundle than the lower sternal head. The transfer of the pedicle flap is begun by detaching the upper part of the sternal head and the entirety of the clavicular head from the sternum and clavicle with careful attention to preserve its neurovascular pedicle. The pedicle is located distal to the mid-clavicle, and the muscle belly must be elevated prior to dissection of the muscle from the bone distal to the mid-clavicle. Once the muscle is detached from its origin, the insertion into the humerus is detached and the muscle elevated, allowing for visualization and mobilization of the pedicle proximally to the level of the axillary artery and vein (Fig. 7.3b–d). Once the muscle has been mobilized and prepared, it is protected with moist gauze during the RSA.

The RSA is then performed in the standard fashion. In preparation to perform the pedicled pectoralis transfer, the anterior atrophic deltoid is excised, and the lateral one-third of the clavicle and anterior aspect of the acromion are debrided. Multiple #2 nonabsorbable sutures are placed through transosseous tunnels in the prepared clavicle and acromion. The pectoralis muscle is then flipped (like turning a page in a book) so that the most medial portion is transposed laterally. While keeping the shoulder in approximately 60° of flexion, the proximal aspect is repaired to the clavicle and acromion, and the distal tendon is repaired using cortical button fixation with soft tissue reinforcement. A drain is placed prior to a layered subcuticular incision closure.

Postoperatively, the patient has pre-made custom shoulder brace that is aimed to position the shoulder in 60° of flexion with resting internal rotation. If tendon transfer is performed for external rotation, then the brace is adjusted to have 60°

of flexion in addition to 40° of external rotation. The patient is strictly in the brace for 8 weeks followed by active-assisted range of motion for another 8 weeks. After these 4 months, the patient is started on gentle strengthening for 8 weeks followed by activity as tolerated with a limitation of 15 pounds maximum in any direction. Passive stretching of the shoulder in any direction should be avoided for at least 5 months after surgery to avoid damaging the muscle transfer.

Conclusion

In patients with deltoid deficiency or paralysis, reconstruction of the deltoid with either nerve restoration or tendon transfer yields good results for restoring motion and stability. This can be combined with shoulder arthroplasty in patients with glenohumeral joint or rotator cuff pathology with promising results for pain relief and functional shoulder improvement.

Bibliography

1. Howell SM, Kraft TA. The role of the supraspinatus and infraspinatus muscles in glenohumeral kinematics of anterior should instability. Clin Orthop Relat Res. 1991;(263):128–34.
2. Yang X, Xu B, Tong JS, Zhang CG, Dong Z, Liu JB. Triceps motor branch transfer for isolated axillary nerve injury: outcomes in 9 patients. Orthop Traumatol Surg Res. 2017;103:1283.
3. Perlmutter GS. Axillary nerve injury. Clin Orthop Relat Res. 1999;(368):28–36.
4. Steinmann SP, Moran EA. Axillary nerve injury: diagnosis and treatment. J Am Acad Orthop Surg. 2001;9(5):328–35.
5. Narakas AO. Paralytic disorders of the shoulder girdle. Hand Clin. 1988;4(4):619–32.
6. Chang H, Park JB, Hwang JY, Song KJ. Clinical analysis of cervical radiculopathy causing deltoid paralysis. Eur Spine J. 2003;12(5):517–21.
7. Rosso C, Mueller AM, McKenzie B, Entezari V, Cereatti A, Della Croce U, et al. Bulk effect of the deltoid muscle on the glenohumeral joint. J Exp Orthop. 2014;1(1):14.
8. Werthel JD, Bertelli J, Elhassan BT. Shoulder function in patients with deltoid paralysis and intact rotator cuff. Orthop Traumatol Surg Res. 2017;103(6):869–73.
9. Selim NM. Trapezius tendon transfer according to Saha after neglected complete axillary nerve injury. Acta Orthop Belg. 2012;78(4):436–41.
10. Cofield RH, Briggs BT. Glenohumeral arthrodesis. Operative and long-term functional results. J Bone Joint Surg Am. 1979;61(5):668–77.
11. Witoonchart K, Leechavengvongs S, Uerpairojkit C, Thuvasethakul P, Wongnopsuwan V. Nerve transfer to deltoid muscle using the nerve to the long head of the triceps, part I: an anatomic feasibility study. J Hand Surg Am. 2003;28(4):628–32.
12. Leechavengvongs S, Witoonchart K, Uerpairojkit C, Thuvasethakul P. Nerve transfer to deltoid muscle using the nerve to the long head of the triceps, part II: a report of 7 cases. J Hand Surg Am. 2003;28(4):633–8.
13. Leechavengvongs S, Malungpaishorpe K, Uerpairojkit C, Ng CY, Witoonchart K. Nerve transfers to restore shoulder function. Hand Clin. 2016;32(2):153–64.
14. Baltzer HL, Kircher MF, Spinner RJ, Bishop AT, Shin AY. A comparison of outcomes of triceps motor branch-to-axillary nerve transfer or sural nerve interpositional grafting for isolated axillary nerve injury. Plast Reconstr Surg. 2016;138(2):256e–64e.
15. Salazar DH, Chalmers PN, Mackinnon SE, Keener JD. Reverse shoulder arthroplasty after radial-to-axillary nerve transfer for axillary nerve palsy with concomitant irreparable rotator cuff tear. J Shoulder Elb Surg. 2017;26(1):e23–e8.
16. Kotwal PP, Mittal R, Malhotra R. Trapezius transfer for deltoid paralysis. J Bone Joint Surg Br. 1998;80(1):114–6.
17. Saha AK. Surgery of the paralysed and flail shoulder. Acta Orthop Scand. 1967;(Suppl 97):5–90.
18. Ruhmann O, Schmolke S, Bohnsack M, Carls J, Wirth CJ. Trapezius transfer in brachial plexus palsy. Correlation of the outcome with muscle power and operative technique. J Bone Joint Surg Br. 2005;87(2):184–90.
19. Aziz W, Singer RM, Wolff TW. Transfer of the trapezius for flail shoulder after brachial plexus injury. J Bone Joint Surg Br. 1990;72(4):701–4.
20. Mir-Bullo X, Hinarejos P, Mir-Batlle P, Busquets R, Carrera L, Navarro A. Trapezius transfer for shoulder paralysis. 6 patients with brachial plexus injuries followed for 1 year. Acta Orthop Scand. 1998;69(1):69–72.
21. Itoh Y, Sasaki T, Ishiguro T, Uchinishi K, Yabe Y, Fukuda H. Transfer of latissimus dorsi to replace a paralysed anterior deltoid. A new technique using an inverted pedicled graft. J Bone Joint Surg Br. 1987;69(4):647–51.
22. Muramatsu K, Ihara K, Tominaga Y, Hashimoto T, Taguchi T. Functional reconstruction of the deltoid muscle following complete resection of musculoskeletal sarcoma. J Plast Reconstr Aesthet Surg. 2014;67(7):916–20.
23. Narakas AO. Muscle transpositions in the shoulder and upper arm for sequelae of brachial plexus palsy. Clin Neurol Neurosurg. 1993;95(Suppl):S89–91.
24. Resch H, Povacz P, Maurer H, Koller H, Tauber M. Pectoralis major inverse plasty for functional reconstruction in patients with anterolateral deltoid deficiency. J Bone Joint Surg Br. 2008;90(6):757–63.

25. Hou CL, Tai YH. Transfer of upper pectoralis major flap for functional reconstruction of deltoid muscle. Chin Med J. 1991;104(9):753–7.
26. Lin H, Hou C, Xu Z. Transfer of the superior portion of the pectoralis major flap for restoration of shoulder abduction. J Reconstr Microsurg. 2009;25(4):255–60.
27. Elhassan BT, Wagner ER, Werthel JD, Lehanneur M, Lee J. Outcome of reverse shoulder arthroplasty with pedicled pectoralis transfer in patients with deltoid paralysis. J Shoulder Elb Surg. 2018;27(1):96–103.
28. Dosari M, Hameed S, Mukhtar K, Elmhiregh A. Reverse shoulder arthroplasty for deltoid-deficient shoulder following latissimus dorsi flap transfer. Case report. Int J Surg Case Rep. 2017;39: 256–9.
29. Goel DP, Ross DC, Drosdowech DS. Rotator cuff tear arthropathy and deltoid avulsion treated with reverse total shoulder arthroplasty and latissimus dorsi transfer: case report and review of the literature. J Shoulder Elb Surg. 2012;21(5):e1–7.

Part II

Revision Shoulder Arthroplasty: Diagnosis and Management

8 General Approach to the Painful Shoulder Arthroplasty

Vahid Entezari and Surena Namdari

Introduction

Arthritis affects more than 54 million (~23%) adults in the United States and results in pain, loss of function, and significant disability [1]. Arthroplasty is an effective treatment for end-stage arthritis, providing pain relief, increased range of motion, and improved quality of life. Although, the number of shoulder arthroplasty procedures is still small compared to hip and knee arthroplasty [2], the past few decades have seen a surge in the number of primary and revision shoulder arthroplasty cases. For instance, between 2000 and 2008, the number of shoulder arthroplasties in the United States increased 12% per year [3]. This increase in utilization is mainly due to an aging population, better diagnostic modalities, improvement in implant material and design, expanded indications, and more widespread surgical training in shoulder replacement [3–5]. According to national trends, the utilization of hemiarthroplasties is falling drastically, while the utilization of reverse total shoulder arthroplasty increases yearly since its introduction to US market in 2004 [6, 7].

Increasing utilization and expanding indications of total shoulder arthroplasty (TSA) have huge implications for the future burden of revision arthroplasty [5]. While several studies have shown that surgeon and hospital case volume have a direct correlation with the outcome and complications after shoulder arthroplasty, still, the majority of shoulder arthroplasties are done by low-volume surgeons [8]. Expanding indications for arthroplasty, especially to younger patients, is going to increase the burden and complexity of revision arthroplasty in the future [9, 10]. Denard et al. studied the long-term outcome of shoulder arthroplasty in patients under 55 years of age and reported 98% implant survival at 5 years but only 63% survival at 10 years [11].

Because of the projected revision burden, an understanding of the work-up, diagnosis, and management of the failed shoulder arthroplasty is critical for the shoulder and elbow surgeon caring for this complex patient population. This section of chapters will review the etiology, diagnosis, and management of painful shoulder arthroplasty and report evidence-based and systematic approaches to common challenges.

Painful Shoulder Arthroplasty

Shoulder arthroplasty provides predictable pain relief, improved function, and good longevity for the majority of patients [12–16]. Carter et al.

V. Entezari · S. Namdari (✉)
Department of Orthopaedic Surgery, Rothman Institute at Thomas Jefferson University, Philadelphia, PA, USA
e-mail: vahid.entezari@rothmaninstitute.com; Surena.namdari@rothmaninstitute.com

R. Z. Tashjian (ed.), *Complex and Revision Shoulder Arthroplasty*,
https://doi.org/10.1007/978-3-030-02756-8_8

[17] performed a systematic review of 20 studies with a total of 1576 TSAs and showed significant improvement in pain level and generic and shoulder-specific patient-reported outcomes. Despite these impressive results, pain after shoulder arthroplasty is not uncommon. For example, Deshmukh et al. [14] reported on 320 TSA patients at a minimum of 10 years follow-up and, despite low revision rates (6.9%), reported some level of persistent pain in 32% of patients.

The painful shoulder has been cited as the most common reason for revision shoulder arthroplasty [18]. Hasan et al. [8] reviewed 141 shoulder arthroplasties who were evaluated for unsatisfactory results and found that 82% had pain and 74% had stiffness. In their cohort, major factors that were associated with failed arthroplasty included instability, glenoid loosening, component malposition, tuberosity malunion, rotator cuff tear, glenoid erosion, and infection.

Etiology of Painful Shoulder Arthroplasty

Although having pain immediately after surgery is expected, persistent pain or development of new pain after recovering from surgery is considered abnormal and warrants further investigation. Because of the non-weight-bearing nature of the shoulder joint and high capacity of the upper extremity to compensate for loss of motion, many patients with a less than optimal result may delay their presentation and/or choose not to have revision surgery. Regardless, persistent pain after shoulder arthroplasty should trigger a comprehensive work-up to address both the patients' concerns and need for revision surgery.

A systematic approach to a painful arthroplasty requires the surgeon to consider early- and late-onset causes for a failed shoulder arthroplasty (Table 8.1). Unfortunately, there is no universal definition of "early" or "late" timing of presentation. As a general rule, if a patient did not have a pain-free period after surgery, early-onset etiologies should be given more consideration in the work-up as opposed to a patient whose shoulder becomes painful after functioning well for several years. Some complications, such as instability, can happen at any time in postoperative course and may have different mechanical causes. While early-onset instability can be associated with implant malposition, poor soft tissue balancing, or traumatic subscapularis failure, late-onset instability might be a result of implant failure, polyethylene wear, or attritional rotator cuff tear.

Table 8.1 Etiology of painful shoulder arthroplasty

Early onset	Late onset
Acute infection	Subacute/chronic infection
Hematoma	Rotator cuff failure
Stiffness	Aseptic loosening
Nerve injury	Heterotopic ossification
Scapular fracture (reverse TSA)	Glenoid erosion (Hemi)
Subscapularis failure	Implant failure
Deltoid detachment	Instability
Metal allergy	Periprosthetic fracture
Instability	
Periprosthetic fracture	

The causes of a painful shoulder arthroplasty may vary based on patient demographics, primary etiology for surgery, and the type of implant (Table 8.2). For instance, glenoid erosion is the most common cited cause of failure of hemiarthroplasty for osteoarthritis [8], while tuberosity nonunion or malunion is the most common cause of failure after hemiarthroplasty for proximal humerus fracture [21]. While stiffness and glenoid loosening are the most common cause of failure in anatomic TSA [18], instability is the number one cause of revision after reverse TSA [22]. Bohsali et al. [19] reviewed the complication rates after shoulder arthroplasty in the past decade and reported that the overall rate of complications is trending down from 14.7% to 11.0%. Some etiologies such as scapular stress fracture are unique to reverse TSA and commonly happen in osteoporotic female patients [23]. Surgeons should adopt an individualized approach to the work-up of the painful shoulder arthroplasty to take into account patient history, physical examination, radiographs, laboratory testing, and implant-specific characteristics.

Table 8.2 Common causes of complication after shoulder arthroplasty for each type of implant

	HA			
	For OA	For proximal humerus fracture	aTSA	rTSA
Complication rate (short to mid- term) [19, 20]	2.9–17%	5.0–64.0%	10.3%	16.1%
Complications	Glenoid erosion Rotator cuff failure Nerve injury Infection	Tuberosity nonunion/ malunion Technical error in implant height and version Nerve injury Infection	Implant loosening Instability Periprosthetic fracture Rotator cuff tear Nerve injury Infection	Instability Scapular fracture Periprosthetic fracture Nerve injury Infection

Diagnosis of Painful Shoulder Arthroplasty

History

A complete and focused history is perhaps the most important part of the work-up of a painful shoulder arthroplasty. The history should start with delineating the nature, severity, and anatomic location of the pain, its relationship with joint movement, and the timing of symptoms in relation to surgery. Any associated symptoms including stiffness, mechanical symptoms of clicking and popping, sense of instability, numbness or weakness in the upper extremity, neck pain, and radicular pain should be recorded. Although typical signs of infection are rare in shoulder periprosthetic infection, patients should be asked about constitutional symptoms including fever, chills, and night sweats and any difficulty with wound healing, excessive drainage, and being on prolonged antibiotics postoperatively. Information about the postoperative course, rehabilitation regimen, and history of a fall or direct trauma to the upper extremity are very valuable. Past medical history including diabetes, osteoporosis, coagulopathy, and prior infection as well as information regarding use of certain medications, such as chronic antibiotics, corticosteroids, systemic immunosuppressors, and anticoagulant medication, should be obtained. History of prior surgeries both before and after the index arthroplasty, recent dental work, urologic or GI procedure, and details of each surgery such as date, name of the surgeon, and hospital should be collected in case operative reports need to be obtained for revision surgery.

Physical Examination

Inspection is the first step to a thorough physical examination and requires complete exposure of the shoulder girdle. The examiner should look for asymmetry, muscle atrophy, deltoid detachment and locations of prior incisions, delayed wound healing, and signs of infection (erythema, swelling, or drainage). Palpation is the next step and involves an evaluation for tenderness around the incision, glenohumeral joint line, acromioclavicular and sternoclavicular joints, and posterior border of the acromion and scapular spine. The evaluation of motion in all planes should be conducted, and the examiner should pay particular attention to whether passive range of motion and active range of motion are equal to one another. If passive range of motion and active range of motion are equally limited, possible causes include extensive scar formation or mechanical impingement from the implant or bony abnormalities. If passive motion is preserved but active motion is limited, muscle weakness, tendon rupture, or nerve deficit should be considered. Patients should be asked to reproduce mechanical symptoms such as crepitation or clicking, if possible. A neurovascular examination should be performed to assess nerve function and vascular perfusion of the upper extremity.

Imaging

The goal of imaging in the assessment of a painful shoulder arthroplasty is to assess bone, soft tissue, implants, and their relationships [24] (Table 8.3). Plain X-ray and computed tomography (CT) scan are main modalities in assessing bone quality, fractures, tuberosity healing, implant position, dislocation, and loosening. When it comes to soft tissue assessment, ultrasound (US) and CT arthrogram are modalities of choice to assess soft tissue reaction, fluid collection, and integrity of rotator cuff tendon and muscles around the shoulder. In our experience, the utility of magnetic resonance imaging (MRI) is limited due to artifact caused by the metallic implant and limited soft tissue evaluation even with metal subtraction imaging.

X-Ray

Plain radiographs are inexpensive, readily available in most clinical settings, and provide information about the bone, soft tissue, and implants. Therefore, they are the initial modality of choice for evaluation of a painful shoulder arthroplasty [25, 26]. Radiographic studies should, at minimum, include anteroposterior (AP), true AP or Grashey, and axillary views. Images should be taken as such that the glenohumeral joint, medial border of the scapula and entirety of the implant, including the humeral stem is visible. Generally, changes are subtle, and comparisons between serial radiographs enhance the examiner's ability to discern bone loss and implant loosening or migration [26].

The AP and true AP views allow evaluation of overall bone quality, focal bone resorption, fracture or notching, and presence of heterotopic ossification. On the humeral side, implant alignment, humeral head size, tuberosity height, cement mantle, and osteolysis are evaluated for "overstuffing" [27], possible stem loosening, or subsidence (Fig. 8.1). The axillary view is useful to assess glenoid version, anteroposterior relationship of the implant to the glenoid, and implant subluxation or dislocation (Fig. 8.2). The axillary view is also useful to assess the position and possible displacement of the lesser tuberosity osteotomy (Fig. 8.3). Examiner should specifically look for acromial and scapular spine fractures in a painful reverse total shoulder arthroplasty and compare preoperative and postoperative radiographs for evidence of displacement.

Radiographs are also important tool for preoperative planning. They are used to assess overall bone stock, amount of joint line medialization,

Table 8.3 Imaging modalities in assessing bone, soft tissue, and implant in painful shoulder arthroplasty

Imaging	Bone	Soft tissue	Implant
XRAY	Bone quality Bone resorption Glenoid erosion Tuberosity malunion Periprosthetic fracture Scapular fracture Overstuffing Notching	Swelling Air in the joint Foreign body Heterotopic ossification	Implant loosening Implant failure/dissociation Subluxation/dislocation
US	–	Joint effusion Hematoma Deltoid detachment Rotator cuff integrity	–
CT/CT arthrogram/MARS CT	Bone quality Humeral bone loss Glenoid erosion Fracture healing Tuberosity position Periprosthetic fracture Scapular fracture	Integrity of soft tissue envelop Muscle atrophy Calcification Air in the joint Foreign body	Implant integrity Implant loosening

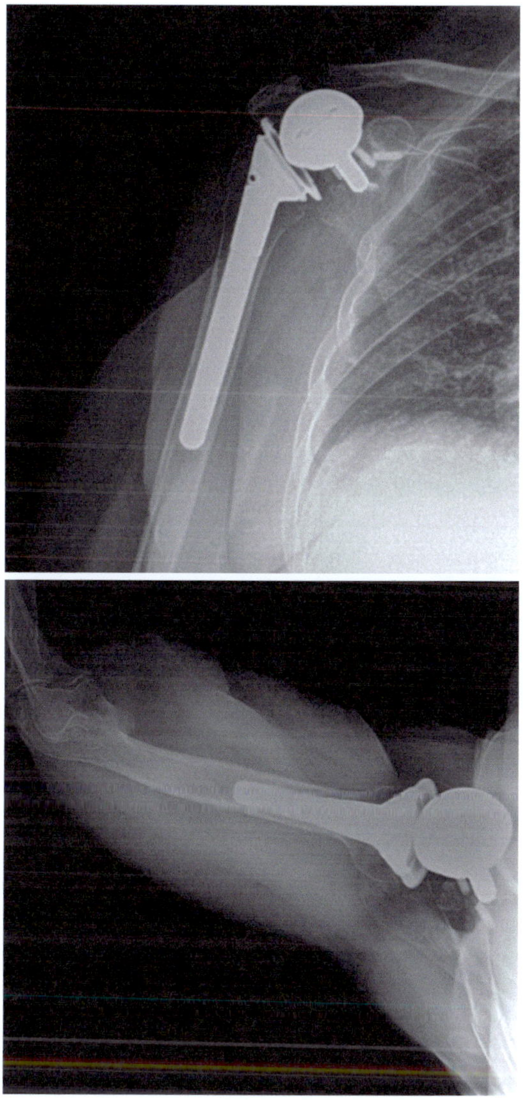

Fig. 8.1 78-year-old male who presented 1 year after pain and stiffness following reverse total shoulder arthroplasty with AP and axillary X-ray revealing a failed baseplate due to aseptic loosening

location of tuberosities, and presence and location of heterotopic ossifications. We know that under- or over-tensioning of the deltoid may lead to instability or possible scapular spine fracture in reverse arthroplasty implants. Avascular necrosis, malunion, or proximal humerus bone loss makes it difficult to assess bony landmarks and the amount of lengthening based on the affected shoulder. Bilateral full-length arm X-ray with a scale included in the image will provide an objective preoperative tool to accurately measure arm lengthening and optimize soft tissue tensioning [28].

Ultrasound

Ultrasound is another low-cost modality that allows evaluation of soft tissue derangements including rotator cuff tear, muscle detachment or atrophy, and fluid collections around the implant [29]. Ultrasound is not affected by metal artifact from the implant and allows dynamic evaluation of the joint [25]. The feasibility of ultrasound in evaluating posterior-superior rotator cuff tears or subscapularis failure in shoulder arthroplasty has been established [29]. Ultrasound is also commonly used in the guided diagnostic aspiration of the painful shoulder arthroplasty. The main limitations of ultrasound are its dependence on the experience and skill of the operator, difficulty in patients with large body habitus, and the inability to assess bone and implant loosening.

CT Scan

CT scan plays an important role as an advanced imaging modality in the evaluation of the painful shoulder arthroplasty. CT scan provides granular evaluation of bone stock, implant loosening, and migration [30]. CT arthrogram can be used to assess rotator cuff integrity and glenoid implant loosening [31]. Mallo et al. [32] studied the accuracy of CT arthrography to assess implant loosening in the setting of painful shoulder arthroplasty and found that this technique can underestimate glenoid loosening and cautioned against its use. Application of CT to quantify glenoid loosening in anatomic TSA was limited due to metal artifact generated by the humeral head implant [33]. New metal artifact reduction protocols have improved the quality of CT images [34] and, along with simple patient positioning techniques [30], have made reproducible evaluation of glenoid loosening possible [35]. Metal artifact reduction protocols have their own limitations, and, although they visually create

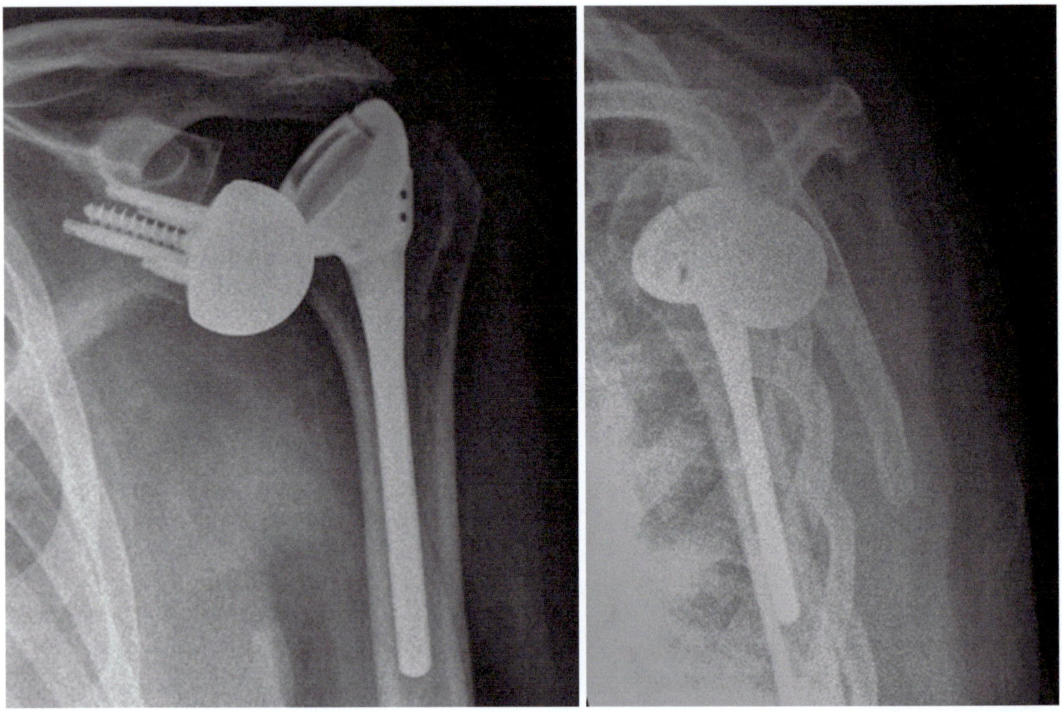

Fig. 8.2 74-year-old female who underwent a reverse total shoulder arthroplasty presented 6 months later with pain, inability to raise the arm, and deformity of the upper arm. Radiographs show anterosuperior dislocation of the prosthesis

better images with less streaking, they can affect sizing of the metal implant and the quality of trabecular bone images [36, 37]. Using 3D reconstruction of CT images in recent year has become a powerful tool for preoperative planning for revision surgery.

MRI

MRI has high soft tissue resolution, but, given its high cost and vulnerability to metal artifact, its use has been limited in evaluation of painful shoulder arthroplasty [24]. The main advantage of MRI in the setting of arthroplasty, especially if metal artifact reduction protocols are applied, [38] is its ability to assess for rotator cuff tearing, rotator cuff muscle atrophy, brachial plexus injury, and surrounding soft tissue injury [39]. Sperling et al. [40] reported that, despite metal artifact, MRI was able to correctly identify 10 out of 11 cases that had a full-thickness rotator cuff tear and 8 of 10 who did not have a rotator cuff tear after shoulder arthroplasty. With these findings, selective application of MRI with metal artifact reduction protocols in patients who are high risk for a rotator cuff tear might be justified.

Nuclear Medicine

Application of nuclear medicine in work-up of the painful shoulder arthroplasty has focused on prosthetic joint infection, assessment of implant loosening, and occult fracture [24]. X-ray imaging is usually negative in early stages of infection, implant loosening, and stress fracture, and ability to detect a biologic response is valuable and can lead to early diagnosis. The challenges of

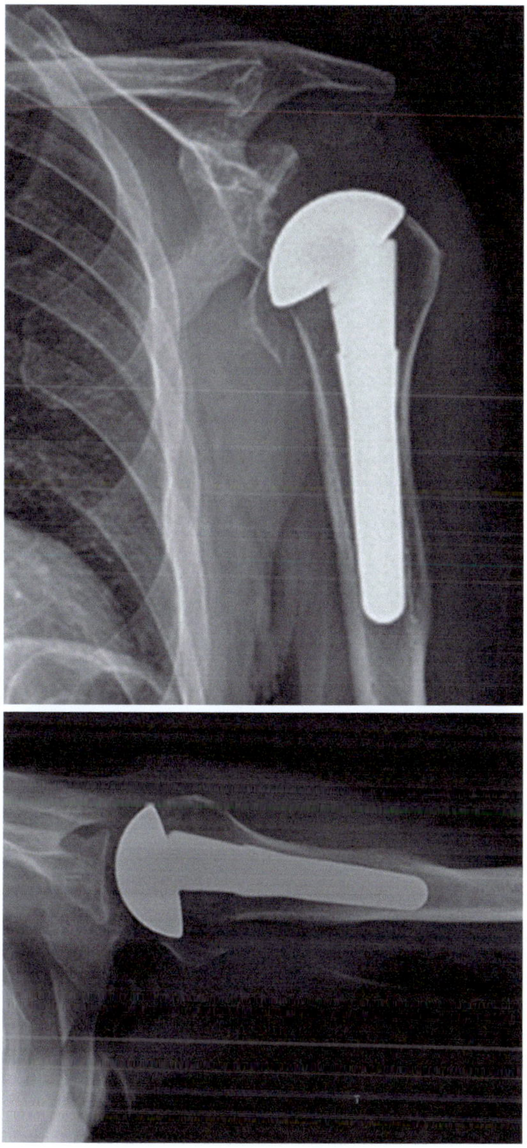

Fig. 8.3 72-year-old male who presented 6 weeks after an anatomic total shoulder arthroplasty with a failed lesser tuberosity osteotomy repair resulting in subscapularis dysfunction and implant subluxation

conventional technetium bone scan are its lack of specificity in diagnosing prosthetic shoulder infection [25]. Because of their nonspecific nature, the role of nuclear medicine scans in the work-up of the painful shoulder arthroplasty remains undetermined.

Electromyography (EMG)

Nerve injury is reported in 0.1–4.3% of shoulder arthroplasties with the majority involving the axillary nerve. There is a high rate of spontaneous recovery in the first 3 months postoperatively [41–43]. Involvement of the brachial plexus, radial nerve, and ulnar nerve has also been reported with far less frequency [18]. In reverse TSA, excess arm lengthening >2 cm and placement of arm in extreme positions during the surgery may stretch brachial plexus and lead to nerve injury [44, 45]. Ladermann et al. [46] reported that prevalence of nerve injury detected by EMG at 3.6 weeks was 10.5 times higher after reverse than anatomic TSA. If neurologic recovery did not start by 12 weeks after surgery, an EMG study is warranted to assess integrity and function of the upper extremity nerves.

Laboratory Studies

Infection is one of the important differential diagnoses in any painful shoulder arthroplasty, and, at minimum, laboratory markers including white blood cell count and inflammatory markers such as erythrocyte sedimentation rate (ESR) and C-reactive protein (CRP) should be ordered to screen for infection. Unfortunately, most periprosthetic shoulder infections are caused by indolent organisms, and laboratory markers are commonly normal [47, 48]. There is poor correlation between positive intraoperative cultures and elevated laboratory markers in failed arthroplasty cases [49]. Villacis et al. showed that WBC count had poor sensitivity and only predicted 7% of cases with positive cultures [50]. In a cohort of 193 revision shoulder arthroplasties, Pottinger et al. [51] showed that only 17% of patients with positive culture for *Propionibacterium acnes* had elevated ESR levels. Similarly, Grosso et al. [52] reported 33% sensitivity for CRP in detecting positive cultures in revision shoulder arthroplasty. Preoperative inflammatory markers and WBC count are commonly normal in painful shoulder arthroplasty, but positive results are useful and in most cases should be taken seriously. Chalmers et al. looked at a large national insurance database and identified patients who developed infection 1 year following revision shoulder arthroplasty and found that besides male gender (OR = 3.8, $P < 0.001$), elevated preoperative ESR significantly increased the odds of developing infection following revision arthroplasty (OR = 2.4, $P < 0.05$) [53]. Analysis of cytokine profiles of the serum and joint aspirate such as IL-6 and α-defensin has shown promising results [54–56], but their application have been limited due to cost, lack of sensitivity for blood samples [48], limited availability, and lack of a well-developed infection work-up algorithm to interpret results.

Allergy Testing

Metal allergy is a poorly understood cause of painful arthroplasty. Data available on this topic in the hip and knee literature is inconclusive. Bravo et al. compared 161 total knee arthroplasty cases with positive metal allergy history (56 patients had positive skin test) with 161 matched controls with no history of metal allergy [57]. After 5.3 years of follow-up, there were no differences in pain level, complications, or revision rate among any of the groups. The most commonly reported allergy is to nickel, and there is limited data available to assess the extent of this problem in shoulder arthroplasty. Ko et al. [58] reported ten female patients who presented with persistent pain on average 2 months after surgery and found that eight cases were positive for nickel allergy and two were positive for cobalt allergy. The challenge is the unclear relevance of skin testing to deep tissue reaction to metal implants and lack of consistency and standardization of blood testing for metal allergy [59]. Morwood et al. reviewed the current literature on shoulder arthroplasty in patients with metal allergy and found no evidence supporting routine preoperative testing for metal allergy [60]. They recommend screening patients for history of metal/jewelry hypersensitivity and change the implant system to nickel-/cobalt-free implants in patients with positive history. In the setting of a painful shoulder arthroplasty, it is reasonable to screen patients for possible metal allergy using either skin patch or lymphocyte transformation test after other causes such as infection or mechanical failure are ruled out.

Joint Aspiration

Aspiration of joint fluid can be an effective means to directly collect fluid for culture from a painful shoulder arthroplasty, but its utility for diagnosis of periprosthetic infection has not yet been established. Blind aspiration of a shoulder arthroplasty may fail due to distorted anatomy and postoperative scar formation [61]. Image-guided aspiration may have better success rates in targeting loculated fluid around the implant and can also lavage the joint in cases of a dry tap. Even when aspirations are successful, it is unclear whether they correlate with tissue cultures [62]. Dilisio et al. [63] compared the results of fluoroscopically guided joint aspiration with arthroscopically obtained tissue biopsies in 19 patients with painful shoulder arthroplasty and showed sensitivity of 16.7% and negative predictive values of 58.3%. The accuracy of the synovial fluid cell count for diagnosing periprosthetic joint infection in the shoulder is much lower than hip and knee arthroplasty. We recommend preoperative aspiration to be attempted under sterile conditions in all patients with atraumatic, painful shoulder arthroplasty. Although the majority of arthroplasty aspirations will result in a dry tap or a negative result, positive aspiration has high specificity for infection. Overall, even with a negative aspiration, infection cannot be ruled out in the setting of a painful shoulder arthroplasty.

Examination Under Anesthesia (EUA)

Examination under anesthesia in the setting of painful shoulder arthroplasty can provide useful information about implant loosening, frank or subclinical instability, and possible bony and soft tissue impingement. Surgeons can utilize live fluoroscopy to gain a better understanding of the stability of the implant prior to undertaking an arthroscopic or open surgery. Gee et al. [64] reported cases of posterior instability after TSA that failed conservative management and was evaluated with EUA and addressed through arthroscopic capsular imbrication. The surgeon should be mindful of the possibility of iatrogenic periprosthetic fracture, dislocation, or nerve injury during manipulation of a stiff or unstable shoulder arthroplasty.

Arthroscopic Evaluation and Tissue Biopsy

When a patient presents with an unexplained painful shoulder arthroplasty and negative infection work-up, an arthroscopic evaluation of the joint will allow for assessment of bony and soft tissue structures, glenoid component fixation, and the opportunity to obtain synovial fluid and multiple tissue biopsies. One study showed that diagnostic arthroscopy has a much higher success rate in identifying pathogens than joint aspiration [63]. Tashjian et al. [65], in their analysis of 17 patients with failed shoulder arthroplasty, showed that sensitivity and specificity of pre-revision biopsies taken arthroscopically or open in predicting final cultures at the time of revision were 90% and 86%, respectively. Also assessment of implant stability through arthroscopy is more accurate than CT arthrogram [32].

Diagnostic Injections

Although stiffness, glenoid loosening, and instability are commonly cited causes of painful shoulder arthroplasty, the source of the patient's pain can be challenging to identify. Diagnostic injections of local anesthetic in the subacromial space or AC joint can provide insight into the source of pain. The use of diagnostic injections after shoulder arthroplasty is controversial due to the potential risk of causing a periprosthetic joint infection.

Authors' Preferred Work-Up for Painful Arthroplasty

Painful shoulder arthroplasty represents a wide range of pathologies with a long list of etiologies. There is little consensus in the literature on how this complex entity should be evaluated and what set of laboratory tests, imaging studies, or diagnostic procedures should be ordered to reach a final diagnosis. Moreover, it is common that majority, if not all, of the preoperative diagnostic tests are negative, leaving clinicians without a clear explanation for a patient's continued pain and dysfunction. Our preferred approach is shown in Flowchart 8.1.

Summary

This chapter provides an overview of the diagnostic approaches to the painful shoulder arthroplasty. The diagnostic evaluation includes a comprehensive history, physical examination, laboratory evaluation, and review of diagnostic studies. The chapters that follow will further evaluate the causes of pain and dysfunction after shoulder arthroplasty with a focus on diagnostic algorithms and management options.

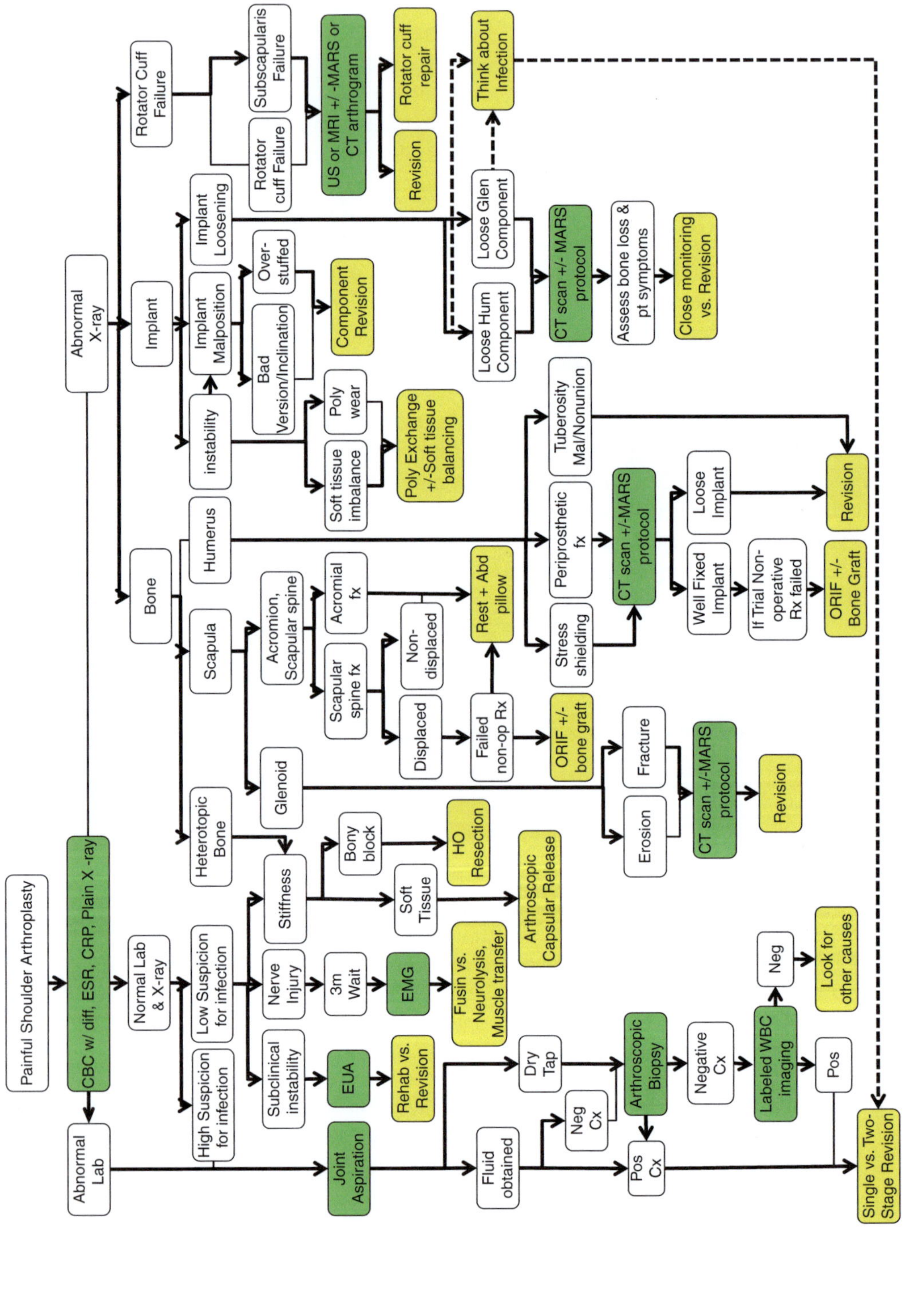

Flowchart 8.1 Work-up of painful shoulder arthroplasty

References

1. Ma VY, Chan L, Carruthers KJ. Incidence, prevalence, costs, and impact on disability of common conditions requiring rehabilitation in the United States: stroke, spinal cord injury, traumatic brain injury, multiple sclerosis, osteoarthritis, rheumatoid arthritis, limb loss, and back pain. Arch Phys Med Rehabil. 2014;95:986–95. e981.
2. Jain NB, Higgins LD, Guller U, Pietrobon R, Katz JN. Trends in the epidemiology of total shoulder arthroplasty in the United States from 1990-2000. Arthritis Rheum. 2006;55:591–7.
3. Kim SH, Wise BL, Zhang Y, Szabo RM. Increasing incidence of shoulder arthroplasty in the United States. J Bone Joint Surg Am. 2011;93:2249–54.
4. Dillon MT, Chan PH, Inacio MCS, Singh A, Yian EH, Navarro RA. Yearly trends in elective shoulder arthroplasty, 2005–2013. Arthritis Care Res (Hoboken). 2017;69:1574–81.
5. Schwartz BE, Savin DD, Youderian AR, Mossad D, Goldberg BA. National trends and perioperative outcomes in primary and revision total shoulder arthroplasty: trends in total shoulder arthroplasty. Int Orthop. 2015;39:271–6.
6. Jain NB, Yamaguchi K. The contribution of reverse shoulder arthroplasty to utilization of primary shoulder arthroplasty. J Shoulder Elb Surg. 2014;23:1905–12.
7. Trofa D, Rajaee SS, Smith EL. Nationwide trends in total shoulder arthroplasty and hemiarthroplasty for osteoarthritis. Am J Orthop (Belle Mead NJ). 2014;43:166–72.
8. Hasan SS, Leith JM, Smith KL, Matsen FA 3rd. The distribution of shoulder replacement among surgeons and hospitals is significantly different than that of hip or knee replacement. J Shoulder Elb Surg. 2003;12:164–9.
9. Bansal A, Khatib ON, Zuckerman JD. Revision total joint arthroplasty: the epidemiology of 63,140 cases in New York state. J Arthroplast. 2014;29:23–7.
10. Day JS, Lau E, Ong KL, Williams GR, Ramsey ML, Kurtz SM. Prevalence and projections of total shoulder and elbow arthroplasty in the United States to 2015. J Shoulder Elb Surg. 2010;19:1115–20.
11. Denard PJ, Raiss P, Sowa B, Walch G. Mid- to long-term follow-up of total shoulder arthroplasty using a keeled glenoid in young adults with primary glenohumeral arthritis. J Shoulder Elb Surg. 2013;22:894–900.
12. Walch G, Young AA, Melis B, Gazielly D, Loew M, Boileau P. Results of a convex-back cemented keeled glenoid component in primary osteoarthritis: multicenter study with a follow-up greater than 5 years. J Shoulder Elb Surg. 2011;20:385–94.
13. Lo IK, Litchfield RB, Griffin S, Faber K, Patterson SD, Kirkley A. Quality-of-life outcome following hemiarthroplasty or total shoulder arthroplasty in patients with osteoarthritis. A prospective, randomized trial. J Bone Joint Surg Am. 2005;87:2178–85.
14. Deshmukh AV, Koris M, Zurakowski D, Thornhill TS. Total shoulder arthroplasty: long-term survivorship, functional outcome, and quality of life. J Shoulder Elb Surg. 2005;14:471–9.
15. Torchia ME, Cofield RH, Settergren CR. Total shoulder arthroplasty with the Neer prosthesis: long-term results. J Shoulder Elb Surg. 1997;6:495–505.
16. Hawkins RJ, Bell RH, Jallay B. Total shoulder arthroplasty. Clin Orthop Relat Res. 1989;242:188–94.
17. Carter MJ, Mikuls TR, Nayak S, Fehringer EV, Michaud K. Impact of total shoulder arthroplasty on generic and shoulder-specific health-related quality-of-life measures: a systematic literature review and meta-analysis. J Bone Joint Surg Am. 2012;94:e127.
18. Franta AK, Lenters TR, Mounce D, Neradilek B, Matsen FA 3rd. The complex characteristics of 282 unsatisfactory shoulder arthroplasties. J Shoulder Elb Surg. 2007;16:555–62.
19. Bohsali KI, Bois AJ, Wirth MA. Complications of shoulder arthroplasty. J Bone Joint Surg Am. 2017;99:256–69.
20. Bohsali KI, Wirth MA, Rockwood CA Jr. Complications of total shoulder arthroplasty. J Bone Joint Surg Am. 2006;88:2279–92.
21. Boileau P, Krishnan SG, Tinsi L, Walch G, Coste JS, Mole D. Tuberosity malposition and migration: reasons for poor outcomes after hemiarthroplasty for displaced fractures of the proximal humerus. J Shoulder Elb Surg. 2002;11:401–12.
22. Boileau P. Complications and revision of reverse total shoulder arthroplasty. Orthop Traumatol Surg Res. 2016;102:S33–43.
23. Otto RJ, Virani NA, Levy JC, Nigro PT, Cuff DJ, Frankle MA. Scapular fractures after reverse shoulder arthroplasty: evaluation of risk factors and the reliability of a proposed classification. J Shoulder Elb Surg. 2013;22:1514–21.
24. Gyftopoulos S, Rosenberg ZS, Roberts CC, Bencardino JT, Appel M, Baccei SJ, et al. ACR appropriateness criteria imaging after shoulder arthroplasty. J Am Coll Radiol. 2016;13:1324–36.
25. Wiater BP, Moravek JE Jr, Wiater JM. The evaluation of the failed shoulder arthroplasty. J Shoulder Elb Surg. 2014;23:745–58.
26. Sheridan BD, Ahearn N, Tasker A, Wakeley C, Sarangi P. Shoulder arthroplasty. Part 2: normal and abnormal radiographic findings. Clin Radiol. 2012;67:716–21.
27. Alolabi B, Youderian AR, Napolitano L, Szerlip BW, Evans PJ, Nowinski RJ, et al. Radiographic assessment of prosthetic humeral head size after anatomic shoulder arthroplasty. J Shoulder Elb Surg. 2014;23:1740–6.
28. Ladermann A, Williams MD, Melis B, Hoffmeyer P, Walch G. Objective evaluation of lengthening in reverse shoulder arthroplasty. J Shoulder Elb Surg. 2009;18:588–95.
29. Sofka CM, Adler RS. Original report. Sonographic evaluation of shoulder arthroplasty. AJR Am J Roentgenol. 2003;180:1117–20.

30. Gregory T, Hansen U, Khanna M, Mutchler C, Urien S, Amis AA, et al. A CT scan protocol for the detection of radiographic loosening of the glenoid component after total shoulder arthroplasty. Acta Orthop. 2014;85:91–6.
31. Arican P, Okudan Tekin B, Sefizade R, Naldoken S, Bastug A, Ozkurt B. The role of bone SPECT/CT in the evaluation of painful joint prostheses. Nucl Med Commun. 2015;36:931–40.
32. Mallo GC, Burton L, Coats-Thomas M, Daniels SD, Sinz NJ, Warner JJ. Assessment of painful total shoulder arthroplasty using computed tomography arthrography. J Shoulder Elb Surg. 2015;24:1507–11.
33. Yian EH, Werner CM, Nyffeler RW, Pfirrmann CW, Ramappa A, Sukthankar A, et al. Radiographic and computed tomography analysis of cemented pegged polyethylene glenoid components in total shoulder replacement. J Bone Joint Surg Am. 2005;87:1928–36.
34. Pessis E, Sverzut JM, Campagna R, Guerini H, Feydy A, Drape JL. Reduction of metal artifact with dual-energy CT: virtual monospectral imaging with fast kilovoltage switching and metal artifact reduction software. Semin Musculoskelet Radiol. 2015;19:446–55.
35. Vidil A, Valenti P, Guichoux F, Barthas JH. CT scan evaluation of glenoid component fixation: a prospective study of 27 minimally cemented shoulder arthroplasties. Eur J Orthop Surg Traumatol. 2013;23:521–5.
36. Huang JY, Kerns JR, Nute JL, Liu X, Balter PA, Stingo FC, et al. An evaluation of three commercially available metal artifact reduction methods for CT imaging. Phys Med Biol. 2015;60:1047–67.
37. Shim E, Kang Y, Ahn JM, Lee E, Lee JW, Oh JH, et al. Metal artifact reduction for orthopedic implants (O-MAR): usefulness in CT evaluation of reverse total shoulder arthroplasty. AJR Am J Roentgenol. 2017;209:860–6.
38. Jungmann PM, Agten CA, Pfirrmann CW, Sutter R. Advances in MRI around metal. J Magn Reson Imaging. 2017;46:972–91.
39. Petscavage-Thomas J. Preoperative planning and postoperative imaging in shoulder arthroplasty. Semin Musculoskelet Radiol. 2014;18:448–62.
40. Sperling JW, Potter HG, Craig EV, Flatow E, Warren RF. Magnetic resonance imaging of painful shoulder arthroplasty. J Shoulder Elb Surg. 2002;11:315–21.
41. Aldinger PR, Raiss P, Rickert M, Loew M. Complications in shoulder arthroplasty: an analysis of 485 cases. Int Orthop. 2010;34:517–24.
42. Gonzalez JF, Alami GB, Baque F, Walch G, Boileau P. Complications of unconstrained shoulder prostheses. J Shoulder Elb Surg. 2011;20:666–82.
43. Lynch NM, Cofield RH, Silbert PL, Hermann RC. Neurologic complications after total shoulder arthroplasty. J Shoulder Elb Surg. 1996;5:53–61.
44. Barco R, Savvidou OD, Sperling JW, Sanchez-Sotelo J, Cofield RH. Complications in reverse shoulder arthroplasty. EFORT Open Rev. 2016;1:72–80.
45. Ladermann A, Edwards TB, Walch G. Arm lengthening after reverse shoulder arthroplasty: a review. Int Orthop. 2014;38:991–1000.
46. Ladermann A, Lubbeke A, Melis B, Stern R, Christofilopoulos P, Bacle G, et al. Prevalence of neurologic lesions after total shoulder arthroplasty. J Bone Joint Surg Am. 2011;93:1288–93.
47. Dodson CC, Craig EV, Cordasco FA, Dines DM, Dines JS, Dicarlo E, et al. Propionibacterium acnes infection after shoulder arthroplasty: a diagnostic challenge. J Shoulder Elb Surg. 2010;19:303–7.
48. Shields MV, Abdullah L, Namdari S. The challenge of Propionibacterium acnes and revision shoulder arthroplasty: a review of current diagnostic options. J Shoulder Elb Surg. 2016;25:1034–40.
49. Topolski MS, Chin PY, Sperling JW, Cofield RH. Revision shoulder arthroplasty with positive intraoperative cultures: the value of preoperative studies and intraoperative histology. J Shoulder Elb Surg. 2006;15:402–6.
50. Villacis D, Merriman JA, Yalamanchili R, Omid R, Itamura J, Rick Hatch GF 3rd. Serum interleukin-6 as a marker of periprosthetic shoulder infection. J Bone Joint Surg Am. 2014;96:41–5.
51. Pottinger P, Butler-Wu S, Neradilek MB, Merritt A, Bertelsen A, Jette JL, et al. Prognostic factors for bacterial cultures positive for Propionibacterium acnes and other organisms in a large series of revision shoulder arthroplasties performed for stiffness, pain, or loosening. J Bone Joint Surg Am. 2012;94:2075–83.
52. Grosso MJ, Frangiamore SJ, Ricchetti ET, Bauer TW, Iannotti JP. Sensitivity of frozen section histology for identifying Propionibacterium acnes infections in revision shoulder arthroplasty. J Bone Joint Surg Am. 2014;96:442–7.
53. Chalmers P, Sumner S, Romeo A, Tashjian R. Do elevated inflammatory markers associate with infection in revision shoulder arthroplasty? J Shoulder Elbow Arthroplasty. 2018;2:1–5.
54. Frangiamore SJ, Saleh A, Grosso MJ, Kovac MF, Higuera CA, Iannotti JP, et al. Alpha-Defensin as a predictor of periprosthetic shoulder infection. J Shoulder Elb Surg. 2015;24:1021–7.
55. Frangiamore SJ, Gajewski ND, Saleh A, Farias-Kovac M, Barsoum WK, Higuera CA. Alpha-Defensin accuracy to diagnose Periprosthetic joint infection-best available test? J Arthroplast. 2016;31:456–60.
56. Berbari E, Mabry T, Tsaras G, Spangehl M, Erwin PJ, Murad MH, et al. Inflammatory blood laboratory levels as markers of prosthetic joint infection: a systematic review and meta-analysis. J Bone Joint Surg Am. 2010;92:2102–9.
57. Bravo D, Wagner ER, Larson DR, Davis MP, Pagnano MW, Sierra RJ. No increased risk of knee arthroplasty failure in patients with positive skin patch testing for metal hypersensitivity: a matched cohort study. J Arthroplast. 2016;31:1717–21.

58. Ko JK, Nicholson TA, Hoffler CE, Williams G Jr, Getz C. Metal allergy as a cause of implant failure in shoulder arthroplasty. Orthopedics. 2017;40:e844–8.
59. Teo WZW, Schalock PC. Metal hypersensitivity reactions to orthopedic implants. Dermatol Ther (Heidelb). 2017;7:53–64.
60. Morwood MP, Garrigues GE. Shoulder arthroplasty in the patient with metal hypersensitivity. J Shoulder Elb Surg. 2015;24:1156–64.
61. Ince A, Seemann K, Frommelt L, Katzer A, Loehr JF. One-stage exchange shoulder arthroplasty for peri-prosthetic infection. J Bone Joint Surg Br. 2005;87:814–8.
62. Coste JS, Reig S, Trojani C, Berg M, Walch G, Boileau P. The management of infection in arthroplasty of the shoulder. J Bone Joint Surg Br. 2004;86:65–9.
63. Dilisio MF, Miller LR, Warner JJ, Higgins LD. Arthroscopic tissue culture for the evaluation of periprosthetic shoulder infection. J Bone Joint Surg Am. 2014;96:1952–8.
64. Gee AO, Angeline ME, Dines JS, Dines DM. Shoulder instability after total shoulder arthroplasty: a case of arthroscopic repair. HSS J. 2014;10:88–91.
65. Tashjian RZ, Granger EK, Zhang Y. Utility of prerevision tissue biopsy sample to predict revision shoulder arthroplasty culture results in at-risk patients. J Shoulder Elb Surg. 2017;26:197–203.

Management of the Failed Hemiarthroplasty

9

Manesha Lankachandra and Anand M. Murthi

Hemiarthroplasty has a long and varied history in the treatment of different shoulder pathologies. Neer's first description of shoulder arthroplasty in 1955 involved replacement of the humeral head with a Vitallium implant for seven cases of severe proximal humeral fracture [1]. This unconstrained, monoblock prosthesis offered better pain relief and function when compared to the resection arthroplasty of that time. Over the past 70 years, the indications for shoulder hemiarthroplasty have grown and changed, from comminuted and unreconstructable proximal humerus fractures and their sequelae to osteoarthritis in young, active patients to patterns of nonconcentric glenoid wear in patients who are not candidates for reverse total shoulder arthroplasty.

Despite its increasingly common use, the failure rate of hemiarthroplasty is high, in both arthritis and fracture settings. The most common causes of hemiarthroplasty failure include prosthesis instability, glenoid erosion, rotator cuff dysfunction, and, in the case of fracture, tuberosity malposition and resorption.

Hemiarthroplasty has been used instead of total shoulder arthroplasty in patients with osteoarthritis because of concern over early glenoid loosening, especially in younger and more active patients. Although early results for hemiarthroplasty were promising in this subset of patients, multiple studies have shown unsatisfactory results. Especially as time of follow-up increases, durability and patient satisfaction decrease. Levine et al. [2] reported a series of 28 patients followed for an average of 17 years. Eight of these patients underwent revision, and the overall Neer satisfaction rating was 25% [2]. Sandow et al. compared long-term outcomes of anatomic total shoulder arthroplasty and hemiarthroplasty after a minimum of 10 years and found that none of the patients in the hemiarthroplasty group were pain-free at final follow-up with a revision rate of 31% [3].

The most common cause for revision in hemiarthroplasty patients is painful glenoid arthritis. The radiographic finding of glenoid erosion is routinely found after shoulder hemiarthroplasty. Recently in a review of 118 shoulders, Herschel et al. found some degree of glenoid erosion in all but 13 shoulders [4]. In a review of both total shoulder arthroplasty and hemiarthroplasty in the setting of rheumatoid arthritis, Sperling et al. found glenoid erosion in 58 of 59 shoulders [5]. When this finding manifests as painful glenoid arthritis, it often leads to a deterioration in functional outcome and requires revision surgery [4–6].

Radiographic findings in patients with glenoid erosion show characteristic wear patterns ranging from mild erosion into subchondral bone to medialization of subchondral bone with

M. Lankachandra · A. M. Murthi (✉)
Department of Orthopaedic Surgery, MedStar Union Memorial Hospital, Baltimore, MD, USA

R. Z. Tashjian (ed.), *Complex and Revision Shoulder Arthroplasty*,
https://doi.org/10.1007/978-3-030-02756-8_9

hemispheric deformation up to and beyond the level of the coracoid. The role of factors such as implant positioning is unclear in terms of the degree of erosion and its clinical findings, although it is generally thought that better preoperative bone stock and better glenoid condition are protective [4].

Rotator cuff dysfunction in hemiarthroplasty patients manifests as anterosuperior escape with coracoacromial arch incompetence. Clinically, this is evident as functional decline and progressive loss of active motion. In severe cases, physical exam can show subcutaneous displacement of the prosthesis (Fig. 9.1). A recent series showed rotator cuff insufficiency and instability as a reason for revision in 127 of 157 patients undergoing revision surgery [7]. As with glenoid erosion, it is unclear what factors such as implant positioning have on the natural history of rotator cuff wear in these patients, though overstuffing, increased lateral offset, and large humeral head are certain contributors. In our own experience, we have most commonly revised hemiarthroplasties due to rotator cuff insufficiency and resulting loss of function (Figs. 9.2, 9.3, 9.4 and 9.5). These patients had characteristic proximal migration of their prosthesis on radiographs and physical examination, and both cases showed

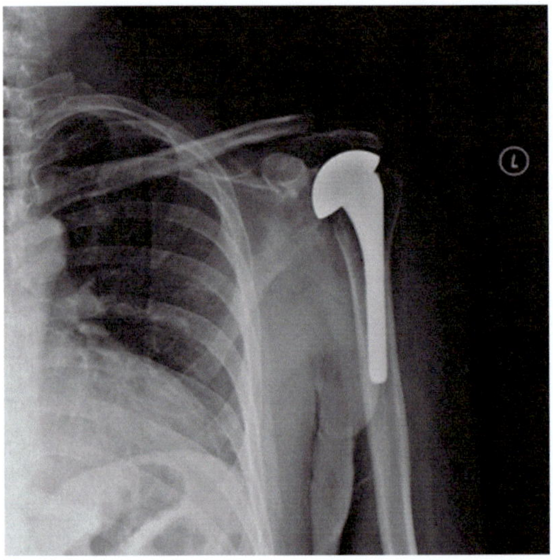

Fig. 9.2 Anteroposterior x-ray of a failed hemiarthroplasty with proximal migration of the implant and clinical rotator cuff insufficiency

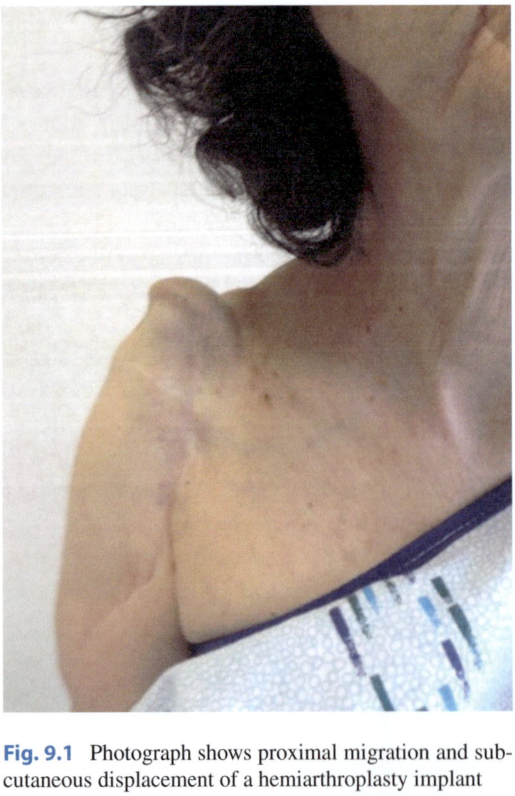

Fig. 9.1 Photograph shows proximal migration and subcutaneous displacement of a hemiarthroplasty implant

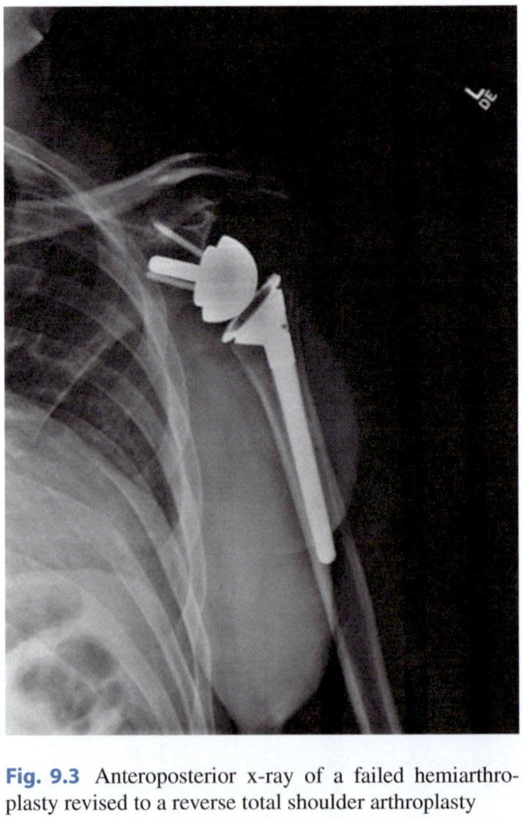

Fig. 9.3 Anteroposterior x-ray of a failed hemiarthroplasty revised to a reverse total shoulder arthroplasty

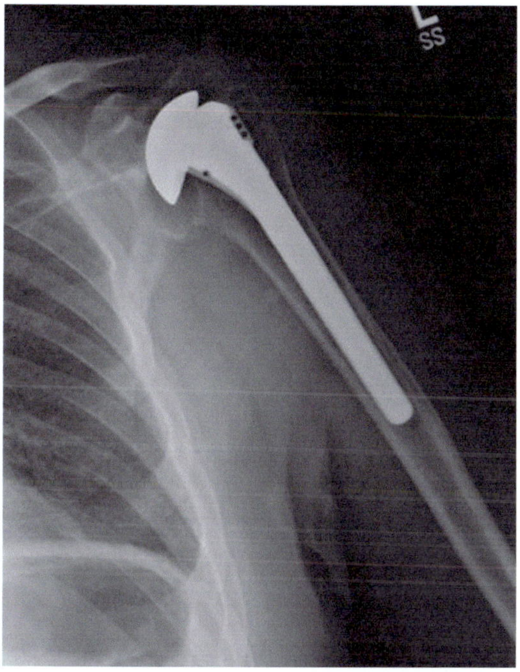

Fig. 9.4 Anteroposterior x-ray of a failed hemiarthroplasty with proximal migration of the implant and clinical rotator cuff insufficiency

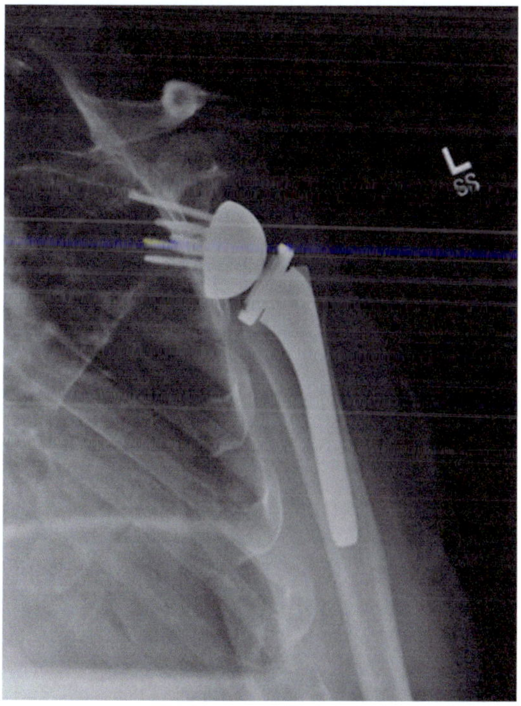

Fig. 9.5 Anteroposterior x-ray of a failed hemiarthroplasty revised to a reverse total shoulder arthroplasty

pseudoparalysis. They were both revised to reverse total shoulder arthroplasty with good results of pain relief and improved function.

In patients who have undergone hemiarthroplasty for fracture, the status of the rotator cuff is closely tied to the position and function of the tuberosities [8]. This can present as both initial tuberosity malposition or tuberosity detachment and subsequent migration and resorption. Tuberosity malposition and loss of fixation are also related to initial implant position and poor bone quality. Prevention is paramount. Careful tuberosity reconstruction with cerclage techniques is useful to prevent these complications.

Multiple studies have shown that tuberosity malposition correlates with an unsatisfactory result, including stiffness, weakness, and persistent pain. In a series of 66 patients, Boileau et al. found that final tuberosity malposition occurred in 33 patients and correlated with an unsatisfactory clinic result [9]. In a study of 167 patients, Kralinger et al. found the only factor significantly influencing the outcome was healing of the tuberosity in an anatomical position. Patients in whom the tuberosity healed with displacement were only slightly better than those in whom it did not heal or resorbed [10].

A tuberosity that remains displaced can lead to decreased range of movement because of bony impingement, causing a mechanical block to motion as well as pain. Nonanatomic stresses on the attached rotator cuff can also cause pain and weakness. Unsurprisingly, revision surgery performed for soft tissue concerns yields worse outcomes than does revision surgery for glenoid erosion [11].

The options for revision implants with a failed hemiarthroplasty are an anatomic total shoulder arthroplasty (TSA), a reverse total shoulder arthroplasty (RSA), and, rarely, another hemiarthroplasty with or without glenoid interposition. This decision depends largely on the status of the rotator cuff. If the cuff is deficient, then anatomic total shoulder arthroplasty is contraindicated. Because the indication for each of these procedures is based on two different clinical scenarios, it is difficult to compare reverse total shoulder arthroplasty and anatomic shoulder arthroplasty in this setting. Other factors that can influence the decision between anatomic and reverse total shoulder arthroplasty include the age of the patient, the pattern of glenoid bone loss (concentric versus eccentric and contained versus uncontained), and the modularity and status of the humeral implant (loose or well fixed).

Studies done prior to the widespread popularity of reverse total shoulder arthroplasty showed generally poor results with revision of failed hemiarthroplasty to anatomic total shoulder arthroplasty. In a series of 16 patients who underwent revision from hemiarthroplasty to anatomic total shoulder arthroplasty, Carroll et al. observed an unsatisfactory result in 7 based on Neer's criteria [12]. Sperling et al. reported unsatisfactory results in 7 of 18 revision patients [13]. The patients in the study by Carroll et al. were mostly treated with hemiarthroplasty initially for osteoarthritis, whereas those in the Sperling et al. study were more often treated with hemiarthroplasty for fracture, but results in both groups of patients were variable and sometimes unpredictable.

As the popularity of reverse total shoulder arthroplasty has increased and its indications have expanded, so too has its use in the revision setting. There is a paucity of data regarding revision of hemiarthroplasty to reverse total shoulder arthroplasty, but most studies show reasonable clinical outcomes with satisfactory pain relief and functional improvement. Levy et al. reported significant improvement in pain and function for 19 patients treated with RSA for failed hemiarthroplasty due to osteoarthritis and cuff deficiency. The complication rate in this series was relatively high, with six shoulders having prosthesis-related complications including failure of the polyethylene and baseplate loosening. The rate of prosthesis complications was significantly higher in patients with severe bone loss of the glenoid and humerus [14]. In another study, Levy et al. showed significant improvement in range of motion and patient satisfaction in patients treated with RSA after failure of hemiarthroplasty for fracture. The complication rate in this group of patients was 28%. Poorer outcomes were again associated with severe proximal humeral bone deficiency [15].

Faced with the question of glenoid erosion, there are multiple options for reconstruction. Many of these are designed for revision in the setting of prior TSA, with glenoid bone loss related to a cemented polyethylene glenoid component. The pattern of bone loss in failed hemiarthroplasty usually reflects wear-related erosion rather than the cavitary bone loss associated with polyethylene wear generally seen with failed TSA. Nonetheless, the medialization seen in both scenarios often requires some type of additional mechanical support beyond that of a standard implant. In the setting of extreme bone loss, most surgeons choose to use an RSA versus an anatomic TSA because the rigid fixation of an RSA baseplate allows improved implant stability. Multiple studies have demonstrated the failures of traditional TSA glenoid fixation in cases of nonconcentric or severe wear [16–18].

The exact indications for glenoid bone grafting or a custom implant are not entirely clear, but in general, if there is less than 50% backside coverage of an RSA baseplate, some type of additional fixation is used. Wagner et al. reported on the use of both structural and nonstructural grafts in patients undergoing revision shoulder arthroplasty. As in other similar studies, they reported moderate levels of improvement. Factors related to failure were varied. Structural versus nonstructural bone graft did not affect outcomes [19].

Another option for treatment of large glenoid defects is the use of patient-specific implants that have been designed to fill glenoid defects. This "vault reconstruction system" involves making a preoperative plan based on a patient's three-dimensional CT scan with a customized implant and instrumentation. Our experience with this type of implant has been largely with failed TSA and the resulting cavitary bone loss, but it is described in cases of failed hemiarthroplasty as well. The benefits of this system are that there is no need for structural or nonstructural bone graft and the implant is designed to rigidly fixate to whatever bony support is left in the native glenoid. This system relies heavily on the accuracy of the preoperative CT scan [20].

Indications for component removal can include loosening, malposition or mechanical failure and instability, or infection. Hemiarthroplasty prostheses are often cemented, and the presence of any of these complications can necessitate the removal of the humeral component and cement mantel. If it's not possible to remove the prosthesis through the prior proximal humeral osteotomy, both humeral windows and longitudinal splits have been described to gain access to and release the implant [21–23].

If the humeral component is well fixed and in acceptable position, it is sometimes possible to keep the previous humeral implant and take advantage of modular systems that allow for conversion from a hemiarthroplasty or anatomic total shoulder arthroplasty to reverse total shoulder design. Wieser et al. found that patients who did not have to undergo stem exchange had less operative time and less blood loss as well as fewer intraoperative complications than those who did have to undergo stem removal [24]. This is logical, but it also underlies the importance of being prepared for and adapting to, within reason, whatever implant was initially used. Data regarding the functional outcomes of patients who undergo modular conversion of hemiarthroplasty to total or reverse total shoulder arthroplasty is limited, but overall function appears improved [25].

Authors' Preferred Algorithm

In these situations the authors prefer to maximize bone preservation and understand that revision surgery is usually dependent on the status of the rotator cuff and its functional use after surgery. If the shoulder is cuff or tuberosity deficient, then conversion to reverse shoulder replacement is necessary. If the patient is healthy and relatively young with an intact rotator cuff and arthritic glenoid, then conversion from hemiarthroplasty to total shoulder replacement is warranted. However, intraoperative factors are also important, such as the quality of the subscapularis tendon, which will require a second detachment and secure repair. Also, the quality and quantity of glenoid bone are important and are crucial to revision surgery. A stable polyethylene glenoid with good fixation is paramount to success. The authors will always consent these patients for both conversion to total shoulder and reverse shoulder replacement in cases where stable glenoid fixation and subscapularis repair are not possible. The use of platform humeral stems for conversion to reverse shoulder replacement is purely an intraoperative decision as the stem positioning, especially height, may make it difficult if not impossible to implant the glenoid baseplate/sphere. Therefore, the removal of the entire hemiarthroplasty stem is often performed with revision humeral neck cut and possibly a humeral osteotomy as well. Furthermore, glenoid bone grafting may be necessary either bulk allograft (utilizing femoral head allograft) or demineralized bone matrix and cancellous chips for contained cavitary defects. On the humeral side, cortical strut grafts (medial and/or lateral) may be applied to support weakened humeral shaft bone after revision humeral replacement with shaft bone loss.

Conclusions

Revision of the failed hemiarthroplasty is a complex multifactorial problem in shoulder surgery. The correct diagnosis for failure must be made, and then proper history, physical examination, and imaging studies must be done. Revision surgery must be carefully planned with all support instrumentation and prostheses available to enable the surgeon to obtain a good functional outcome.

References

1. Neer CS. Articular replacement for the humeral head. J Bone Joint Surg Am. 1955;37-A:215–28.
2. Levine WN, Fischer CR, Nguyen D, Flatow EL, Ahmad CS, Bigliani LU. Long-term follow-up of shoulder hemiarthroplasty for glenohumeral osteoarthritis. J Bone Joint Surg Am. 2012;94:e164.
3. Sandow MJ, David H, Bentall SJ. Hemiarthroplasty vs total shoulder replacement for rotator cuff intact osteoarthritis: how do they fare after a decade? J Shoulder Elb Surg. 2013;22:877–85.
4. Herschel R, Wieser K, Morrey ME, Ramos CH, Gerber C, Meyer DC. Risk factors for glenoid erosion in patients with shoulder hemiarthroplasty: an analysis of 118 cases. J Shoulder Elb Surg. 2017;26:246–52.

5. Sperling JW, Cofield RH, Schleck CD, Harmsen WS. Total shoulder arthroplasty versus hemiarthroplasty for rheumatoid arthritis of the shoulder: results of 303 consecutive cases. J Shoulder Elb Surg. 2007;16:683–90.
6. Rispoli DM, Sperling JW, Athwal GS, Schleck CD, Cofield RH. Humeral head replacement for the treatment of osteoarthritis. J Bone Joint Surg Am. 2006;88:2637–44.
7. Merolla G, Wagner E, Sperling JW, Paladini P, Fabbri E, Porcellini G. Revision of failed shoulder hemiarthroplasty to reverse total arthroplasty: analysis of 157 revision implants. J Shoulder Elb Surg. 2018;27:75–81.
8. Hashiguchi H, Iwashita S, Ohkubo A, Takai S. The outcome of hemiarthroplasty for proximal humeral fractures is dependent on the status of the rotator cuff. Int Orthop. 2015;39:1115–9.
9. Boileau P, Krishnan SG, Tinsi L, Walch G, Coste JS, Mole D. Tuberosity malposition and migration: reasons for poor outcomes after hemiarthroplasty for displaced fractures of the proximal humerus. J Shoulder Elb Surg. 2002;11:401–12.
10. Kralinger F, Schwaiger R, Wambacher M, Farrell E, Menth-Chiari W, Lajtai G, et al. Outcome after primary hemiarthroplasty for fracture of the head of the humerus. A retrospective multicentre study of 167 patients. J Bone Joint Surg Br. 2004;86:217–9.
11. Sajadi KR, Kwon YW, Zuckerman JD. Revision shoulder arthroplasty: an analysis of indications and outcomes. J Shoulder Elb Surg. 2010;19:308–13.
12. Carroll RM, Izquierdo R, Vazquez M, Blaine TA, Levine WN, Bigliani LU. Conversion of painful hemiarthroplasty to total shoulder arthroplasty: long-term results. J Shoulder Elb Surg. 2004;13:599–603.
13. Sperling JW, Cofield RH. Revision total shoulder arthroplasty for the treatment of glenoid arthrosis. J Bone Joint Surg Am. 1998;80:860–7.
14. Levy JC, Virani N, Pupello D, Frankle M. Use of the reverse shoulder prosthesis for the treatment of failed hemiarthroplasty in patients with glenohumeral arthritis and rotator cuff deficiency. J Bone Joint Surg Br. 2007;89:189–95.
15. Levy J, Frankle M, Mighell M, Pupello D. The use of the reverse shoulder prosthesis for the treatment of failed hemiarthroplasty for proximal humeral fracture. J Bone Joint Surg Am. 2007;89:292–300.
16. Allen B, Schoch B, Sperling JW, Cofield RH. Shoulder arthroplasty for osteoarthritis secondary to glenoid dysplasia: an update. J Shoulder Elb Surg. 2014;23:214–20.
17. Farron A, Terrier A, Buchler P. Risks of loosening of a prosthetic glenoid implanted in retroversion. J Shoulder Elb Surg. 2006;15:521–6.
18. Iannotti JP, Norris TR. Influence of preoperative factors on outcome of shoulder arthroplasty for glenohumeral osteoarthritis. J Bone Joint Surg Am. 2003;85-A:251–8.
19. Wagner E, Houdek MT, Griffith T, Elhassan BT, Sanchez-Sotelo J, Sperling JW, et al. Glenoid bone-grafting in revision to a reverse total shoulder arthroplasty. J Bone Joint Surg Am. 2015;97:1653–60.
20. Dines DM, Gulotta L, Craig EV, Dines JS. Novel solution for massive glenoid defects in shoulder arthroplasty: a patient-specific glenoid vault reconstruction system. Am J Orthop (Belle Mead NJ). 2017;46:104–8.
21. Johnston PS, Creighton RA, Romeo AA. Humeral component revision arthroplasty: outcomes of a split osteotomy technique. J Shoulder Elb Surg. 2012;21:502–6.
22. Sahota S, Sperling JW, Cofield RH. Humeral windows and longitudinal splits for component removal in revision shoulder arthroplasty. J Shoulder Elb Surg. 2014;23:1485–91.
23. Wright TW, Glowczewskie F, Wheeler D, Miller G, Cowin D. Excursion and strain of the median nerve. J Bone Joint Surg Am. 1996;78:1897–903.
24. Wieser K, Borbas P, Ek ET, Meyer DC, Gerber C. Conversion of stemmed hemi- or total to reverse total shoulder arthroplasty: advantages of a modular stem design. Clin Orthop Relat Res. 2015;473:651–60.
25. Williams PN, Trehan SK, Tsouris N, Dines JS, Dines DM, Craig EV, et al. Functional outcomes of modular conversion of hemiarthroplasty or total to reverse total shoulder arthroplasty. HSS J. 2017;13:102–7.

Management of the Failed Anatomic Total Shoulder Arthroplasty

10

John Wu, Catherine M. Rapp, Edward J. Shields, and J. Michael Wiater

Introduction

Total shoulder arthroplasty is now the third most commonly performed joint replacement surgery in the United States, behind the hip and knee [1]. Over the past 20 years, there has been a rapid and exponential increase in the number of total shoulder replacements performed. During the 1990s, annual total shoulder arthroplasty rates were less than 10,000 per year; however, in 2011, roughly 67,000 shoulder arthroplasties were performed [1, 2]. The most common indication for an anatomic total shoulder arthroplasty (aTSA) is osteoarthritis of the glenohumeral joint, with an intact rotator cuff and adequate glenoid bone stock [3].

As the prevalence of aTSA continues to increase, a wide spectrum of potential failure mechanisms can be expected to occur. Knowing the common modes of aTSA failure, how they are diagnosed, and how to manage the different failure mechanisms is important not only in managing these complex cases but also preventing them from occurring. This chapter will review the most common mechanisms of aTSA failure, discuss the various diagnostic tools, and review the literature for evidence regarding the best method for revision surgery. Recommendations for treatment including a decision algorithm will be reviewed (Fig. 10.1).

Mechanisms for Failure

Bohsali et al. have twice performed a systematic review of the literature regarding aTSA complications. Their first review covered publications from 1996 to 2005 and included over 30 studies with more than 2500 patients [5]; their second review of the literature is from 2006 to 2015 and included another 30 studies and over 3300 patients [6]. While the overall rates of complications appear to be declining, component failure, specifically of the glenoid, continues to be a significant problem affecting implant longevity.

Component Failure

The most common mechanism of failure after aTSA is component loosening and wear and fracture [5–7]. Prosthetic loosening accounts for roughly 39% of all complications, affecting 4–6.3% of all shoulders [5, 6]. The mode and cause of component failure is important to understand as these factors will ultimately affect treatment decisions.

Glenoid Component Failure

The glenoid is the most common site of failure (Fig. 10.2) [5, 6]. Glenoid component loosening

J. Wu · C. M. Rapp · E. J. Shields
J. Michael Wiater (✉)
Department of Orthopaedic Surgery, Beaumont Health System, Royal Oak, MI, USA
e-mail: J.Michael.Wiater@beaumont.org

R. Z. Tashjian (ed.), *Complex and Revision Shoulder Arthroplasty*,
https://doi.org/10.1007/978-3-030-02756-8_10

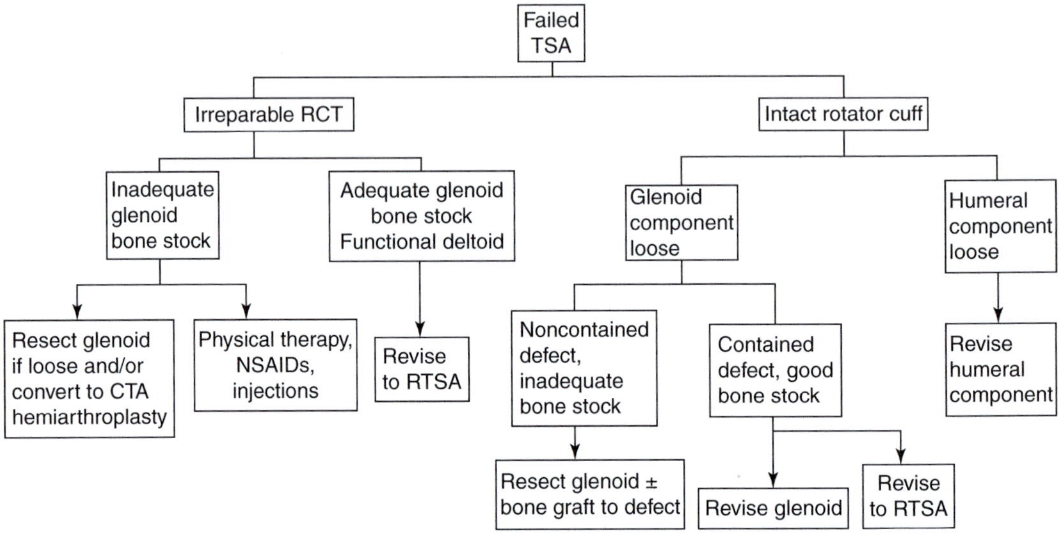

Fig. 10.1 Treatment algorithm for management of the failed anatomic total shoulder arthroplasty without infection or fracture. (Revised and reused with permission from *JAAOS* [4])

was found to account for 32–37.7% of all complications, with 3.9–5.3% of all patients experiencing some degree of loosening [5, 6]. Individual studies have reported glenoid loosening rates as low as 1.1% [8] up to 14% [9]. It is important to note that glenoid loosening may be asymptomatic, not requiring further treatment but only observation. In a systematic review of glenoid failure in aTSA, Papadonikolakis et al. found that the annualized rate of asymptomatic loosening was 7.3%, while symptomatic loosening was lower at only 1.2% and revision even lower at 0.8% [7]. They did not find a correlation between asymptomatic loosening and revision ($r = 0.03$), although symptomatic loosening was correlated with revision ($r = 0.77$) [7]. Thus, asymptomatic loosening may be carefully followed without the need for further workup or treatment. The variability in the literature may be partially explained by a number of design factors that have been linked with glenoid component survival.

There have been numerous reports of inferior outcomes of metal-backed and metal ingrowth glenoids compared to all-polyethylene components due to increased loosening and implant fractures (Fig. 10.3) [10–14]. Rates of loosening of metal-backed components have been reported as 5–42% [10–15]. Fractures of metal-backed implants have been reported to occur in 9.4–21% of cases [11–13]. In addition, biomechanical testing has also favored cemented all-polyethylene components over metal-backed for initial fixation strength and micromotion [16]. Consequently, early designs of true metal-backed glenoids have largely been abandoned [10, 11]. However, the success of ingrowth components in total hip arthroplasty as well as on the humeral side of the shoulder makes the addition of an ingrowth component to the glenoid alluring. Thus, newer designs combining a central ingrowth peg with peripherally cemented pegs attempt to combine the best of both worlds (Comprehensive Total Shoulder System, Zimmer Biomet, Warsaw, IN). Long-term data regarding the success or failure of this implant is currently unavailable.

Another design component that may play a role in longevity is radial mismatch or conformity between the glenoid and humeral head. Decreasing radial mismatch or increasing conformity limits contact stresses at the humeral interface, decreasing glenoid polyethylene wear and improving joint stability; it also decreases the ability for humeral head translation leading to increased contact stresses at the bone-implant interface and the potential for component loosen-

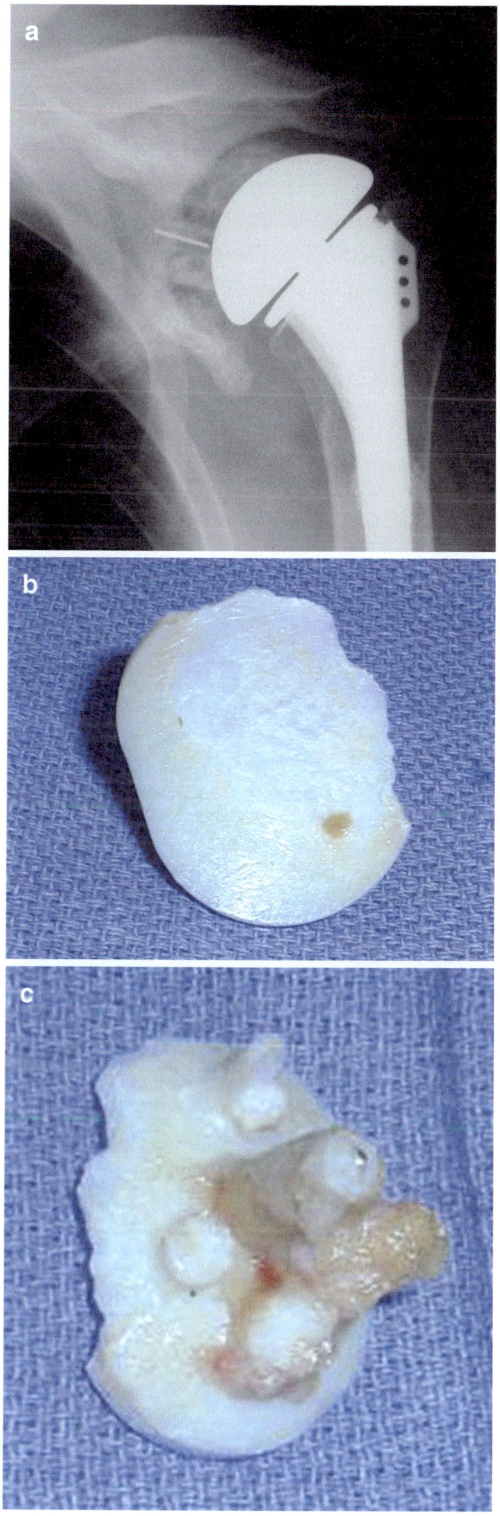

Fig. 10.2 Failed all-polyethylene glenoid. AP radiograph (**a**) demonstrating a loose glenoid component. Glenoid component showing posterior superior wear after removal including articulating surface (**b**) and backside (**c**)

ing [17, 18]. Thus, some radial mismatch, with a glenoid radius of curvature greater than that of the humeral head, may be desirable to balance the risks of wear and instability to the risk of loosening. In a multicenter case series review of 1542 aTSAs using all-polyethylene, cemented, flat-backed glenoids (Tornier Aequalis) followed for 24–110 months, Walch et al. found that glenohumeral radial mismatch between 5.5 and 10 mm resulted in the least amount of radiolucent changes and mismatch of 4.5–7 mm was associated with better active external rotation of the arm at the side [17]. However, a biomechanical study of a cementless, metal-backed, round, posterior-curved, central screw glenoid implant (Multiplex; ESKA, Lübeck, Germany) by Suárez et al. found that increasing mismatch from 0 mm to 6 mm led to significantly increased micromotion at the bone-implant interface. The authors contributed this finding to increased humeral head translation resulting in the rocking-horse phenomenon [18]. While some relative micromotion between the bone and the component of less than 150 μm allows for bone ingrowth in a cementless design, too much is detrimental and may be one reason for early component failure in metal-backed designs [18, 19]. Additional research is needed to understand the optimal radial mismatch for aTSA which will likely affect the method of glenoid fixation.

Currently used cemented glenoids are designed with a keel or a peg on the backside for fixation into the glenoid. This is another area of design debate. Early results suggested that keeled designs were at a higher risk for developing radiolucency and ultimate failure. However, more recent data has shown that mid- to long-term results are equivalent for radiolucencies surrounding the implant and the need for revision [20, 21].

The degree of glenoid component retroversion at implantation may also play a role in long-term survivorship with most authors recommending techniques that restore glenoid version under 10 degrees of retroversion. However, data supporting such a recommendation is unclear. A biomechanical model demonstrated greater than 10° of retroversion dramatically increased eccentric load on the posterior implant [22].

Clinically, a 2013 study examined 66 aTSAs from 2 to 7 years postoperatively and correlated over 15° of component retroversion with a significant increase in osteolysis around the center peg of a press fit, bone ingrowth design, although this was not related to worse patient outcomes or an increased rate of reoperation [23]. Conversely presented in 2017, researchers using the same glenoid at a different facility compared 21 aTSA glenoids implanted with 15° or greater of retroversion to 50 implanted in less than 15° between 18 and 36 months postoperatively and found no significant difference between groups regarding osteolysis, outcomes, or reoperation [24].

Humeral Component Failure

The humeral component in aTSA loosens infrequently. According to Bohsali et al., the rate of humeral loosening is decreasing from roughly 6.5% of all complications or 1% of all aTSAs in the decade preceding 2005 down to 1.5% or 0.1%, respectively, in the decade up to 2015 [5, 6]. There is limited evidence from a small ($n = 40$

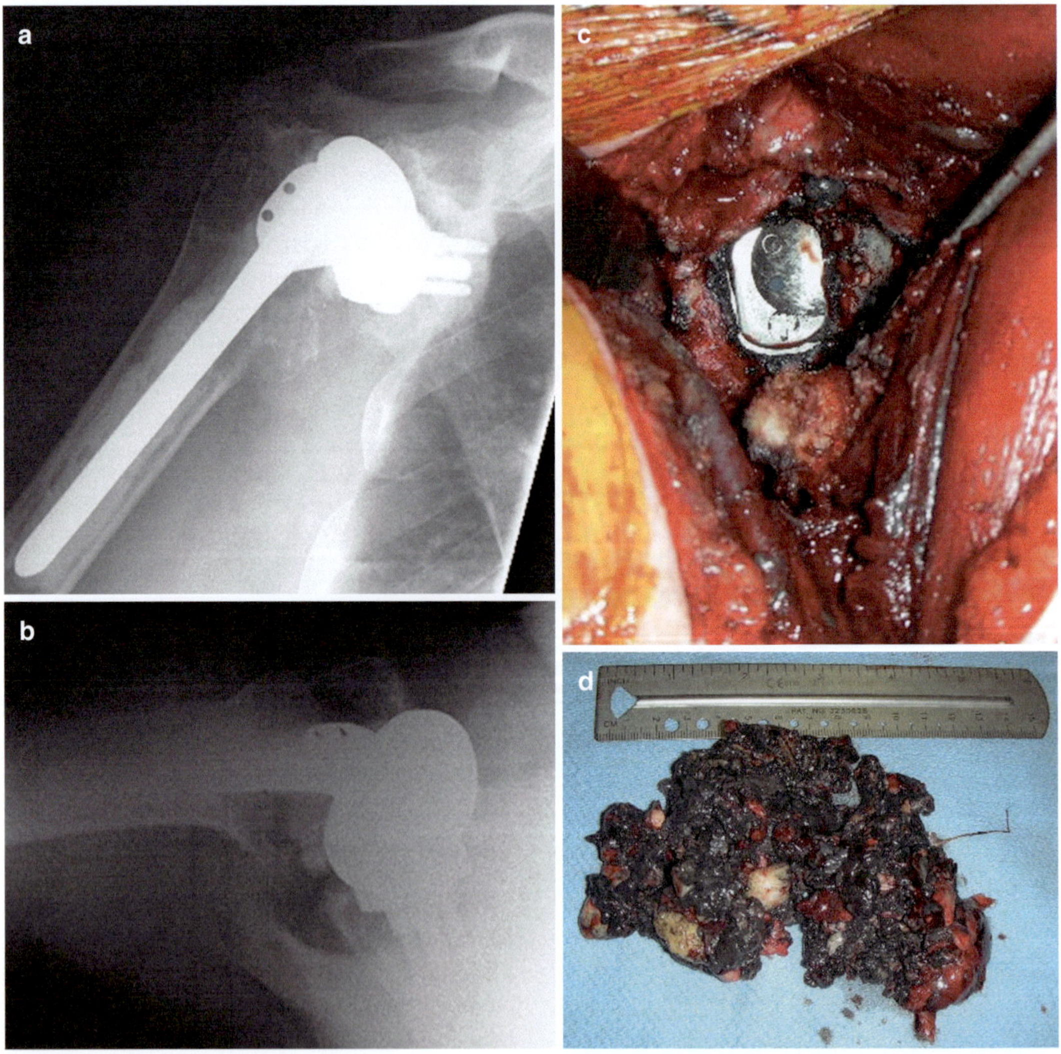

Fig. 10.3 Failed metal-backed glenoid. AP (**a**) and lateral (**b**) radiographs demonstrating a failed glenoid component. Intraoperative photo demonstrating metal debris in situ (**c**) and after debridement (**d**). Glenoid component showing anterior superior wear after removal including articulating surface (**e**) and backside (**f**)

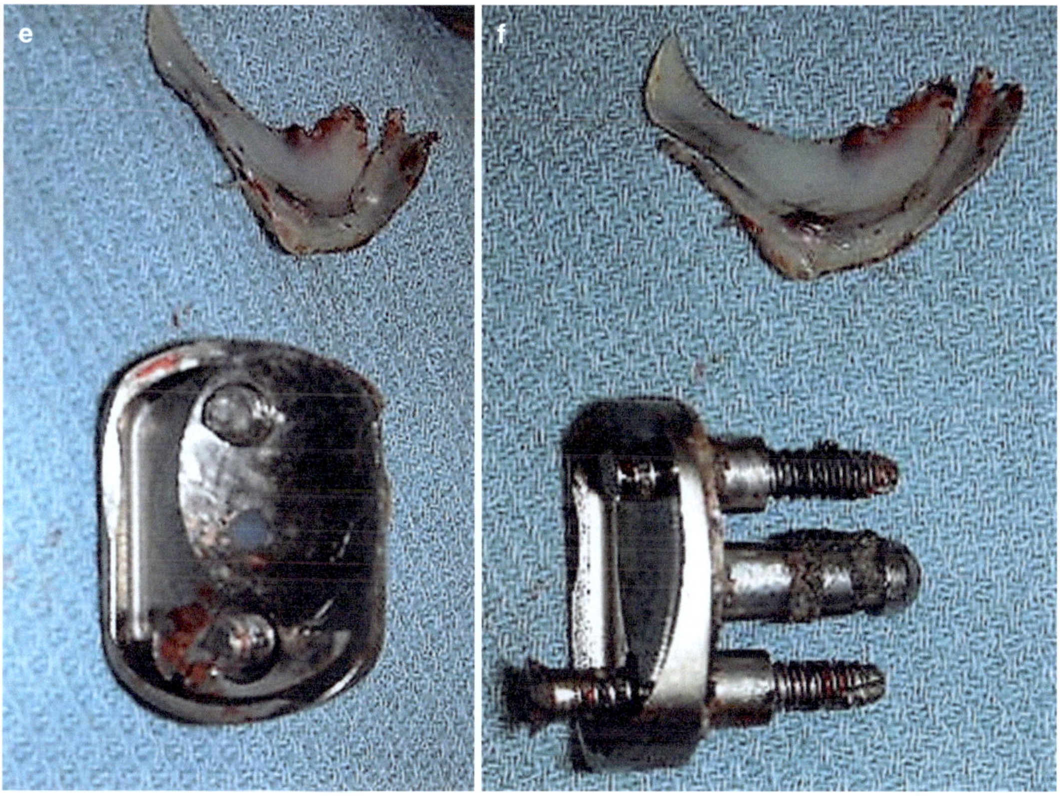

Fig.10. 3 (continued)

aTSAs) level IV study suggesting cemented humeral stems may loosen less frequently than press fit [25]. If loosening occurs, the underlying etiology is an important factor to be addressed during treatment. Causes include glenoid polyethylene wear leading to osteolysis, infection, and fracture [6]. Infection should be ruled out prior to consideration of other etiologies. Improper component positioning or failure to restore anatomic humeral anatomy may be the major source of humeral component failure.

Soft Tissue Dysfunction

Capsular integrity and a competent rotator cuff are critical to the success of aTSA; therefore, soft tissue dysfunction is the second most common cause of aTSA failure [5, 6]. Instability was identified by Bohsali et al. as the second most common aTSA complication, after component failure, albeit with a decreasing incidence from 30% of all complications or 4.9% of all aTSAs down to 10.1% and 1.0% from 1996 to 2015 [5, 6]. Tearing of the rotator cuff has a more stable prevalence, accounting for roughly 7.7–9% of complications (0.9–1.3% of all aTSAs) [5, 6].

The subscapularis tendon is particularly at risk as it is usually taken down to gain access to the joint to perform the procedure and subsequently repaired. Rates of subscapularis failure after aTSA range from 1% to 6% [8, 26] attributing to over half of all rotator cuff dysfunction [5]. Failure of the repair or general subscapularis dysfunction can have devastating consequences to the aTSA patient including anterior instability, pain, internal rotation weakness, and overall poor shoulder function. Such complications have been associated with lengthening procedures of the tendon, an oversized humeral component, poor tissue quality, and early, excessive postoperative external rotation or resisted internal rotation [6, 26].

The superior rotator cuff musculature, including the supraspinatus and infraspinatus, is also at risk of tearing after aTSA. This may be due to poor tissue quality or continued degeneration, muscular atrophy, superior glenoid tilt, or an oversized humeral head [6]. Tearing of the tendons can lead to superior migration of the humeral head, loss of motion and strength for overhead activities, pain, and poor function.

Posterior capsular insufficiency can result in pain and posterior instability. This is associated with significant glenoid retroversion, which results in stretching of the posterior capsule as the humeral head rests in a subluxated position [27]. Correcting the glenoid retroversion and balancing of the soft tissue tension, such as using posterior capsulorrhaphy, at the index procedure can help decrease this risk [28, 29].

Fractures

The third most common cause for aTSA failure is fracture. Periprosthetic fractures have also shown a declining incidence from 11% to 6.7% of all complications, now affecting 0.69% of all aTSA patients down from 1.8% [5, 6]. Higher Charlson comorbidity index scores and female sex have been associated with higher risk for periprosthetic fractures [30]. Fracture is often associated with loosening of the stem, and stem loosening is associated with infection. Therefore periprosthetic fractures should be considered for an infection workup prior to revision.

Infection

Infection is a devastating complication after aTSA. The rate of infection has been reported to range from 0.7% to 2.3% [5, 8, 9, 15, 31–33]. Bohsali et al.'s reviews found that rate of infection has remained stable at 4.6–4.9% of all complications or 0.51–0.7% of all aTSAs [5, 6]. A National Inpatient Sample report by Padegimas et al. found a similar incidence of 0.98% [33]. Infections significantly increase the financial burden for hospital systems and payors [33]. The risk of infection is increased with nutritional deficits, male sex, drug abuse, blood transfusion, and increasing body mass index [33, 34].

Miscellaneous

Other reasons for failed aTSA are much less common. Poor range of motion can result from arthrofibrosis or excessive heterotopic ossification (HO). Studies looking at HO after aTSA have reported rates of 15–45% [35, 36]. Although seen on imaging with some frequency, HO rarely affects the glenohumeral joint or results in functional deficits [36, 37]. Another source of failure is nerve injury. This may manifest in the form of complex regional pain syndrome, pain of unknown origin, or muscle weakness with atrophy including deltoid dysfunction. Nerve injury may affect 0.63–0.8% of all shoulders undergoing aTSA [5, 6].

Treatment Options and Outcomes for the Failed Anatomic Total Shoulder

Treatment of a failed aTSA is dependent on the mode of failure. As previously discussed, failure can be a result of rotator cuff insufficiency, component malpositioning, fracture, infection, and soft tissue dysfunction, all of which can result in pain, instability, and loosening. Therefore, revision surgery, if indicated, must take into account the underlying pathology in order to optimize outcomes.

Treatment for Component Failure

The glenoid component is the most common site of failure. Indications for revision surgery include pain or mechanical symptoms of the shoulder due to glenohumeral joint instability or a loose glenoid component with subsidence and/or tilting. While intrinsic factors such as radial mismatch between the glenoid and humeral component and normal wear resulting in osteolysis can contribute to loosening, other causes such as rotator cuff insufficiency and infection should be investigated prior to revision surgery [38, 39]. Rotator cuff insufficiency, joint instability, and infection can be the primary cause or occur in conjunction with glenoid loosening. Addressing not just the primary cause but the associated pathologies is of utmost importance in gaining a satisfactory outcome.

Glenoid Reimplantation Versus Hemiarthroplasty (Bone Grafting and Glenoid Removal)

A failed glenoid may require surgical removal with revision to another aTSA (glenoid reimplantation), conversion to a hemiarthroplasty, or conversion to a reverse total shoulder arthroplasty (rTSA). Reimplantation with a new glenoid is a good option provided that there is adequate bone stock of the glenoid vault. This can be completed as a single- or two-stage revision with or without bone grafting. Conversion to a hemiarthroplasty can likewise be done with or without bone grafting. Revision to rTSA will be discussed in a later section of this chapter.

Regardless of the chosen revision option, first the failed glenoid must be removed. In the setting of a loose glenoid, this is typically quite simple to perform. Any broken pieces should be removed, and a synovectomy to remove wear particles is frequently necessary. Should revision surgery be undertaken for glenoid malpositioning or polyethylene wear in the setting of good glenoid fixation, removal may be more intensive. It is helpful to know the manufacturer of the implanted system, as many have developed specialized tools to simplify component removal. For an all-polyethylene glenoid (Fig. 10.4), removal begins by cutting the implant into quadrants with a straight, sharp osteotome. Each quadrant can then be disassociated from the bony glenoid with the use of a curved osteotome between the bone and the cement or between the cement and the glenoid. This will leave the pegs or keel from the glenoid as well as cement remaining in the bone. For a trabecular metal ingrowth component, a similar strategy is typically successful. For a true metal-backed glenoid, start with screw removal followed by the use of a small, curved or flexible osteotome between the implant and bone in a progressive fashion. Confirm that you have appropriate screw drivers available as these are usually flat-headed screws to lie behind the poly. Depending on the revision planned, it is only necessary to remove as much or as little of the remaining implant and cement as is necessary for fixation of the new implant. Care should be taken to preserve as much bone stock as possible. It is often possible to drill, burr, or ream through the remaining polyethylene, cement, or trabecular metal only where it is impeding placement of a new component. Care should be taken to collect any debris when using this technique. This can be done by placing lap sponges or a viscous substance, such as sterile ultrasound gel, to protect the peripheral tissues and collect the debris. Sponges can then be removed, while gel can be suctioned. Should conversion to a hemiarthroplasty be done, it may be necessary to perform a more thorough cement removal to prevent its articulation with a metal humeral head and subsequent metal wear. If there is concern for infection, all foreign bodies should be removed which typically requires the use of small curettes and osteotomes (e.g., ¼″) to dislodge cement and remaining polyethylene components from the glenoid. This may lead to significantly greater bone loss.

After implant removal and debridement, there are several reconstructive techniques available to restore anatomic version and offset to allow for appropriate tensioning of the rotator cuff muscles and improve function and stability in the aTSA. Eccentric reaming can help restore anatomic version of the glenoid if correction of only 10–15° is required [40]. Further correction could narrow and compromise the glenoid vault and subsequent glenoid screw or peg fixation while also decreasing offset by further medializing the joint line [41]. While correction of glenoid version to neutral has been advocated as the appro-

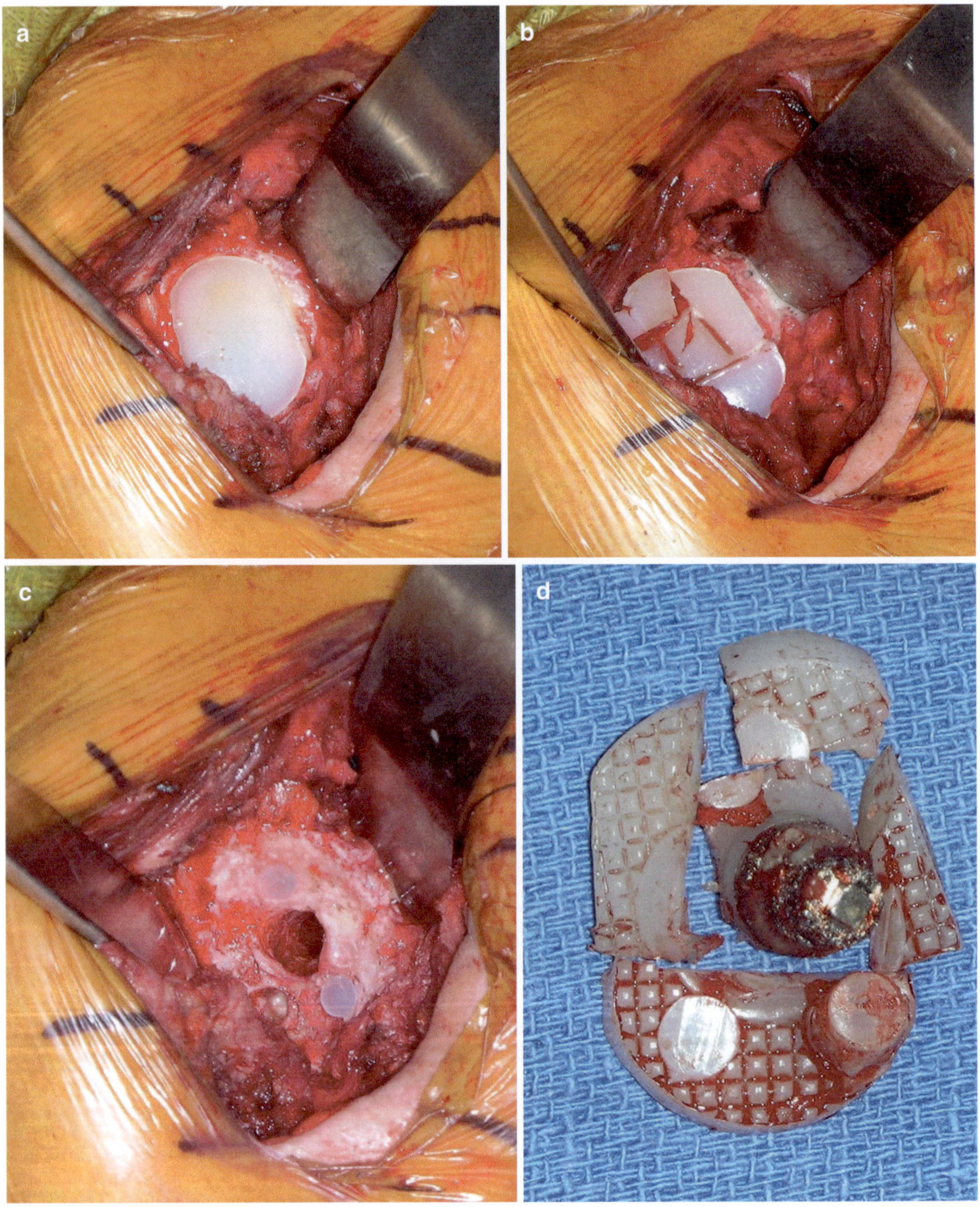

Fig. 10.4 Removal of a well-fixed all-polyethylene glenoid including glenoid exposure (**a**) and in vivo breakdown (**b**). After glenoid removal, if polyethylene pegs are well fixed, they may be left in place (**c**) and drilled through for fixation of a new reverse glenoid baseplate as was done in this case. The glenoid component is thus removed in parts (**d**)

priate technique, more recent literature suggests that retroversion may not be as detrimental as previously thought [24]. Regardless, in the setting of revision surgery, where bone loss is often encountered and the glenoid has already been reamed during the primary procedure, an attempt to neutralize version via reaming alone may further complicate matters. Loss of support from violation of the subchondral plate may lead to instability of the glenoid component and ultimate failure [5]. Therefore, care must be taken to preserve as much bone stock as possible. Bone graft, cancellous or corticocancellous, can be used to fill bony defects and provide structural support for the new glenoid. Alternatively, posterior augments can also be used to compensate for bone loss and help restore anatomic version and offset with minimal reaming [42]. When indicated, eccentric reaming may be preferable over a posteriorly augmented glenoid because of the possibility of accelerated implant loosening when comparing angled augmented glenoid implants to a neutral version glenoid component [43]. The new glenoid is often cemented and should use third-generation cementation techniques [44]. A previous pegged glenoid can be replaced with a new pegged or keeled implant depending on the condition of the peg holes, while a failed keeled component is revised to another keeled glenoid [41]. It is desirable to have at least 50–60% of the new glenoid supported by native glenoid [45].

Hemiarthroplasty with bone graft is an option if the glenoid has significant bone loss [46, 47]. It can be the definitive treatment for an appropriately selected patient or serve as the first stage in a two-stage reimplantation. If the cortical walls of the glenoid vault are relatively intact, allograft cancellous chips can be used to fill any void [46]. Alternatively, an autogenous iliac crest bone graft or femoral head structural allograft can be used to augment the glenoid and prevent medialization of the joint line by positioning the cortical surface laterally to provide structural support [46, 47]. The graft can be impacted with cancellous bone packed behind and around the graft or secured with cortical screws. Care should be taken to position and direct the screws away from the lateral surface to prevent metal-on-metal wear in the setting of conversion to hemiarthroplasty and to allow adequate space for glenoid reimplantation if planned. Complications include failure of graft incorporation, graft resorption, and subsidence. Subsidence was observed to be more severe with structural graft versus cancellous graft which may be a result of the stiffer structural graft in combination with a lack of cortical rim and underlying bony support from the native glenoid [46]. Complete loss of the glenoid vault down to or beyond the scapular confluence (intersection of the coracoid, spine, and body) may preclude the ability to bone graft and require conversion to a hemiarthroplasty.

Hemiarthroplasty without bone grafting should be reserved as a salvage option when addressing a failed glenoid that cannot be reconstructed [41]. During this procedure the glenoid can be reamed (ream and run technique) to a slightly larger radius of curvature than the humeral head implant to allow a more congruent joint surface. However, in cases of significant bone loss, this may be difficult if not impossible to perform and result only in further medialization of the joint line. In these instances, only glenoid removal may be possible.

Outcomes for Glenoid Reimplantation Versus Hemiarthroplasty with Bone Grafting

Glenoid loosening treated with either reimplantation of a new glenoid component or glenoid removal and bone grafting without glenoid reimplantation was previously investigated by Cheung et al. (2008) [48]. There was significant improvement in pain for both groups. Pain improvement occurred in 73% of the new glenoid group ($N = 33$) versus 54% in the bone grafting group ($N = 35$). This difference did not reach significance ($p = 0.65$). Average follow-up was 3.8 years for the new glenoid group and 6.2 years in the bone grafting group. There was also no significant difference in range of motion when comparing preoperative to postoperative exam except for forward elevation in the group treated with a new glenoid ($p = 0.0387$). The rate of survival-free reoperation at 5 years was 91% in the new glenoid group versus 78% in the bone grafting, which was not found to be significant ($p = 0.3$). Interestingly, 20 shoulders had a late positive culture, with *Propionibacterium acnes* being the most common organism isolated. The authors concluded that revision surgery for a loose glenoid component using reimplantation or bone grafting can often provide pain relief and patient satisfaction. Deutsch et al. found that reimplantation of a new glenoid resulted in statistically significant pain relief and increased external rotation compared to conversion to hemiarthroplasty [45]. These authors noted that rotator cuff integrity and glenohumeral joint stability were important components to improve outcomes in terms of motion, function, and pain [45].

Aibinder et al. reported outcomes for glenoid loosening revision surgery comparing the same techniques (reimplantation of a new glenoid component ($N = 20$) versus glenoid removal and bone grafting without glenoid reimplantation ($N = 11$)) with a mean follow-up of 8.3 years [49]. The rate of survival-free reoperation at 10 years was 79% in the new glenoid group versus 84% in the bone grafting group, which was not found to be significant ($p = 0.5$). There was a trend for reoperation in patients with preoperative instability (5/8). Pain relief occurred in 26/31 shoulders regardless of treatment type. Active elevation and external rotation improved in both groups. The authors concluded that reimplantation of a glenoid component is reasonable in an active patient with a sufficient glenoid bone stock, an intact rotator cuff, and a stable glenohumeral articulation. If a new glenoid cannot be secured, conversion to a hemiarthroplasty is also reasonable (Fig. 10.5).

Treatment of the Failed Metal-Backed Glenoid

For a modular metal-backed glenoid with wear or disassociation of the polyethylene component, poly exchange may be possible. For such a scenario, preoperative planning is of utmost importance. The treating surgeon will need to know the manufacturer and exact version of the patient's current implants in order to determine surgical technique for exchange as well as new component availability. Cheung et al. (2007) reported their results on 12 shoulders (11 Smith & Nephew Richards, Memphis, TN; 1 Kirschner Medical, Fair Lawn, NJ) that underwent component exchange prior to 2002. Only four shoulders had a satisfactory result including the only two patients with an intact rotator cuff and stable shoulder. For a successful modular component revision, the integrity of the rotator cuff and glenohumeral stability are of prime importance [50].

Treatment for Soft Tissue Dysfunction

Subscapularis Tendon Repair and Reconstruction

The subscapularis tendon is most susceptible to injury as previously discussed. Treatment options are determined by the chronicity of the tear. For acute injuries, early repair with gentle mobilization is the best treatment option if there is quality tendon present [26]. For chronic tears or poor tendon quality, augmentation has been described [26, 51–54].

Pectoralis major tendon transfer has been described with limited success. Deprey attempted such a reconstruction while also decreasing the humeral head size to allow subscapularis repair with limited functional gains ([52] as cited in [51]). Elhassan et al. also reported poor functional outcome scores in patients after pectoralis major tendon transfer for chronic subscapularis insufficiency after aTSA [53]. Patients with preoperative anterior subluxation were associated with even worse outcomes. This may be due to the difference in vector of the pectoralis major tendon, which is an anterior chest wall structure, versus the vector of the subscapularis as a posterior chest wall structure. As a result, the pectoralis major tendon transfer may act as a static buttress to improve stability rather than a dynamic constraint that can also improve function [53].

The use of a static bone Achilles tendon allograft has also been described to achieve stability [26]. Moeckel et al. treated 7 patients with anterior instability after shoulder replacement [54]. All were treated with primary repair; 3 required a second revision surgery using Achilles tendon allograft. Stability was eventually achieved for all shoulders, although functional outcomes were not reported. Thus, given the lack of reliable outcomes, subscapularis reconstruction should only be considered if the patient is symptomatic and unwilling or unable to undergo the more reliable procedure, conversion to rTSA. Prevention, with meticulous repair and soft tissue handling of the subscapularis tendon during the index procedure, is imperative.

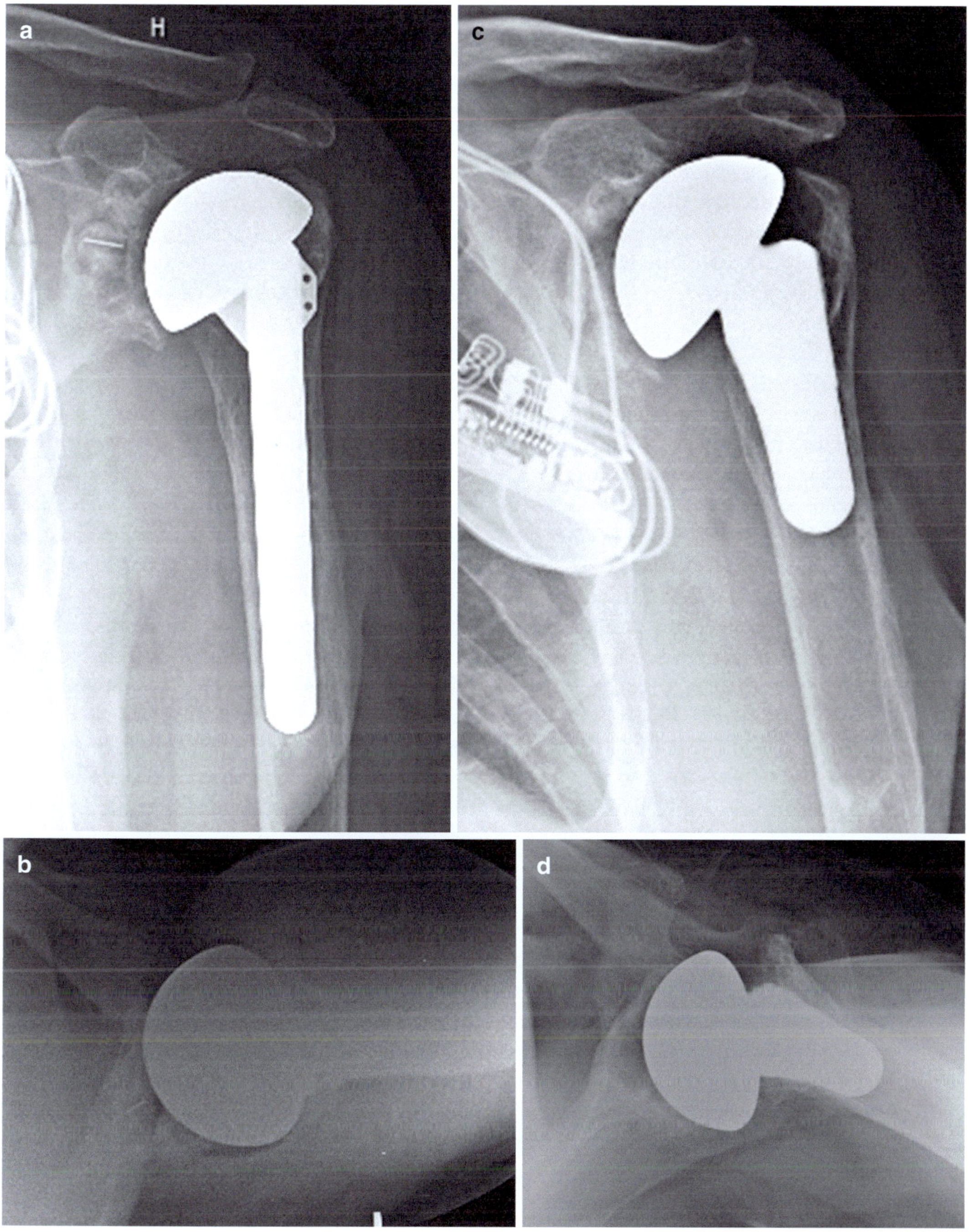

Fig. 10.5 A failed aTSA due to glenoid wear and loosening as seen on AP (**a**) and lateral (**b**) radiographs. The patient had an intact rotator cuff and wished to continue manual labor activities. Therefore, the patient was converted to a hemiarthroplasty as seen on AP (**c**) and lateral (**d**) radiographs

Posterosuperior Rotator Cuff Repair

Supraspinatus and infraspinatus tendon tears can result in weakness in forward elevation and external rotation. Massive disruption of the superior rotator cuff will lead to superior humeral head migration and is more likely to be treated surgically given the associated loss in shoulder function. Initially, conservative treatment should be utilized for minimal symptoms. Primary open rotator cuff repair was reported by Hattrup et al. with only 4/18 considered successful [55]. Pain relief was reliable after repair but restoration of active motion was poor. As a result, the authors recommended careful repair of the rotator cuff during the index arthroplasty and appropriate postoperative therapy to prevent future tears. Early repair did not improve functional results.

Instability

Instability of a failed aTSA can occur anteriorly or posteriorly and is typically due to soft tissue imbalance or component malposition [56, 57]. Superior instability is usually a result of massive tear of the posterosuperior rotator cuff as previously discussed. Component positioning should always be evaluated, and strong consideration for revision should be made if malpositioning is present. Treatment with surgical revision and maintenance of an anatomic design may result in only modest success. Sanchez-Sotelo et al. reported restoration of stability in only 9 of 32 unstable aTSAs or hemiarthroplasties (with an unsatisfactory Neer rating in 23) treated with revision aTSA or hemiarthroplasty for component loosening, component malposition, and/or soft tissue dysfunction [57].

Treatment and Outcomes for Anterior Instability

The most common causes for anterior instability after an aTSA are subscapularis rupture or insufficiency and excessive anteversion of the humeral and/or glenoid components. As previously discussed, revision surgery for chronic subscapularis insufficiency provides poor results. Unfortunately, results are still poor when an aTSA with anterior instability is revised to another aTSA. Sanchez-Sotelo et al. reported results of 19 aTSAs presenting with anterior instability treated with subscapularis repair and component revision with head exchange [57]. Only 5 of the 19 shoulders were stable on follow-up. Ahrens et al. reported similarly poor results where revision surgery consisted of pectoralis major tendon transfer and component revision ([58] as cited by [51]). Approximately half (17/35) of the shoulders had recurrent instability. Three of the shoulders underwent subsequent revision to a rTSA and achieved stability. These results are likely confounded by subscapularis insufficiency. Isolated component malpositioning with an intact subscapularis may have led to improved outcomes with component revision; however evidence-based studies are not available at this time.

Treatment and Outcomes for Posterior Instability

One potential cause of posterior instability is retroversion of the glenoid component. A preoperative biconcave or dysplastic glenoid (Walch classification B2, B3, C) may be a predisposing factor for posterior instability secondary to retroverted glenoid placement during the primary procedure [56]. One theory to address posterior instability due to glenoid retroversion is through isolated revision of the humeral component to a relatively more anteverted position, creating a more combined anteversion. However, this method was brought into question by a cadaveric model that failed to show a significant difference in shoulder stability when a humeral head in anatomic version was compared to one in 15° of relative anteversion on a glenoid implanted at 15° of retroversion [59]. Alternatively, creating anterior offset of the humeral component has also been proposed to address posterior instability and shows promise. In a cadaveric model, researchers demonstrated that anterior offset of the humeral head resulted in an increased resistance to posterior humeral head translation, shifted joint contact pressures anteriorly, and increased joint contact [60]. Subsequent 3D finite analysis confirmed these findings at increasing degrees of glenoid retroversion [61]. These outcomes provide a potential rationale for using such a technique during revision of aTSA for instability with a retroverted glenoid component and intact rotator cuff.

Other causes of posterior instability include posterior capsular laxity or deficiency. Concomitant posterior capsulorrhaphy with primary aTSA is one method recommended to prevent instability [62]. However, there is limited literature, with inconsistent results, regarding the use of this technique during revision of aTSA for posterior instability. Sanchez-Sotelo et al. showed modest results in 8 of 14 posteriorly unstable aTSAs treated with such a technique including posterior capsular plication and case-based component revision [57]. Ahrens et al. reported a series of 29 shoulders treated similarly: 15 achieved good results and 4 were revised to an rTSA with good stability ([58] as cited by [51]). Gee et al. reported a case of arthroscopic posterior capsulorrhaphy in a patient presenting with atraumatic posterior instability after aTSA using two suture anchors to imbricate the posterior capsule; the patient had no further symptoms of instability or pain at 2-year follow-up [63].

Treatment for Fracture

Periprosthetic Humerus Fracture

Treatment of periprosthetic fracture is determined by the fracture location, displacement, and stability of the component. The Wright and Cofield classification may help guide treatment. Type A fractures occur near the tip of the humeral stem and extend proximally. Type B fractures occur near the tip of the stem and extend distally. Type C fractures are located distal to the stem [51]. A thorough history should be performed to determine if any preexisting pathology may affect surgical management, such as infection, component loosening, symptomatic osteolysis, or rotator cuff dysfunction.

Non-operative treatment is indicated for minimally or non-displaced fractures with a well-fixed stem or patients with significant medical comorbidities precluding surgery. Criteria for closed treatment are defined as less than 30° of varus/valgus angulation, 20° of flexion/extension, 20° of rotation, and 3 cm of shortening. Typically, type C fractures with a well-fixed component can be considered for closed treatment. A well-fixed type B fracture can undergo a trial of non-operative treatment; however these fractures are at high risk for failure. One study reported that 4 of 5 well-fixed prostheses with type B fractures initially treated closed eventually required surgery [64]. Close follow-up is important for all fractures to ensure that alignment is maintained in the fracture brace or orthosis. Loss of alignment, intolerance to bracing, failure to achieve fracture union within 3 months, and signs of stem subsidence or loosening are indications for surgical management.

Surgical Management

Type A Fractures Type A fractures with a loose stem should be treated with revision to a long stem implant. The tip of the stem should bypass the fracture by 2 to 3 cortical diameters, if possible [64, 65]. Cortical strut allograft can be used if more bony support is required. The fracture should be treated with AO principles and techniques when possible, with the goal of achieving compression and stability at the fracture site. Fixation can be achieved using cerclage wires alone [66] or in combination with plate and screws. Variable angled unicortical screws can be used proximally in conjunction with cerclage cables to obtain fixation around the stem. As for all fractures, a locking plate should be strongly considered in osteoporotic bone.

Treatment of type A fractures with a well-fixed stem is controversial with concern that a well-fixed stem on radiographs may actually be loose. Fractures with a well-fixed stem and acceptable alignment can be treated closed. Displaced fractures can be treated with open reduction internal fixation (ORIF). However, Steinmann and Cheung recommended using the treatment algorithm of a loose stem even if the stem appears well fixed if there is substantial overlap of the fracture and humeral stem in conjunction with fracture displacement greater than 2 mm and 20° of angulation in any plane [67].

Type B Fractures Treatment of type B fractures with a loose stem is treated similarly to type A fractures. A proximally coated long stem implant can be used. Cementation of the distal canal can be considered to improve fixation at the tip of the long stem revision prosthesis. Care should be taken to avoid extrusion of cement.

Treatment for type B fractures with a well-fixed stem can be considered for closed treatment, although is considered at high risk for failure [64]. Surgical fixation involves ORIF using cerclage wires and plates with screws [68]. Allograft strut and bone graft can be used as needed.

Type C Fractures Treatment of type C fractures with a loose stem is less common with loosening likely present prior to injury. As previously mentioned, obtaining a good history is important to elicit any symptoms suggestive of preexisting loosening. A single-stage revision with ORIF and conversion to a long stem is reasonable for a loose stem with sufficient distal bone. However, a staged procedure with ORIF followed by stem revision can be considered to allow fracture healing and reconstitution of the distal bone stock.

Surgical management of type C fractures with a well-fixed stem involves isolated ORIF using AO principles.

Outcomes of Periprosthetic Humerus Fractures

Kumar et al. reported the largest series (16) investigating postoperative humerus fractures, 10 of which received surgical intervention [64]. The average time to union was 278 days for the fracture fixation group versus 180 days for the non-operative group. As a result, they recommended a trial of closed treatment of fractures with a well-fixed stem, and non-operative criterion is met. Despite achieving union for all fractures, 9 of 16 reported unsatisfactory results using the Neer criteria. Loss of motion was determined to be most responsible for the dissatisfaction. Similarly Wright and Cofield found 6 of 9 patients (5 treated closed, 2 treated with ORIF using screws and cerclage wires, 2 treated with revision arthroplasty) to have unsatisfactory results despite obtaining union in 8 patients [69] The average time to union was 4–6 months. In contrast, Worland et al. reported a series of 6 patients (1 closed treatment, 1 ORIF, 1 revision arthroplasty), all of which healed with satisfactory results [65]. The average time to union was 3.3 months. Overall, complication rates were high including hardware failure, delayed union, frozen shoulder, infection, and axillary and radial nerve neuropraxia [68].

Treatment for Infection

There is minimal data specific to the treatment of an infected aTSA. Evidence-based treatment strategies are often adopted from the total hip and knee arthroplasty literature. As a result, chronicity of infection and time from index surgery often determine the surgical management of a confirmed periprosthetic shoulder infection. Current literature does not show any significant differences in successful eradication when treating an acute (within 3 months of index surgery), subacute (between 3 and 12 months from index surgery), or late infection (presenting over 1 year from index surgery) [70]. Differentiating an acute versus chronic infection is difficult and dependent on patient reliability and history.

Surgical Management

Segawa et al. proposed a classification based on clinical presentation in total knee arthroplasty that has been extrapolated to guide surgical treatment of periprosthetic shoulder infection [71, 72].

Type I Periprosthetic Shoulder Infections

Type I infections have a positive culture after revision surgery for aseptic loosening in a shoulder without previous diagnosis of infection. These patients are treated with an organism-specific antibiotic only [71]. There is limited data regarding recommendations for length of antibiotic treatment.

Type II Periprosthetic Shoulder Infections

Type II infections occur within 30 days of the primary procedure. Immediate surgical debridement and prosthetic retention are preferred in addition to postoperative intravenous antibiotics.

Type III Periprosthetic Shoulder Infections

Type III infections are acute hematogenous infections in a well-functioning joint greater than 30 days from index surgery. Treatment is controversial and determined by surgeon preference.

Options include surgical debridement with prosthetic retention, single stage prosthesis revision, or two-stage revision starting with hardware removal and placement of an antibiotic cement spacer followed by reimplantation surgery. Explantation can be difficult with a well-fixed implant and requires a meticulous approach. Small flexible osteotomes should be available for implant extraction and cement removal. Humeral osteotomy, similar to an extended trochanteric osteotomy, can be used to safely remove a well-fixed humeral component followed by fixation using a cerclage technique and possible allograft augmentation [73]. One-stage revision is reasonable with a well fixed prosthesis and low virulence organism [74]. A course of postoperative intravenous antibiotics with a multidisciplinary approach (infectious disease and microbiology) is recommended regardless of prosthetic retention or removal [75].

In the setting of two-stage revision, reimplantation should be delayed for 8–12 weeks. Inflammatory markers should return to normal after an antibiotic holiday. Reimplantation can be more difficult secondary to loss of bone stock and difficult exposure from soft tissue contractures and scarring.

Type IV Periprosthetic Shoulder Infections

Type IV infections are chronic and should be treated with surgical debridement, two-stage revision, and a course of intravenous antibiotics. Surgical debridement should be thorough with removal of all necrotic tissue and cement present. Reimplantation, if possible, should may be attempted after completion of the antibiotic course presuming inflammatory markers return to normal following an antibiotic holiday.

Resection arthroplasty may be indicated if there is massive bone loss, continued infection, or the patient is medically unable to tolerate prosthesis reimplantation.

Outcomes for Surgical Treatment of Infections

A recent systematic review evaluated the outcomes for surgical treatment of periprosthetic infections after shoulder arthroplasty [70]. Greater than 90% success rate for eradicating infection was found for resection arthroplasty (93.3%), antibiotic spacer-only (90.3%), single-stage excluding unexpected positive cultures (91.7%), and two-stage revisions (93.8%). Success decreased to 90.1% for single-stage revision surgery when a subset of patients who required revision surgery were included. These patients were presumed to have an aseptic etiology during the time of revision but then had an unexpected positive intraoperative culture. Irrigation and debridement with implant retention had only a 69% success rate. However, implant retention also resulted in the best postoperative range of motion in all planes (abduction, forward elevation, and external rotation). Single-stage revisions provided statistically greater abduction when compared to two-stage revisions. Single-stage revisions also demonstrated a trend ($p = 0.06$) for higher constant scores compared to two-stage revisions [70]. A more recent study reported less encouraging results with 19 shoulders that underwent two-stage revision that resulted in a recurrent infection rate of 26% (5/19). Noninfectious complication rates were 16% (3/19), which included aseptic loosening and fracture. The authors noted that these patients had multiple operations prior to their two-stage revision [76].

Revision to Reverse Total Shoulder Arthroplasty

Successful treatment of a failed aTSA hinges upon restoring stability to the glenohumeral joint such that muscular forces can restore motion and strength to the shoulder. Many of the previously mentioned treatment challenges can be addressed with conversion to a rTSA (Fig. 10.6).

In the case of aTSA failure due to glenoid component loosening, fracture, or wear, there is typically inadequate bone stock to support reimplantation of an anatomic, cemented glenoid. Doing so risks a significant decrease in offset, which can result in instability, early failure, repeat loosening, and poor outcomes. For an rTSA glenoid baseplate, bony fixation is achieved through ingrowth rather than cementing, a degree of medialization is well tolerated and preferred in

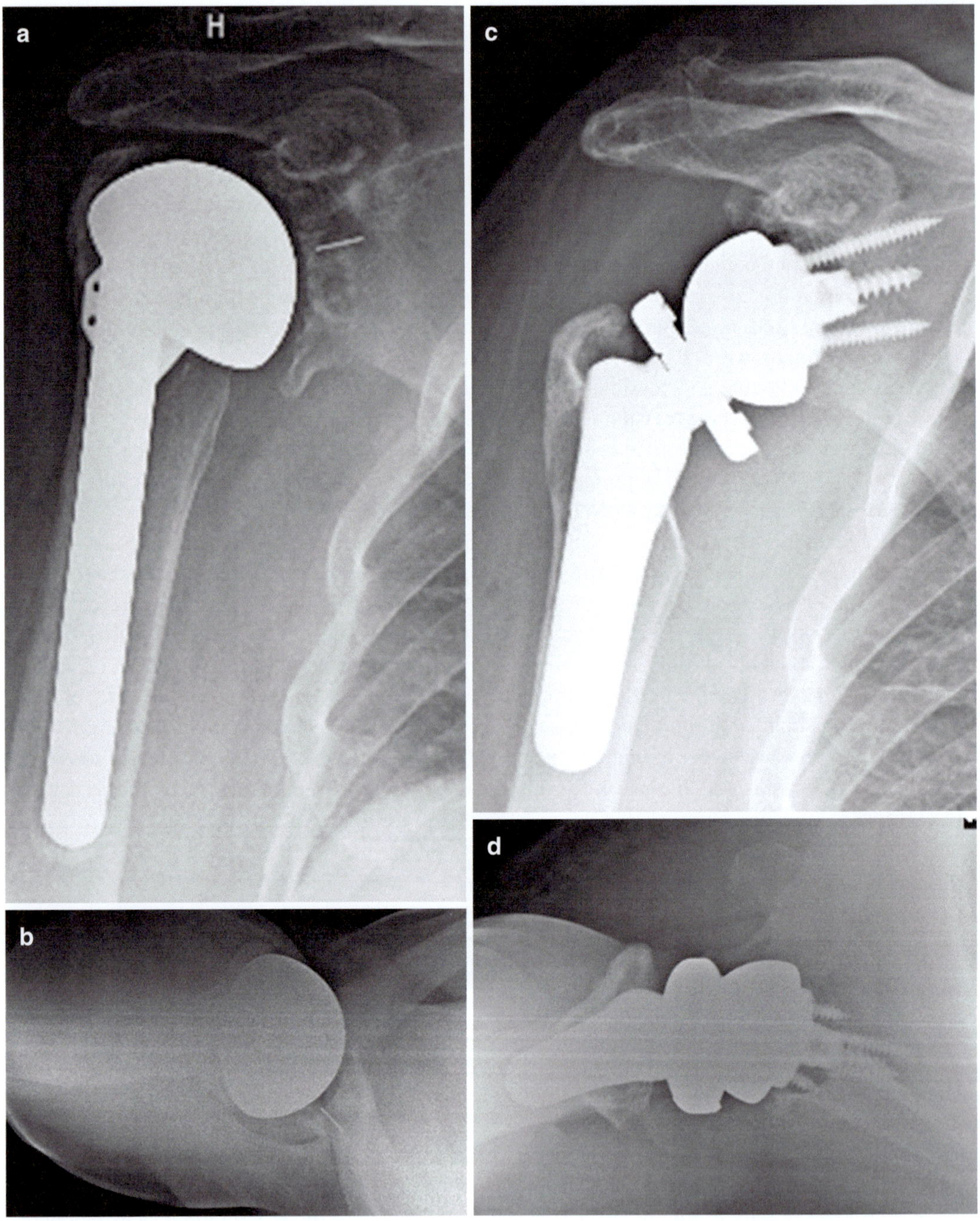

Fig. 10.6 A failed aTSA due to glenoid wear and loosening of both the humeral and glenoid components as seen on AP (**a**) and lateral (**b**) radiographs. Due to glenoid bone loss, the patient was converted to an rTSA as seen on AP (**c**) and lateral (**d**) radiographs

some designs, and placement can vary based on glenoid characteristics. Secure early fixation and optimal placement for bone ingrowth can be chosen by directing the central screw to the best remaining bone stock at the scapular spine, base of the coracoid, or scapular pillar [19]. According to a biomechanical study, as little as 50% bony support of the baseplate is adequate for secure early fixation [77]. One must often be willing to accept a baseplate in a superior position to allow for secure fixation. Implant systems that allow a degree of glenosphere eccentricity on the baseplate can then be used to move the articulation inferiorly.

In the senior author's experience (JMW), a minimum of 20 mm of glenoid depth prior to reaming is needed for stability of the central post/screw on most implant systems. This can be determined with the use of a small diameter drill bit and depth gauge or Lindemann drill to sound the bone and find the optimal location for post-placement and backside bony coverage. If bony support is felt to be questionable, either bone grafting or augmentation may be utilized. In the setting of revision aTSA to rTSA, bone grafting can be accomplished with iliac crest autograft or femoral head allograft fitted to the medial aspect of the baseplate and secured with an extended central post or screw in addition to peripheral screws. Specialized designs exist to simplify the technique (BIO-RSA, Tornier, Wright; Memphis, TN). This should lateralize the joint line to a more anatomic position. Variability in the literature exists as to whether or not doing so improves clinical outcomes such as external rotation after primary rTSA [78–80]. Alternatively, metal-augmented baseplates are being developed for use and have shown early promise [81, 82].

Despite these options, glenoid bone stock may still be insufficient to support a baseplate. Complete loss of the walls of the glenoid vault with a large, cavitary, unconfined defect can be encountered. In these instances, it is unlikely that any form of bone grafting or augmentation will allow for secure baseplate fixation. A hemiarthroplasty, possibly with an extended articulating surface, may be the patient's only option in these cases.

Soft tissue dysfunction due to rotator cuff tear, with anterior or superior instability, is a standard operative indication for primary rTSA [83]. Outcomes of primary reverse total shoulder have been shown to be independent of subscapularis integrity [84]. It is also indicated in the setting of failed aTSA for these diagnoses as well as in the setting of posterior subluxation or instability from glenoid deformity. The versatility of a reverse baseplate location on the remaining glenoid, as described above, makes it an excellent option in these settings.

Conversion to a reverse arthroplasty requires not only revision of the glenoid component but also of the humeral component. Older designs may necessitate complete humerus removal and exchange if no modular component exists to switch from a humeral head to a humeral tray and polyethylene. Newer modular designs may allow for a simple exchange presuming the humeral stem is well-positioned and not loose [85]. However, if the shoulder is unable to be reduced without excessive force, the humeral stem may need to be removed such that the humerus can be cut down and stem seated in a lower position to allow reduction. Alternately, some implant systems allow the tray to be placed in an eccentric position which may allow reduction.

Outcomes for Revision to Reverse Total Shoulder Arthroplasty

Melis reported an 86% satisfaction rate from a multicenter cohort study for patients undergoing aTSA revision to rTSA for glenoid loosening [86]. Eight of 37 shoulders required a reoperation for complications including glenosphere loosening, anterior instability, and humeral subsidence. Repeat revision to a hemiarthroplasty or resection arthroplasty was performed in 2 patients. Shields and Wiater performed a retrospective study of their patient population undergoing conversion of an aTSA to rTSA for component loosening or rotator cuff tear compared to a cohort undergoing primary rTSA [83]. Both groups had significant improvements in VAS pain scores and ASES functional scores that were not significantly different. However, patient satisfaction (74% versus 90%) and subjective shoulder values (63 ± 30 versus 79 ± 21) were significantly lower for the revision group. The authors conjectured that this difference in subjective outcomes despite similar functional outcomes may be a result of patient expectation and psychology associated with revision surgery in addition to reoperation patients in the revision group. In addition to lower subjective scores, complications were also significantly higher in the revision group (31%) versus the primary cohort (13%). Given the high rate of complications associated with aTSA revision to rTSA, patients should be counseled on postoperative complications and high rates of reoperation when converting a failed aTSA to rTSA.

Conclusion

Management of the failed aTSA is one of the most challenging problems a shoulder surgeon will face. Causes of failure are complex and often multifactorial including component failure, soft tissue dysfunction, fracture, infection, and a variety of miscellaneous issues. Treatment must address not only the primary cause of failure but any additional complications or underlying issues. Recognition is the first step to success. Understanding the needs of the individual patient and appropriately tailoring treatment is the second step. While revision to another aTSA has been described, results are poor if the patient is not carefully selected or the shoulder unsuitable for such a revision, meaning unstable or sporting a torn rotator cuff. Most patients that require revision of a failed aTSA will ultimately undergo conversion surgery to either a hemiarthroplasty or an rTSA. Hemiarthroplasty may reliably reduce pain but may not offer a highly functional outcome depending on the patient's needs and desires. Reverse TSA has the potential to successfully address a wide range of etiologies. However, complication rates are high. Regardless of the management choice, both the patient and the surgeon should be prepared for the range of potential outcomes and complications.

References

1. Fisher ES, Bell J-E, Tomek IM, Esty AR, Goodman DC. Trends and regional variation in hip, knee, and shoulder replacement. In: Bronner KK, editor. The Dartmouth Atlas [Internet]. 2010. p. 1–24. Available from: http://www.dartmouthatlas.org/downloads/reports/Joint_Replacement_0410.pdf.
2. Westermann RW, Pugely AJ, Martin CT, Gao Y, Wolf BR, Hettrich CM. Reverse shoulder arthroplasty in the United States: a comparison of national volume, patient demographics, complications, and surgical indications. Iowa Orthop J [Internet]. University of Iowa; 2015;35:1–7. Available from: http://www.ncbi.nlm.nih.gov/pubmed/26361437%5Cn.http://www.pubmedcentral.nih.gov/articlerender.fcgi?artid=PMC4492145.
3. Buck FM, Jost B, Hodler J. Shoulder arthroplasty. Eur Radiol. Springer-Verlag. 2008;18:2937–48.
4. Wiater JM, Fabing MH. Shoulder arthroplasty: prosthetic options and indications. J Am Acad Orthop Surg. 2009;17:415–25.
5. Bohsali KI, Wirth MA, Rockwood CA. Complications of total shoulder arthroplasty. J Bone Joint Surg [Internet]. 2006;88–A:2279–92. Available from: http://jbjs.org/content/88/10/2279.abstract.
6. Bohsali KI, Bois AJ, Wirth MA. Complications of shoulder arthroplasty. J Bone Joint Surg. 2017;99–A:256–69.
7. Papadonikolakis A, Neradilek MB, Matsen FA. Failure of the glenoid component in anatomic total shoulder arthroplasty. J Bone Joint Surg [Internet]. 2013;95–A:2205–12. Available from: http://content.wkhealth.com/linkback/openurl?sid=WKPTLP:landingpage&an=00004623-201312180-00009.
8. Chin PC, Hachadorian ME, Pulido PA, Munro ML, Meric G, Hoenecke HR. Outcomes of anatomic shoulder arthroplasty in primary osteoarthritis in type B glenoids. J Shoulder Elb Surg. 2015;24:1888–93.
9. Gonzalez J-F, Alami GB, Baque F, Walch G, Boileau P. Complications of unconstrained shoulder prostheses. J Shoulder Elb Surg. 2011;20:666–82.
10. Boileau P, Avidor C, Krishnan SG, Walch G, Kempf J-F, Molé D. Cemented polyethylene versus uncemented metal-backed glenoid components in total shoulder arthroplasty: a prospective, double-blind, randomized study. J Shoulder Elb Surg. 2002;11:351–9.
11. Budge MD, Nolan EM, Heisey MH, Baker K, Wiater JM. Results of total shoulder arthroplasty with a monoblock porous tantalum glenoid component: a prospective minimum 2-year follow-up study. J Shoulder Elb Surg. 2013;22:535–41.
12. Fucentese SF, Costouros JG, Kühnel S-P, Gerber C. Total shoulder arthroplasty with an uncemented soft-metal-backed glenoid component. J Shoulder Elb Surg. 2010;19:624–31.
13. Montoya F, Magosch P, Scheiderer B, Lichtenberg S, Melean P, Habermeyer P. Midterm results of a total shoulder prosthesis fixed with a cementless glenoid component. J Shoulder Elb Surg. 2013;22:628–35.
14. Taunton MJ, McIntosh AL, Sperling JW, Cofield RH. Total shoulder arthroplasty with a metal-backed, bone-ingrowth glenoid component. J Bone Joint Surg. 2008;90–A:2180–8.
15. Fox TJ, Cil A, Sperling JW, Sanchez-Sotelo J, Schleck CD, Cofield RH. Survival of the glenoid

component in shoulder arthroplasty. J Shoulder Elb Surg. 2009;18:859–63.
16. Budge MD, Kurdziel MD, Baker KC, Wiater JM. A biomechanical analysis of initial fixation options for porous-tantalum-backed glenoid components. J Shoulder Elb Surg. 2013;22:709–15.
17. Walch G, Edwards TB, Boulahia A, Boileau P, Mole D, Adeleine P. The influence of glenohumeral prosthetic mismatch on glenoid radiolucent lines: results of a multicenter study. J Bone Joint Surg [Internet]. 2002;84–A:2186–91. Available from: http://www.ncbi.nlm.nih.gov/pubmed/12473707.
18. Suárez DR, Nerkens W, Valstar ER, Rozing PM, van Keulen F. Interface micromotions increase with less-conforming cementless glenoid components. J Shoulder Elb Surg. 2012;21:474–82.
19. Walker M, Brooks J, Willis M, Frankle M. How reverse shoulder arthroplasty works. Clin Orthop Relat Res. 2011;469:2440–51.
20. Mclendon PB, Schoch BS, Sperling JW, Sánchez-sotelo J, Schleck CD, Cofield RH. Survival of the pegged glenoid component in shoulder arthroplasty: part II. J Shoulder Elb Surg [Internet]. Elsevier Inc.; 2017;26:1469–76. Available from: https://doi.org/10.1016/j.jse.2016.12.068.
21. Vavken P, Sadoghi P, Von Keudell A, Rosso C, Valderrabano V, Müller AM. Rates of radiolucency and loosening after total shoulder arthroplasty with pegged or keeled glenoid components. J Bone Joint Surg Am. 2013;95–A:215–21.
22. Farron A, Terrier A, Büchler P. Risks of loosening of a prosthetic glenoid implanted in retroversion. J Shoulder Elb Surg. 2006;15:521–6.
23. Ho JC, Sabesan VJ, Iannotti JP. Glenoid component retroversion is associated with osteolysis. J Bone Joint Surg. 2013;95–A:e82(1–8).
24. Service BC, Hsu JE, Somerson JS, Russ SM, Matsen FA III. Does postoperative glenoid retroversion affect the 2-year clinical and radiographic outcomes for total shoulder arthroplasty? Clin Orthop Relat Res. 2017;475:2726–39.
25. Maynou C, Petroff E, Mestdagh H, Dubois HH, Lerue O. Clinical and radiologic outcome of humeral implants in shoulder arthroplasty. Acta Orthop Belg. 1999;65:57–64.
26. Miller BS, Joseph TA, Noonan TJ, Horan MP, Hawkins RJ. Rupture of the subscapularis tendon after shoulder arthroplasty: diagnosis, treatment, and outcome. J Shoulder Elbow Surg Elsevier. 2005;14:492–6.
27. Wirth MA, Rockwood CA. Complications of total shoulder-replacement arthroplasty. J Bone Joint Surg [Internet]. 1996;78–A:603–16. Available from: http://content.wkhealth.com/linkback/openurl?sid=WKPTLP:landingpage&an=00004623-199604000-00018.
28. Hill JM, Norris TR. Long-term results of total shoulder arthroplasty following bone-grafting of the glenoid. J Bone Joint Surg [Internet]. 2001;83–A:877–83. Available from: http://jbjs.org/content/83/6/877.abstract.
29. Namba RS, Thornhill TS. Posterior capsulorrhaphy in total shoulder arthroplasty: a case report. Clin Orthop Relat Res. 1995;313:135–9.
30. Singh JA, Sperling J, Schleck C, Harmsen W, Cofield R. Periprosthetic fractures associated with primary total shoulder arthroplasty and primary humeral head replacement: a thirty-three-year study. J Bone Joint Surg [Internet]. 2012;94–A:1777–85. Available from: http://www.pubmedcentral.nih.gov/articlerender.fcgi?artid=3448303&tool=pmcentrez&rendertype=abstract.
31. Sperling JW, Kozak TKW, Hanssen AD, Cofield RH. Infection after shoulder arthroplasty. Clin Orthop Relat Res. 2001;382:206–16.
32. Florschütz AV, Lane PD, Crosby LA. Infection after primary anatomic versus primary reverse total shoulder arthroplasty. J Shoulder Elb Surg. 2015;24:1296–301.
33. Padegimas EM, Maltenfort M, Ramsey ML, Williams GR, Parvizi J, Namdari S. Periprosthetic shoulder infection in the United States: incidence and economic burden. J Shoulder Elb Surg. 2015;24:741–6.
34. Wagner ER, Houdek MT, Schleck C, Harmsen WS, Sanchez-Sotelo J, Cofield R, et al. Increasing body mass index is associated with worse outcomes after shoulder arthroplasty. J Bone Joint Surg [Internet]. 2017;99:929–37. Available from: http://insights.ovid.com/crossref?an=00004623-201706070-00005%5Cn.http://www.ncbi.nlm.nih.gov/pubmed/28590378.
35. Boehm TD, Wallace WA, Neumann L. Heterotopic ossification after primary shoulder arthroplasty. J Shoulder Elb Surg. 2005;14:6–10.
36. Kjaersgaard-Andersen P, Frich LH, Søjbjerg JO, Sneppen O. Heterotopic bone formation following total shoulder arthroplasty. J Arthroplasty [Internet]. 1989;4:99–104. Available from: http://www.ncbi.nlm.nih.gov/pubmed/2501455.
37. Sperling JW, Cofield RH, Rowland CM. Heterotopic ossification after total shoulder arthroplasty. J Arthroplast. 2000;15:179–82.
38. Sabesan VJ, Ackerman J, Sharma V, Baker KC, Kurdziel MD, Wiater JM. Glenohumeral mismatch affects micromotion of cemented glenoid components in total shoulder arthroplasty. J Shoulder Elbow Surg. Elsevier Ltd. 2015;24:814–22.
39. Walch G, Edwards TB, Boulahia A, Boileau P, Mole D, Adeleine P. The influence of glenohumeral prosthetic mismatch on glenoid radiolucent lines: results of a multicenter study. J Bone Joint Surg. 2002;84–A:2186–91.
40. Gillespie R, Lyons R, Lazarus M. Eccentric reaming in total shoulder arthroplasty: a cadaveric study. Orthopedics. 2009;32:21.
41. Flurin P-H, Janout M, Roche CP, Wright TW, Zuckerman JD. Revision of the loose glenoid component in anatomic total shoulder arthroplasty. Bull Hosp Joint Dis. 2013;71:S68–76.
42. Kersten AD, Flores-Hernandez C, Hoenecke HR, Lima DD. Posterior augmented glenoid designs preserve more bone in biconcave glenoids. J Shoulder Elbow SurgElsevier Ltd. 2015;24:1135–41.

43. Wang T, Abrams GD, Behn AW, Lindsey D, Giori N, Cheung EV. Posterior glenoid wear in total shoulder arthroplasty: eccentric anterior reaming is superior to posterior augment. Clin Orthop Relat Res. Springer US. 2015;473:3928–36.
44. Young AA, Walch G. Fixation of the glenoid component in total shoulder arthroplasty: what is "modern cementing technique?". J Shoulder Elbow Surg. Board of Trustees. 2010;19:1129–36.
45. Deutsch A, Abboud JA, Kelly J, Mody M, Norris T, Ramsey ML, et al. Clinical results of revision shoulder arthroplasty for glenoid component loosening. J Shoulder Elb Surg. 2007;16:706–16.
46. Scalise JJ, Iannotti JP. Bone grafting severe glenoid defects in revision shoulder arthroplasty. Clin Orthop Relat Res. 2008;466:139–45.
47. Neyton L, Walch G, Nové-josserand L, Edwards TB. Glenoid corticocancellous bone grafting after glenoid component removal in the treatment of glenoid loosening. J Shoulder Elb Surg. 2006;15:173–9.
48. Cheung EV, Sperling JW, Cofield RH. Revision shoulder arthroplasty for glenoid component loosening. J Shoulder Elb Surg. 2008;17:371–5.
49. Aibinder WR, Schoch B, Schleck C, Sperling JW, Cofield RH. Revisions for aseptic glenoid component loosening after anatomic shoulder arthroplasty. J Shoulder Elbow Surg. Elsevier Inc. 2017;26:443–9.
50. Cheung EV, Sperling JW, Cofield RH. Polyethylene insert exchange for wear after total shoulder arthroplasty. J Shoulder Elb Surg. 2007;16:574–8.
51. Sperling JW, Hawkins RJ, Walch G, Mahoney AP, Zuckerman JD. Complications in total shoulder arthroplasty. Instr Course Lect. 2013;62:135–41.
52. Deprey F. Problèmes de coiffe après prothèse d'épaule. In: Walch G, Boileau P, Molé D, editors. 2000 shoulder prostheses two to ten year follow. Montpellier: Sauramps Medical; 2001. p. 393–9.
53. Elhassan B, Ozbaydar M, Massimini D, Diller D, Higgins L, Warner JJP. Transfer of pectoralis major for the treatment of irreparable tears of subscapularis: does it work? J Bone Joint Surg. 2008;90–B: 1059–65.
54. Moeckel B, Altchek DW, Warren RF, Wickiewicz TL, Dines DM. Instability of the shoulder after arthroplasty. J Bone Joint Surg. 1993;75–A:492–7.
55. Hattrup SJ, Cofield RH, Cha SS. Rotator cuff repair after shoulder replacement. J Shoulder Elb Surg. 2006;15:78–83.
56. Sperling JW, Hawkins RJ, Walch G, Mahoney AP, Zuckerman JD. Complications in total shoulder arthroplasty. J Bone Joint Surg. 2013;95:562–9.
57. Sanchez-Sotelo J, Sperling JW, Rowland CM, Cofield RH. Instability after shoulder arthroplasty: results of surgical treatment. J Bone Joint Surg. 2003;85–A:622–31.
58. Ahrens P, Boileau P, Walch G. Anterior and posterior instability after unconstrained shoulder arthroplasty. In: Walch G, Boileau P, Mole D, editors. 2000 shoulder prostheses two to ten year follow. Montpellier: Sauramps Medical; 2001. p. 359–93.
59. Spencer EE, Valdevit A, Kambic H, Brems JJ, Iannotti JP. The effect of humeral component anteversion on shoulder stability with glenoid component retroversion. J Bone Joint Surg Am [Internet]. 2005;87: 808–14. Available from: http://www.ncbi.nlm.nih.gov/pubmed/15805211.
60. Kim H-MM, Chacon AC, Andrews SH, Roush EP, Cho E, Conaway WK, et al. Biomechanical benefits of anterior offsetting of humeral head component in posteriorly unstable total shoulder arthroplasty: a cadaveric study. J Orthop Res [Internet]. 2016;34:666–74. Available from: http://www.ncbi.nlm.nih.gov/pubmed/26356804.
61. Lewis GS, Conaway WK, Wee H, Kim HM. Effects of anterior offsetting of humeral head component in posteriorly unstable total shoulder arthroplasty: finite element modeling of cadaver specimens. J Biomech [Internet]. 2017;53:78–83. Available from: http://www.ncbi.nlm.nih.gov/pubmed/28159312.
62. Kontakis GM, Tozakidou M, Karantinos J. Stabilisation of a posteriorly unstable glenohumeral joint during total shoulder arthroplasty: a novel capsulorrhaphy technique. Acta Orthop Belg. 2006;72:353–5.
63. Gee AO, Angeline ME, Dines JS, Dines DM. Shoulder instability after total shoulder arthroplasty: a case of arthroscopic repair. HSS J [Internet]. 2014;10:88–91. Available from: http://www.ncbi.nlm.nih.gov/pubmed/24482628.
64. Kumar S, Sperling JW, Haidukewych GH, Cofield RH. Periprosthetic humeral fractures after shoulder arthroplasty. J Bone Joint Surg. 2004;86–A:680–9.
65. Worland RL, Kim DY, Arredondo J. Periprosthetic humeral fractures: management and classification. J Shoulder Elb Surg. 1999;8:590–4.
66. Campbell JT, Moore RS, Iannotti JP, Norris TR, Williams GR. Periprosthetic humeral fracture: mechanisms of fractures and treatment options. J Shoulder Elb Surg. 1998;7:406–13.
67. Steinmann SP, Cheung EV. Treatment of periprosthetic humerus fractures associated with shoulder arthroplasty. J Am Acad Orthop Surg. 2008;16:199–207.
68. Campbell JT, Richard SM, Williams GR, Joseph P, Norris TR, Francisco CS. Periprosthetic humeral fractures: mechanisms of fracture and treatment options. J Shoulder Elb Surg. 1998;7:406–13.
69. Wright TW, Cofield RH. Humeral fractures after shoulder arthroplasty. J Bone Joint Surg [Internet]. 1995;77–A:1340–6. Available from: http://www.ncbi.nlm.nih.gov/pubmed/7673283.
70. Nelson GN, Davis DE, Namdari S. Outcomes in the treatment of periprosthetic joint infection after shoulder arthroplasty: a systematic review. J Shoulder Elbow Surg. Elsevier Inc. 2016;25:1337–45.
71. Sperling JW, Hawkins RJ, Walch G, Zuckerman JD. Instructional course lectures: complications in total shoulder arthroplasty. J Bone Joint Surg Am. 2013;95A:562–9.
72. Segawa H, Tsukayama DT, Kyle RF, Becker DA, Gustilo RB. Infection after total knee arthroplasty:

a retrospective study of the treatment of eight-one infections. J Bone Joint Surg. 1999;81–A:1434–45.
73. Van Thiel GS, Halloran JP, Twigg S, Romeo AA, Nicholson GP. The vertical humeral osteotomy for stem removal in revision shoulder arthroplasty: Results and technique. J Shoulder Elbow Surg [Internet]. Elsevier Ltd; 2011;20:1248–54. Available from: https://doi.org/10.1016/j.jse.2010.12.013
74. Pinder EM, Ong JCY, Bale RS. Ten questions on prosthetic shoulder infection. Shoulder Elbow. 2016;8:151–7.
75. Coste JS, Reig S, Trojani C, Berg M, Walch G, Boileau P. The management of infection in arthroplasty of the shoulder. J Bone Joint Surg. 2004;86–B:65–9.
76. Buchalter DB, Mahure SA, Mollon B, Yu S, Kwon YW, Zuckerman JD. Two-stage revision for infected shoulder arthroplasty. J Shoulder Elbow Surg. Elsevier Inc. 2017;26:939–47.
77. Martin EJ, Duquin TR, Ehrensberger MT. Reverse total shoulder glenoid baseplate stability with superior glenoid bone loss. J Shoulder Elbow Surg [Internet]. Elsevier Inc.; 2017;26:1748–55. Available from: https://doi.org/10.1016/j.jse.2017.04.020.
78. Collin P, Liu X, Denard PJ, Gain S, Nowak A, Lädermann A. Standard versus bony increased-offset reverse shoulder arthroplasty : a retrospective comparative cohort study. J Shoulder Elbow Surg [Internet]. Elsevier Inc.; 2018;27:59–64. Available from: https://doi.org/10.1016/j.jse.2017.07.020.
79. Athwal GS, Macdermid JC, Reddy KM, Marsh JP, Faber KJ, Drosdowech D. Does bony increased-offset reverse shoulder arthroplasty decrease scapular notching? J Shoulder Elbow Surg [Internet]. Elsevier Ltd; 2017;24:468–73. Available from: https://doi.org/10.1016/j.jse.2014.08.015.
80. Greiner S, Schmidt C, Herrmann S, Pauly S, Perka C. Clinical performance of lateralized versus non-lateralized reverse shoulder arthroplasty: a prospective randomized study. J Shoulder Elbow Surg [Internet]. Elsevier Ltd; 2017;24:1397–404. Available from: https://doi.org/10.1016/j.jse.2015.05.041.
81. Jones RB, Wright TW, Roche CP. Bone grafting the glenoid versus use of augmented glenoid baseplates with reverse shoulder arthroplasty. Bull Hosp Joint Dis. 2015;73:S129–35.
82. Ivaldo N, Mangano T, Caione G, Rossoni M, Ligas A. Customized tantalum-augmented reverse shoulder arthroplasty for glenoid bone defect and excessive medialization : description of the technique. Musculoskelet Surg. Springer Milan. 2016; 100:13–8.
83. Shields EJ, Wiater JM. Patient outcomes after revision of anatomic total shoulder arthroplasty to reverse shoulder arthroplasty for rotator cuff failure or component loosening: a matched cohort study. J Am Acad Orthop Surg. Submitted. 2018. [ahead to print]. https://doi.org/10.5435/JAAOS-D-17-00350.
84. Vourazeris JD, Wright TW, Struk AM, King JJ, Farmer KW. Primary reverse total shoulder arthroplasty outcomes in patients with subscapularis repair versus tenotomy. J Shoulder Elbow Surg. Elsevier Inc. 2017;26:450–7.
85. Crosby LA, Wright TW, Yu S, Zuckerman JD. Conversion to reverse total shoulder arthroplasty with and without humeral stem retention: the role of a convertible-platform stem. J Bone Joint Surg. 2017;99–A:736–42.
86. Melis B, Bonnevialle N, Neyton L, Lévigne C, Favard L, Walch G, et al. Glenoid loosening and failure in anatomical total shoulder arthroplasty: is revision with a reverse shoulder arthroplasty a reliable option? J Shoulder Elb Surg. 2012;21:342–9.

11 Management of Failed Reverse Shoulder Arthroplasty

Eric Michael Padegimas
and Joseph Albert Abboud

Introduction

Reverse shoulder arthroplasty (RSA) was approved by the Food and Drug Administration in the United States in November of 2003. Since that time, utilization of this technique has increased substantially [1–4]. While anatomic shoulder arthroplasty has shown strong durability and functional results [5], this procedure relies on a functional rotator cuff. The RSA implant was originally designed to function in the setting of rotator cuff deficiency and an incongruent glenohumeral joint [6]. However, as results of the RSA implant showed success, the indications and utilization expanded. There has been increased utilization in proximal humerus fractures especially with poor bone quality and unreliable fixation of the tuberosities [7–9], failed previous shoulder reconstruction [10, 11], and rheumatoid arthritis [12–14].

As the incidence of RSA increases with expanding indications, management of the failed RSA will become increasingly important. The purpose of this chapter is to:

- Describe the initial evaluation of a patient with a failed RSA.
- Present the appropriate diagnostic testing.
- Describe the common mechanisms of failure for RSA.
- Define surgical strategies for management of the failed RSA for each mechanism of failure.

Presentation

The first step in evaluation of a patient with a painful RSA is a careful history of the patient's symptoms. Distinguishing whether the chief complaint is pain, loss of function, or both is important for both preoperative planning and management of patient expectations. Any antecedent trauma, whether low or high energy, should be noted. Patients should be asked directly about any potential systemic infectious history. Additionally, patient factors that may confer an increased risk of infection (previous surgery, immune-modulating agents, poor glycemic control in diabetics, etc.) should be defined. Any early complications of the index surgery (persistent wound drainage, early dislocation, etc.) should be assessed. If the failed RSA was performed at an outside institution, obtaining the records of the patient's initial presentation and details of the index surgical procedure is important for preoperative planning.

E. M. Padegimas (✉) · J. A. Abboud
The Rothman Institute-Thomas Jefferson University Hospital, Department of Orthopaedics, Philadelphia, PA, USA

R. Z. Tashjian (ed.), *Complex and Revision Shoulder Arthroplasty*,
https://doi.org/10.1007/978-3-030-02756-8_11

Physical examination should include evaluation of the previous incisions for noting the prior surgical approach as well as assessing the quality of the incisional tissue. Any deformity or muscular atrophy should be determined on initial inspection as well. A thorough evaluation of the patient's neurovascular status is important to note with particular emphasis on axillary nerve dysfunction. While complete deltoid dysfunction is a contraindication to RSA placement, recent analysis by Gulotta et al. suggests that more subtle and common anterior deltoid insufficiency may not be an absolute contraindication to RSA utilization [15]. Complete deltoid dysfunction or axillary nerve palsy should be identified as either an iatrogenic injury from surgery or a persistent palsy from a trauma. Following initial clinical assessment, a thorough diagnostic evaluation should be undertaken.

Diagnostic Evaluation

Standard anteroposterior (AP), true AP, scapular Y, and axillary radiographs are the first diagnostic test of choice. The AP radiographs can be used to assess for periprosthetic fracture (Fig. 11.1) [16], implant dislocation (Fig. 11.2), humeral loosening, glenoid loosening (Fig. 11.3), scapular notching (Fig. 11.4) [17], or catastrophic implant failure. Humeral shortening between the two implants can be measured on comparative bilateral measured humeral radiographs as described by Läderman et al. [18]. Additionally,

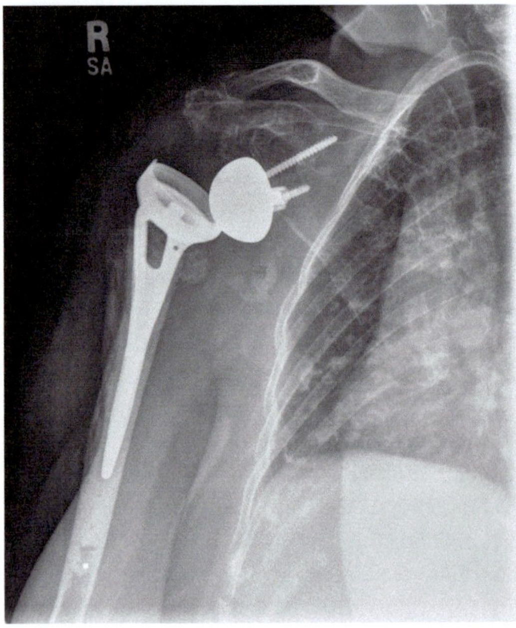

Fig. 11.2 Dislocation after RSA

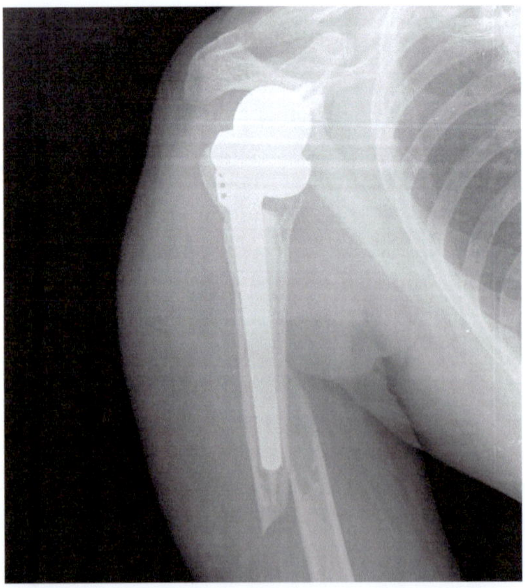

Fig. 11.1 Periprosthetic fracture after RSA

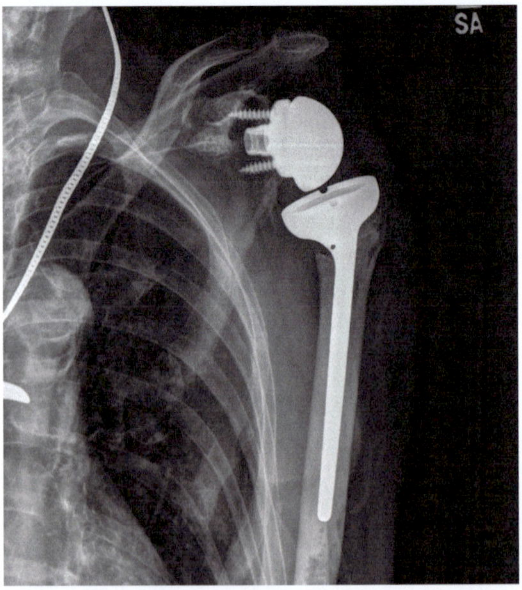

Fig. 11.3 Glenoid loosening after RSA

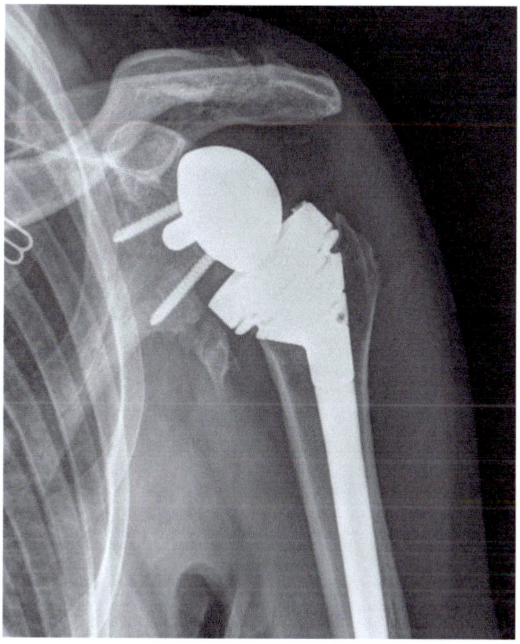

Fig. 11.4 Scapular notching after RSA

comparative AP shoulder radiographs with neutral shoulder rotation can be utilized for evaluation of medialization by comparing the horizontal acromiohumeral distance (the distance between the lateral edge of the acromion and the intramedullary humeral axis) [19].

Shoulder computed tomography (CT) is an important tool to assess the overall bone stock of the RSA implant. Medialization of the glenoid component, the amount of bone available on the glenoid and humeral side, and the orientation of the implants can be assessed. Additionally, three-dimensional CT can be utilized in conjunction with patient-specific guides in complex RSA as described by Walch et al. [20]. While magnetic resonance imaging (MRI) can be used to assess any atrophy of the rotator cuff, this may be limited by metal artifact, and CT can also be used to assess the quality of the rotator cuff [21]. In the setting of a patient who had preservation (through a superior approach) or repair of the subscapularis with the index RSA, ultrasound can be utilized to assess for subsequent subscapularis failure [22]. Finally, for those patients in whom an axillary nerve injury is suspected, electromyography should be performed to determine severity of injury [23, 24]. These patients should be monitored for return of axillary nerve function from 6 months to 1 year from the initial injury before revision RSA is planned if possible.

In addition to radiographic evaluation, serologic evaluation by complete blood count, erythrocyte sedimentation rate (ESR), and C-reactive protein (CRP) can be utilized in the setting of suspected latent infection. It is important to recognize the limitations of these tests in diagnosis of shoulder periprosthetic joint infection (PJI) as the sensitivity and specificity of ESR is 21–42% and 65–93% while the sensitivity and specificity of CRP is 0–63% and 73–95% [25]. While serum interleukin-6 has shown 97% sensitivity in diagnosis of hip and knee PJI [26], it has shown limited utility in diagnosis of shoulder PJI with a sensitivity of 12–14% [27, 28]. For patients in which there is a high suspicion of PJI preoperatively, aspiration should be attempted as part of surgical planning; however the limitations of arthrocentesis must also be considered [29–31]. If suspicion is high and all evaluation for PJI has been negative, arthroscopic tissue biopsy is an option that has shown 100% sensitivity and specificity in a case series of 19 patients [31]. Additionally, open biopsy may have a role in determining clearance of infection before reimplantation [32].

Mechanisms of Failure and Surgical Planning

Infection

Infection rate after RSA ranges from 1.3% to 12% [6, 33–38] compared to 0.98% [39] for the general shoulder arthroplasty population. Postoperative PJI is defined as either early (within 3 months of the index surgery) or late (beyond 3 months of the index surgery). Early PJI has traditionally been treated with surgical debridement with mixed results. Coste et al. found a re-revision rate of 63% in patients treated with an isolated debridement; however this was without controlling for time to diagnosis or treatment [40]. In analyses focusing on early PJI, debridement was sufficient at achieving remission of infection but ineffective in the setting of late diagnosis [29, 41, 42].

Regarding late infection, both one- and two-stage revisions have been described. For one-stage revision, advocates reference low recurrence rates and concern over both glenoid- and humeral-sided bone loss with two-stage revision [43, 44]. Beekman et al. reported 2-year results of 11 patients (3 early, 8 late) treated by one-stage revision of all components with only one recurrence [44]. However, in the setting of late PJI, the standard of care remains two-stage revision as this has shown more widely reproducible results [29, 45–48]. Regarding technique of two-stage revision, there are both stemmed and stemless antibiotic spacers. Institutionally, outcomes of both a stemmed and stemless antibiotic spacer population were evaluated with 22 stemless implants (Fig. 11.5) placed and 15 stemmed implants (Fig. 11.6) placed [49]. There was no significant difference in operative time, complication rates, or outcomes among these two groups, and there were no reinfections in the 27/37 that went on to reimplantation [49]. It must be noted that this antibiotic spacer data is for all PJI patients, not simply those who had an index RSA.

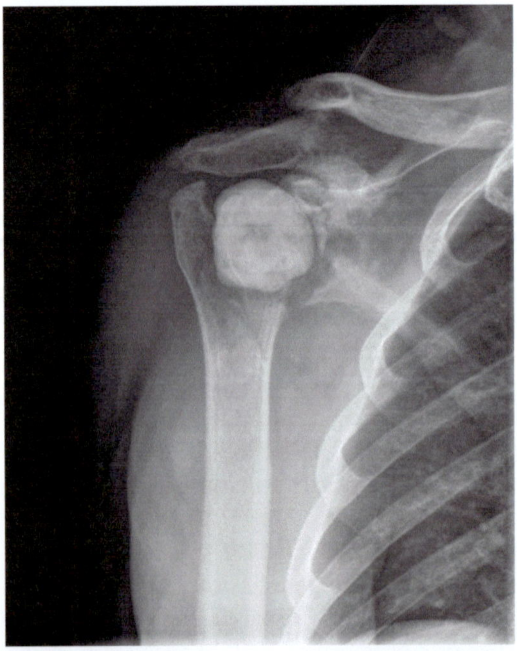

Fig. 11.5 Stemless antibiotic spacer

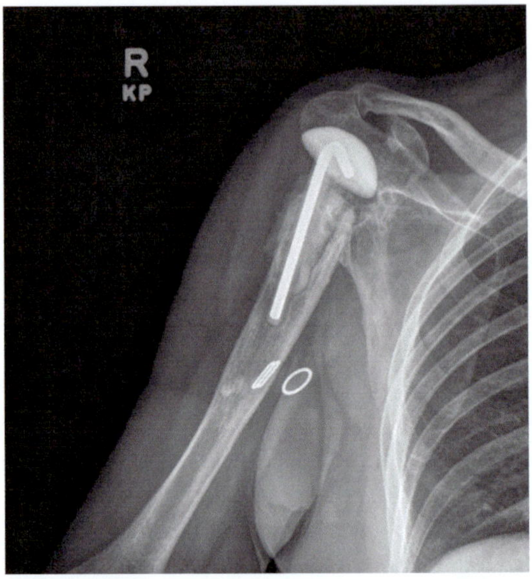

Fig. 11.6 Stemmed antibiotic spacer

Dislocation/Instability

Dislocation rate after RSA has been reported between 2.9% and 15.8% [50–52]. Male patients, malunions, revision RSA, and increased body mass index (BMI) have all been described as risk factors for dislocation [50–52]. Conversely, patients undergoing primary RSA for cuff tear arthropathy have a low rate of dislocation (0.4%) [50]. Institutionally, 510 RSAs were analyzed (393 primaries and 117 revisions) with 15 dislocations identified. All of these 15 patients failed closed reduction in isolation and required a return to the operating room with 10 undergoing an increase in constraint of the components through a combination of humeral stem augment (2 patients), increasing the polyethylene size (6 patients), increasing the glenosphere size (2 patients), or utilization of a retentive polyethylene (2 patients) [50]. This stands in contrast to previous analyses by Chalmers et al. [51] and Teusink et al. [53] that identified a 44% and 62% success rate respectively with closed reduction.

In our experience, dislocation after RSA requires operative intervention often with an increase in the constraint of the implants.

The authors' personal experience with instability management after RSA takes into consideration multiple factors. Surgeon must carefully reassess the index operation's preoperative imaging and intraoperative decision-making to define possible errors in judgment or technique. Of course this assumes there is not an infectious etiology. Timing of instability relative to the index operation as well as associated activity is relevant in the decision process as well. Assuming the shoulder is not reducible in the office, then an evaluation under anesthesia and fluoroscopy is deemed necessary. Under general anesthesia one can easily assess the ability to reduce the shoulder, direction of instability, and ease of recurrent instability. The incision utilized previously is again utilized if it is deemed acceptable. Upon identification of the components, assessment is made as to the implants used for positioning, size, impingement, and range of motion. Almost universally the glenosphere size is increased, and lateralization of the glenoid component is considered if the system allows for such modularity. On the humeral side using a thicker polyethylene liner and possibly a retentive liner may be necessary. In cases where there are gross errors in baseplate placement (too high, superior inclination) or humeral component placement (version, seating of the stem), then revision of these components will be considered; however the risk-benefit ratio of an extensively more involved intervention must be considered. Finally upon completion of this algorithmic approach, meticulous hemostasis is ensured to minimize the risk of instability associated with hematoma formation. In addition the strict adherence to abduction pillow use postoperatively for 4 weeks can help with residual subtle intraoperative instability.

Humeral-Sided Failure

Boileau et al. found humeral-sided failure of RSA to be more common than glenoid-sided failure (21% compared to 3%) [19]. This is attributed to medialization of the center of rotation of the glenohumeral joint thus shifting stress to the humeral implant rather than the glenosphere [19, 54]. In humeral-sided failure, there are two subcategories: those with humeral component loosening and those with a well-fixed humeral component.

Humeral loosening after RSA is uncommon radiographically [55] but is more common in those with proximal humeral bone loss secondary to greater tuberosity lysis [19, 54, 56]. In those with a loose humeral component, explantation should not require osteotomy. However, the accompanying proximal humeral bone loss must be accounted for during the revision. In smaller humeral defects (<5 cm), this can be accounted for by utilization of a cement collar proximally or proximal humeral augmented implants [54]. In larger humeral defects (>5 cm), reconstruction with humeral allograft and a long-stem revision (Fig. 11.7) has been described by Chacon et al. [57] and utilized by Boileau et al. [54]. The implant is typically cemented into the graft proximally and press-fit distally in this technique. Chacon et al. reported good or excellent results in 76% of their patients, satisfactory results in 20%, and unsatisfactory results in only 4% of their patients [57].

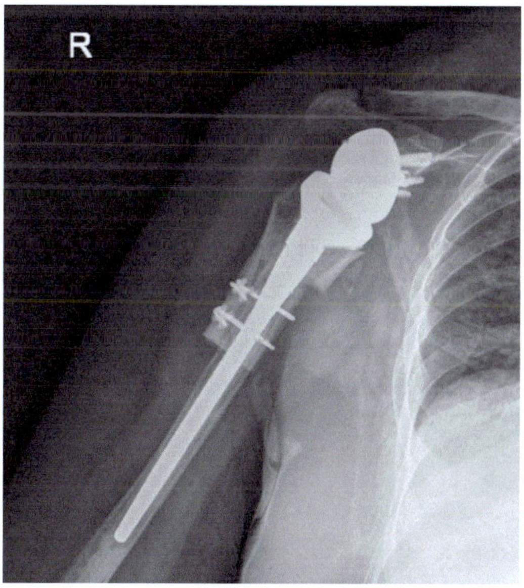

Fig. 11.7 Humeral reconstruction with allograft and long-stem revision

The authors' personal preference for allograft reconstruction of proximal humerus is to use proximal humeral allograft as this better restores the humeral anatomy. In a similar fashion to Chacon et al. [57], the authors first cut the humeral head on the allograft at the anatomic neck. Next, the authors remove any cancellous bone from the allograft canal. Appropriate height is determined by inspecting the remaining amount of diaphyseal bone and estimating how much of the proximal portion requires replacement. A step cut is then made in the allograft leaving a 5 cm strip of cortex laterally and 1 cm of bone medially. Soft tissue is removed from the allograft with the exception of the native subscapularis insertion for potential repair of the native subscapularis to it. The overlapping lateral graft is then secured to the native humeral diaphysis with cable fixation. An intramedullary guide is utilized to determine appropriate version. The authors use a long-stem implant that spans at least 2 to 3 cortical diameters into the native humeral diaphysis. The decision of whether or not to use cement is based on the quality of remaining native bone.

Patients with a humeral implant that is malpositioned but well-fixed have the increased morbidity of extraction of the humeral component. In order to limit the risk of iatrogenic humeral fracture, multiple techniques have been described. Boileau et al. [19] and Van Thiel et al. [58] describe a lateral humeral osteotomy performed lateral to the bicipital groove. Sahota et al. [59] describe utilization of a rectangular anterior humeral window 1 cm wide made 3 cm distal to the humeral neck cut. Institutionally, we prefer an episiotomy if possible, if not we utilize a window as described by Sahota et al. [59] or Wright et al. [60].

The authors' personal preference for removal of a well-fixed humeral stem is similar in fashion to the technique described by Wright et al. [60]. The first step is to extend the deltopectoral approach into the proximal portion of the anterolateral approach. The pectoralis major insertion is maintained with the window. The brachialis attachment is maintained with the exception of the lateral portion in an effort to maintain vascularity to the humeral window. A high-speed burr is then used to make a series of holes from the proximal humerus down to the distal aspect of the cement mantle or stem on the anterolateral cortex. A 2.5 mm drill is then utilized to make a series of holes 1–1.5 cm medially as the hinge for the window. These drill holes should be approximately 0.5 cm apart. The lateral burr holes are then connected with a narrow blade oscillating saw connecting the proximal humerus to the distal aspect of the cement mantle or implant. Then multiple curved osteotomes are placed in this lateral split to open the humeral window around the medial hinge and thus expose the canal. After clearing the cement, extracting the stem, and preparing the canal, a new implant is introduced. The author's preferred technique is to utilize a long stemmed, cementless implant. The implant should bypass the distal aspect of the window by at least 2 cortical diameters. A cemented implant will only be utilized in cases of poor bone quality. The humeral window is fixed with fiberwire or Dacron sutures through the lateral aspect of the window and the lateral cortex. If the fixation of the humeral window is compromised or the bone quality poor, closure of the window can be augmented with strut allograft placed on the lateral aspect of the window and secured with cables. When passing cables, it is important to pass under the radial nerve.

Glenoid-Sided Failure

Glenoid-sided failure is less common than humeral-sided failure and is often a result of component malpositioning [19, 54, 61, 62]. A glenosphere with superior inclination or superior placement is subject to an increase in shear forces that negatively impact fixation [19, 54, 61, 62]. If the patient had a substantial glenoid defect at the time of index RSA that required grafting, poor index fixation into the native bone and/or resultant graft resorption may lend itself to accelerated loosening of the glenoid component [19, 54].

Glenoid-sided failure is often associated with bony defect behind the glenoid component [63]. In patients with smaller bony defects, the defect can be bypassed by placement of the central screw along the scapular center line as described by Klein et al. [64]. This technique can be augmented by use of either a longer central screw or larger diameter peripheral locking screws [65–67]. Central glenoid bone defects with an intact glenoid rim can be treated with cancellous impaction grafting [68, 69]. If the central defect is large, structural graft may be helpful to prevent medialization of the revised glenoid baseplate [68]. Those with a peripheral or uncontained defect can be treated with a structural graft such as tricortical iliac crest graft as described by Norris et al. [70] and Boileau et al. [54]. Additionally, either allograft cancellous chips or structural allograft are options for large uncontained defects, as described by Scalise and Iannotti [71], without the donor site morbidity associated with iliac crest graft harvest.

The authors' preferred method for contained defects is to impact cancellous allograft into the defect. The authors' preferred method for uncontained defects is to use structural allograft. The authors do not prefer tricortical iliac crest autograft because of donor site morbidity. The authors shape the graft for placement into the defect with an oscillating saw, high-speed burr, and rongeur. This is contoured to fit the defect. The graft is then impacted into the defect. If impaction does not hold the graft in place securely during baseplate placement, the graft is provisionally secured with k-wire fixation. The graft is then fixed into the glenoid by the screws from the baseplate if possible. If the graft is not able to be captured primarily by the fixation of the glenoid baseplate, ancillary fixation with 3.5 mm cortical screws is utilized. Implant positioning in the revision setting is based off of the inferior rim of the glenoid and scapular neck. A long post is utilized in patients that have poor glenoid bone stock in order to gain more secure fixation into the scapular body. Determination of graft thickness can be difficult in the setting of severe bone loss. Boileau et al. demonstrated improved radiographic and clinical results in this setting with utilization of an angled bony-increased offset reverse shoulder arthroplasty [72].

Additionally, early experience with augmented glenoid baseplates has recently been described [73, 74]. Early clinical results for patients treated with an augmented glenoid baseplate have found lower rates of scapular notching, lower complication rates, and similar patient-reported outcomes compared to those treated with glenoid bone grafting [74]. The authors follow a more conservative rehabilitation strategy with bone grafting, generally holding glenohumeral motion for 4 weeks to allow for early bony integration followed by initiation of our typical rehab protocol in a delayed fashion.

Conclusions

Utilization of RSA is increasing [1–4] as indications have expanded to include proximal humerus fractures especially with poor bone quality and unreliable fixation of the tuberosities [7–9], failed previous shoulder reconstruction [10, 11], and rheumatoid arthritis [12–14]. As the incidence of RSA increases with expanding indications, management of the failed RSA will become increasingly important. An evidence-based algorithmic approach to initial examination, diagnostic evaluation, and surgical management of a failed RSA will help optimize outcomes of this difficult clinical problem.

References

1. Day JS, Lau E, Ong KL, Williams GR, Ramsey ML, Kurtz SM. Prevalence and projections of total shoulder and elbow arthroplasty in the United States to 2015. J Shoulder Elb Surg. 2010;19(8):1115–20.
2. Kim SH, Wise BL, Zhang Y, Szabo RM. Increasing incidence of shoulder arthroplasty in the United States. J Bone Joint Surg Am. 2011;93(24):2249–54.
3. Padegimas EM, Maltenfort M, Lazarus MD, Ramsey ML, Williams GR, Namdari S. Future patient demand for shoulder arthroplasty by younger patients: national projections. Clin Orthop. 2015;473(6):1860–7.
4. Westermann RW, Pugely AJ, Martin CT, Gao Y, Wolf BR, Hettrich CM. Reverse shoulder arthroplasty in the United States: a comparison of national volume, patient demographics, complications, and surgical indications. Iowa Orthop J. 2015;35:1–7.

5. Sperling JW, Cofield RH, Rowland CM. Minimum fifteen-year follow-up of Neer hemiarthroplasty and total shoulder arthroplasty in patients aged fifty years or younger. J Shoulder Elb Surg. 2004;13(6):604–13.
6. Boileau P, Watkinson D, Hatzidakis AM, Hovorka I. Neer Award 2005: the Grammont reverse shoulder prosthesis: results in cuff tear arthritis, fracture sequelae, and revision arthroplasty. J Shoulder Elb Surg. 2006;15(5):527–40.
7. Acevedo DC, Vanbeek C, Lazarus MD, Williams GR, Abboud JA. Reverse shoulder arthroplasty for proximal humeral fractures: update on indications, technique, and results. J Shoulder Elbow Surg. 2014;23(2):279–89.
8. Bufquin T, Hersan A, Hubert L, Massin P. Reverse shoulder arthroplasty for the treatment of three- and four-part fractures of the proximal humerus in the elderly: a prospective review of 43 cases with a short-term follow-up. J Bone Joint Surg Br. 2007;89-B(4):516–20.
9. Cuff DJ, Pupello DR. Comparison of hemiarthroplasty and reverse shoulder arthroplasty for the treatment of proximal humeral fractures in elderly patients. J Bone Joint Surg Am. 2013;95(22):2050–5.
10. Walker M, Willis MP, Brooks JP, Pupello D, Mulieri PJ, Frankle MA. The use of the reverse shoulder arthroplasty for treatment of failed total shoulder arthroplasty. J Shoulder Elb Surg. 2012;21(4):514–22.
11. Valenti P, Kilinc AS, Sauzières P, Katz D. Results of 30 reverse shoulder prostheses for revision of failed hemi- or total shoulder arthroplasty. Eur J Orthop Surg Traumatol. 2014;24(8):1375–82.
12. Young AA, Smith MM, Bacle G, Moraga C, Walch G. Early results of reverse shoulder arthroplasty in patients with rheumatoid arthritis. J Bone Joint Surg Am. 2011;93(20):1915–23.
13. Hedtmann A, Werner A. Shoulder arthroplasty in rheumatoid arthritis. Orthopade. 2007;36(11):1050–61.
14. Rittmeister M, Kerschbaumer F. Grammont reverse total shoulder arthroplasty in patients with rheumatoid arthritis and nonreconstructible rotator cuff lesions. J Shoulder Elbow Surg. 2001;10(1):17–22.
15. Gulotta LV, Choi D, Marinello P, Wright T, Cordasco FA, Craig EV, et al. Anterior deltoid deficiency in reverse total shoulder replacement: a biomechanical study with cadavers. J Bone Joint Surg Br. 2012;94(12):1666–9.
16. Wright TW, Cofield RH. Humeral fractures after shoulder arthroplasty. J Bone Joint Surg Am. 1995;77(9):1340–6.
17. Sirveaux F, Favard L, Oudet D, Huquet D, Walch G, Molé D. Grammont inverted total shoulder arthroplasty in the treatment of glenohumeral osteoarthritis with massive rupture of the cuff. Results of a multicentre study of 80 shoulders. J Bone Joint Surg Br. 2004;86(3):388–95.
18. Lädermann A, Williams MD, Melis B, Hoffmeyer P, Walch G. Objective evaluation of lengthening in reverse shoulder arthroplasty. J Shoulder Elb Surg. 2009;18(4):588–95.
19. Boileau P, Melis B, Duperron D, Moineau G, Rumian AP, Han Y. Revision surgery of reverse shoulder arthroplasty. J Shoulder Elb Surg. 2013;22(10):1359–70.
20. Walch G, Vezeridis PS, Boileau P, Deransart P, Chaoui J. Three-dimensional planning and use of patient-specific guides improve glenoid component position: an in vitro study. J Shoulder Elb Surg. 2015;24(2):302–9.
21. Goutallier D, Postel JM, Bernageau J, Lavau L, Voisin MC. Fatty muscle degeneration in cuff ruptures. Pre- and postoperative evaluation by CT scan. Clin Orthop. 1994;304:78–83.
22. Armstrong A, Lashgari C, Teefey S, Menendez J, Yamaguchi K, Galatz LM. Ultrasound evaluation and clinical correlation of subscapularis repair after total shoulder arthroplasty. J Shoulder Elb Surg. 2006;15(5):541–8.
23. Cheung E, Willis M, Walker M, Clark R, Frankle MA. Complications in reverse total shoulder arthroplasty. J Am Acad Orthop Surg. 2011;19(7):439–49.
24. Scarlat MM. Complications with reverse total shoulder arthroplasty and recent evolutions. Int Orthop. 2013;37(5):843–51.
25. Piper KE, Fernandez-Sampedro M, Steckelberg KE, Mandrekar JN, Karau MJ, Steckelberg JM, et al. C-reactive protein, erythrocyte sedimentation rate and orthopedic implant infection. PLoS One. 2010;5(2):e9358.
26. Berbari E, Mabry T, Tsaras G, Spangehl M, Erwin PJ, Murad MH, et al. Inflammatory blood laboratory levels as markers of prosthetic joint infection: a systematic review and meta-analysis. J Bone Joint Surg Am. 2010;92(11):2102–9.
27. Grosso MJ, Frangiamore SJ, Saleh A, Kovac MF, Hayashi R, Ricchetti ET, et al. Poor utility of serum interleukin-6 levels to predict indolent periprosthetic shoulder infections. J Shoulder Elb Surg. 2014;23(9):1277–81.
28. Villacis D, Merriman JA, Yalamanchili R, Omid R, Itamura J, Rick Hatch GF. Serum interleukin-6 as a marker of periprosthetic shoulder infection. J Bone Joint Surg Am. 2014;96(1):41–5.
29. Sperling JW, Kozak TK, Hanssen AD, Cofield RH. Infection after shoulder arthroplasty. Clin Orthop. 2001;382:206–16.
30. Ricchetti ET, Frangiamore SJ, Grosso MJ, Alolabi B, Saleh A, Bauer TW, et al. Diagnosis of periprosthetic infection after shoulder arthroplasty: a critical analysis review. JBJS Rev. 2013;1(1):1.
31. Dilisio MF, Miller LR, Warner JJP, Higgins LD. Arthroscopic tissue culture for the evaluation of periprosthetic shoulder infection. J Bone Joint Surg Am. 2014;96(23):1952–8.
32. Zhang AL, Feeley BT, Schwartz BS, Chung TT, Ma CB. Management of deep postoperative shoulder infections: is there a role for open biopsy during staged treatment? J Shoulder Elb Surg. 2015;24(1):e15–20.
33. Sirveaux F, Favard L, Oudet D, Huquet D, Walch G, Molé D. Grammont inverted total shoulder arthroplasty in the treatment of glenohumeral osteoarthritis

with massive rupture of the cuff. J Bone Joint Surg. 2004;86(3):388–95.
34. Werner CML. Treatment of painful pseudoparesis due to irreparable rotator cuff dysfunction with the delta III reverse-ball-and-socket total shoulder prosthesis. J Bone Joint Surg Am. 2005;87(7):1476.
35. Frankle M. The Reverse shoulder prosthesis for glenohumeral arthritis associated with severe rotator cuff deficiency a minimum two-year follow-up study of sixty patients. J Bone Joint Surg Am. 2005;87(8):1697.
36. Guery J. Reverse total shoulder arthroplasty: survivorship analysis of eighty replacements followed for five to ten years. J Bone Joint Surg Am. 2006;88(8):1742.
37. Levy J. The use of the reverse shoulder prosthesis for the treatment of failed hemiarthroplasty for proximal humeral fracture. J Bone Joint Surg Am. 2007;89(2):292.
38. Cuff D, Pupello D, Virani N, Levy J, Frankle M. Reverse shoulder arthroplasty for the treatment of rotator cuff deficiency. J Bone Joint Surg Am. 2008;90(6):1244–51.
39. Padegimas EM, Maltenfort M, Ramsey ML, Williams GR, Parvizi J, Namdari S. Periprosthetic shoulder infection in the United States: incidence and economic burden. J Shoulder Elb Surg. 2015;24(5):741–6.
40. Coste JS, Reig S, Trojani C, Berg M, Walch G, Boileau P. The management of infection in arthroplasty of the shoulder. J Bone Joint Surg Br. 2004;86(1):65–9.
41. Bicknell R, Boileau P, Chuinard C, Jacquot N. Results of deep infection after reverse shoulder arthroplasty. Orthop Proc. 2009;91(SUPP II):245–6.
42. Jerosch J, Schneppenheim M. Management of infected shoulder replacement. Arch Orthop Trauma Surg. 2003;123(5):209–14.
43. Zavala JA, Clark JC, Kissenberth MJ, Tolan SJ, Hawkins RJ. Management of deep infection after reverse total shoulder arthroplasty: a case series. J Shoulder Elb Surg. 2012;21(10):1310–5.
44. Beekman PDA, Katusic D, Berghs BM, Karelse A, De Wilde L. One-stage revision for patients with a chronically infected reverse total shoulder replacement. J Bone Joint Surg-Br. 2010;92-B(6):817–22.
45. Sabesan VJ, Ho JC, Kovacevic D, Iannotti JP. Two-stage reimplantation for treating prosthetic shoulder infections. Clin Orthop. 2011;469(9):2538–43.
46. Loebenberg MI, Zuckerman JD. An articulating interval spacer in the treatment of an infected total shoulder arthroplasty. J Shoulder Elb Surg. 2004;13(4):476–8.
47. Stine IA, Lee B, Zalavras CG, Hatch G, Itamura JM. Management of chronic shoulder infections utilizing a fixed articulating antibiotic-loaded spacer. J Shoulder Elb Surg. 2010;19(5):739–48.
48. Muh SJ, Streit JJ, Lenarz CJ, McCrum C, Wanner JP, Shishani Y, et al. Resection arthroplasty for failed shoulder arthroplasty. J Shoulder Elb Surg. 2013;22(2):247–52.
49. Padegimas E, Narzikul A, Lawrence C, Hendy B, Abboud J, Ramsey M, et al. Antibiotic spacers in shoulder arthroplasty: comparison of stem and stemless implants. Clin Orthop Surg. 2017;9:e52.
50. Padegimas EM, Zmistowski BM, Restrepo C, Abboud JA, Lazarus MD, Ramsey ML, et al. Instability after reverse total shoulder arthroplasty: which patients dislocate? Am J Orthop (Belle Mead NJ). 2016;45(7):E444–50.
51. Chalmers PN, Rahman Z, Romeo AA, Nicholson GP. Early dislocation after reverse total shoulder arthroplasty. J Shoulder Elb Surg. 2014;23(5):737–44.
52. Gallo RA, Gamradt SC, Mattern CJ, Cordasco FA, Craig EV, Dines DM, et al. Instability after reverse total shoulder replacement. J Shoulder Elb Surg. 2011;20(4):584–90.
53. Teusink MJ, Pappou IP, Schwartz DG, Cottrell BJ, Frankle MA. Results of closed management of acute dislocation after reverse shoulder arthroplasty. J Shoulder Elb Surg. 2015;24(4):621–7.
54. Boileau P. Complications and revision of reverse total shoulder arthroplasty. Orthop Traumatol Surg Res OTSR. 2016;102(1 Suppl):S33–43.
55. Gilot G, Alvarez-Pinzon AM, Wright TW, Flurin P-H, Krill M, Routman HD, et al. The incidence of radiographic aseptic loosening of the humeral component in reverse total shoulder arthroplasty. J Shoulder Elb Surg. 2015;24(10):1555–9.
56. Cuff D, Levy JC, Gutiérrez S, Frankle MA. Torsional stability of modular and non-modular reverse shoulder humeral components in a proximal humeral bone loss model. J Shoulder Elb Surg. 2011;20(4):646–51.
57. Chacon A, Virani N, Shannon R, Levy JC, Pupello D, Frankle M. Revision arthroplasty with use of a reverse shoulder prosthesis-allograft composite. J Bone Joint Surg Am. 2009;91(1):119–27.
58. Van Thiel G, Piasecki D, Nicholson GS. Vertical humeral osteotomy for revision of well-fixed humeral components: case report and operative technique. Am J Orthop (Belle Mead NJ). 2009;38(2):67–71.
59. Sahota S, Sperling JW, Cofield RH. Humeral windows and longitudinal splits for component removal in revision shoulder arthroplasty. J Shoulder Elb Surg. 2014;23(10):1485–91.
60. Wright TW. Revision of humeral components in shoulder arthroplasty. Bull Hosp Joint Dis. 2013;71(Suppl 2):77–81.
61. Gutiérrez S, Greiwe RM, Frankle MA, Siegal S, Lee WE. Biomechanical comparison of component position and hardware failure in the reverse shoulder prosthesis. J Shoulder Elb Surg. 2007;16(3):S9–12.
62. Wall BT, Mottier F, Walch G. Complications and revision of the reverse prosthesis: a multicenter study of 457 cases. J Shoulder Elb Surg. 2007;16(2):e55.
63. Antuna SA, Sperling JW, Cofield RH, Rowland CM. Glenoid revision surgery after total shoulder arthroplasty. J Shoulder Elb Surg. 2001;10(3):217–24.
64. Klein SM, Dunning P, Mulieri P, Pupello D, Downes K, Frankle MA. Effects of acquired glenoid bone defects on surgical technique and clinical outcomes in reverse shoulder arthroplasty. J Bone Joint Surg Am. 2010;92(5):1144–54.
65. Melis B, Bonnevialle N, Neyton L, Lévigne C, Favard L, Walch G, et al. Glenoid loosening and failure in

anatomical total shoulder arthroplasty: is revision with a reverse shoulder arthroplasty a reliable option? J Shoulder Elb Surg. 2012;21(3):342–9.
66. Kelly JD, Zhao JX, Hobgood ER, Norris TR. Clinical results of revision shoulder arthroplasty using the reverse prosthesis. J Shoulder Elb Surg. 2012;21(11):1516–25.
67. Holcomb JO, Cuff D, Petersen SA, Pupello DR, Frankle MA. Revision reverse shoulder arthroplasty for glenoid baseplate failure after primary reverse shoulder arthroplasty. J Shoulder Elb Surg. 2009;18(5):717–23.
68. Neyton L, Walch G, Nové-Josserand L, Edwards TB. Glenoid corticocancellous bone grafting after glenoid component removal in the treatment of glenoid loosening. J Shoulder Elb Surg. 2006;15(2):173–9.
69. Elhassan B, Ozbaydar M, Higgins LD, Warner JJP. Glenoid reconstruction in revision shoulder arthroplasty. Clin Orthop. 2008;466(3):599–607.
70. Norris TR, Kelly JD, Humphrey CS. Management of glenoid bone defects in revision shoulder arthroplasty: a new application of the reverse total shoulder prosthesis. Tech Should Elbow Surg. 2007;8(1):37–46.
71. Scalise JJ, Iannotti JP. Bone grafting severe glenoid defects in revision shoulder arthroplasty. Clin Orthop. 2008;466(1):139–45.
72. Boileau P, Morin-Salvo N, Gauci M-O, Seeto BL, Chalmers PN, Holzer N, et al. Angled BIO-RSA (bony-increased offset–reverse shoulder arthroplasty): a solution for the management of glenoid bone loss and erosion. J Shoulder Elb Surg. 2017;26(12):2133–42.
73. Michael RJ, Schoch BS, King JJ, Wright TW. Managing glenoid bone deficiency-the augment experience in anatomic and reverse shoulder arthroplasty. Am J Orthop (Belle Mead NJ). 2018; 47(3): 1–12.
74. Jones RB, Wright TW, Roche CP. Bone grafting the glenoid versus use of augmented glenoid baseplates with reverse shoulder arthroplasty. Bull Hosp Joint Dis. 2015;73(Suppl 1):S129–35.

12 Diagnosis and Management of the Infected Shoulder Arthroplasty

Ryan L. Eschbaugh, Joseph P. Iannotti, and Eric T. Ricchetti

Introduction

The number of total shoulder arthroplasties performed in the United States is rapidly increasing [1, 2]. A recent review of the NIS database estimated that the number of primary shoulder arthroplasties in the United States more than tripled from 2002 to 2011 [2]. During this same time period, the incidence of infection after primary total shoulder arthroplasty (TSA) remained constant, at just under 1% [2]. This number is consistent with other published data showing the infection rate in primary TSA ranging from 0.7% to 1.8%, accounting for approximately 3–5% of all complications after unconstrained TSA [3, 4]. Infection in the setting of reverse total shoulder arthroplasty (RSA) has been reported to be higher than that for unconstrained TSA. Zumstein et al. performed a systematic review of 21 studies (782 patients) and reported a deep infection rate of 3.8% (2.9% primary, 5.8% revision) at a minimum 2-year follow-up after RSA [5]. In 2011, Trappey et al. found a 3% infection rate after RSA in their cohort of 284 patients [6]. Recently, Walch et al. have challenged these findings, noting a decreased infection rate (0.9% versus 4%) when comparing a recent series of RSA cases to a series from the early use of the prosthesis [7]. They conclude that surgeon experience likely plays a key role in this complication. Though the incidence of infection after shoulder arthroplasty remains low, periprosthetic joint infection (PJI) continues to be a burden to patients, surgeons, hospitals, and the healthcare system, with a median institutional cost of $17,163.57 for each shoulder PJI hospitalization, based on estimates from the Hospital Cost Utilization Project (HCUP) data from 2011 [2].

Despite an increasing number of infected shoulder arthroplasties, the diagnosis and management of this problem is still evolving. Recent literature has demonstrated that the most common cultured organisms are *Propionibacterium acnes* (*P. acnes*) and *coagulase-negative Staphylococcus species*. The indolent nature of these organisms makes clinical presentation subtle and diagnosis elusive. Standard diagnostic testing used for hip and knee PJI do not perform as well in the shoulder, most commonly from lower sensitivity of these tests in the shoulder. After diagnosis is made, there is a lack of evidence available to guide decision-making on optimal treatment. This chapter will review the diagnosis and management of the infected shoulder arthroplasty, particularly indolent infections, including patient evaluation and diagnostic strategies, along with current management options and outcomes.

R. L. Eschbaugh · J. P. Iannotti · E. T. Ricchetti (✉)
Orthopaedic and Rheumatologic Institute,
Cleveland Clinic, Cleveland, OH, USA
e-mail: ricchee@ccf.org

R. Z. Tashjian (ed.), *Complex and Revision Shoulder Arthroplasty*,
https://doi.org/10.1007/978-3-030-02756-8_12

Diagnosis

History and Physical Examination

Infections in total joint arthroplasty (TJA) are often classified by chronicity as acute (less than 3 months after surgery), subacute (3–12 months after surgery), and late/chronic (more than 1 year after surgery) [3, 8]. Infections caused by non-virulent organisms, such as *P. acnes*, are typically present since the time of primary arthroplasty but are often chronic by the time of diagnosis, as the paucity of clinical signs of infection leads to a delay in diagnosis. For this reason, the surgeon needs to be vigilant and maintain a high index of suspicion for infection in any patient with persistent pain after shoulder arthroplasty.

A thorough history and focused shoulder examination is critical to diagnosing infection after shoulder arthroplasty. The physician should inquire about fever, warmth at the incision, erythema, and purulent drainage from the wound. Most often, however, these symptoms are not present with shoulder infections given the indolent nature of the infecting organisms, particularly *P. acnes*. Key portions of the history when evaluating a potential PJI of the shoulder include duration of pain relief before recurrence of symptoms, postoperative stiffness, hematoma formation, postoperative wound drainage, history of multiple previous shoulder surgeries, use of antibiotics, and smoking history. Hematoma formation after shoulder arthroplasty, particularly if necessitating an irrigation and debridement procedure, has been associated with the development of positive cultures and subsequent deep infection [9]. Smoking history has also been directly associated with shoulder PJI. A recent study evaluated infection risk associated with smoking and found a hazard ratio of 7.27 for patients who had smoked within 1 month of their shoulder arthroplasty. Interestingly, patients who were former smokers (no smoking within 1 month of surgery) still had a 4.5 times greater chance of developing a postoperative deep infection following shoulder arthroplasty when compared to non-smokers [10]. Werthel et al. also recently found that patients who had a non-arthroplasty shoulder surgery prior to shoulder arthroplasty developed deep infections twice as often [11]. Finally, the overall health of the patient is also important, as periprosthetic shoulder infections occur more commonly in patients with chronic systemic diseases and those who cannot mount an immune response. A recent study by Bala and colleagues showed that patients who were HIV positive had a higher risk of developing a shoulder PJI compared to healthy controls [12].

Pain is the most common complaint of patients with an infected shoulder arthroplasty [13–16]. Determining the onset, duration, and frequency may help determine the chronicity of the infection. The pattern of pain may also help distinguish infection from other aseptic causes of pain such as loosening or instability. Patients may describe pain that is present in the immediate postoperative period and does not improve over time in the setting of shoulder PJI, or they may have a period of initial improvement after surgery followed by the development of pain. While loosening or instability typically causes pain with activity only, patients with infection often report pain at rest or describe it as constant but worse with activity. Excessive stiffness can be associated with pain and with infection [14, 15]. Patients may note inability to regain motion after surgery, and this stiffness can increase symptoms of pain.

Physical examination of the shoulder should start with inspection of the patient's prior incision(s). Overtly concerning signs include redness or cellulitis, swelling, purulent drainage, or a chronic sinus tract. Most often the incision(s) will look benign in a low-grade or subclinical infection. Specifically, *P. acnes* infections are very rarely associated with purulent drainage [17–19] or abnormal-appearing wounds but occasionally present with a non-blanching, erythematous rash. Signs of muscle atrophy, particularly in the deltoid and rotator cuff muscles, should also be noted as possible evidence of another problem, such as a rotator cuff tear or nerve injury. Tenderness can be noted when palpating about the shoulder, particularly along the glenohumeral joint line. Range of motion of the shoulder will demonstrate signs of stiffness, which is typically present in all planes. End-range pain is usually associated with loss of motion. Discrepancies in passive and active range of motion should also be determined and can raise concern for an associated rotator cuff or nerve injury. Strength testing of the shoulder will also bring out evidence of a possible rotator cuff problem or nerve injury.

Diagnostic Testing

Currently, there is no single diagnostic test that is reliable enough to detect shoulder PJI, particularly in the setting of an indolent infection. The diagnosis can be challenging in this setting and must utilize a combination of pre- and intraoperative laboratory tests and imaging modalities. The most common preoperative tests that are obtained include serum markers; paticularly white blood cell (WBC) count, C-reactive protein (CRP), and Erythrocyte sedimentation rate (ESR); joint aspiration, plain radiographs, advanced imaging studies [3]. Recent studies have also looked into the utility of synovial markers, including leukocyte esterase, alpha-defensin, and several cytokines in the diagnosis of shoulder PJI [20–24]. Intraoperatively, if revision surgery is indicated, multiple tissue specimens should be obtained from around the prosthetic components for analysis by both microbiology and pathology.

In the early postoperative period, serum CRP and ESR may normally be elevated rendering them less useful. It is not known when these levels normalize after shoulder arthroplasty; however, in the hip and knee literature, it has been reported that CRP typically peaks on the second postoperative day and normalizes within 2 weeks of an uncomplicated surgery [25, 26]. ESR declines more slowly, and one or both may remain elevated for longer periods in patient with inflammatory arthropathy, such as rheumatoid arthritis. In this subset of patients with inflammatory disease, it is important to consider a rise from baseline, as they often have a CRP/ESR that is elevated above normal limits even in the absence of surgery or infection. Though serum CRP and ESR have been shown to have a high negative predictive value in hip and knee arthroplasty, this cannot be extrapolated to the shoulder. Both tests are inconsistently elevated in the presence of shoulder PJI, likely due to the indolent nature of the most commonly isolated organisms. Topolski et al. and Kelly and Hobgood demonstrated a large percentage of patients with positive intraoperative cultures at revision surgery that had negative preoperative serum markers, including WBC count, ESR, and CRP [27, 28]. Nodzo and colleagues also recently found that serum ESR and CRP elevation was significantly less common in the setting of *P. acnes*-associated shoulder PJI compared to *P. acnes* hip and knee PJI at the same institution [29]. Serum interleukin-6 (IL-6) has received attention in hip and knee PJI due to increased sensitivity and specificity in diagnosis [30] and has subsequently been evaluated in the shoulder. Villacis et al. prospectively evaluated the utility of serum IL-6 levels and showed that there was no difference in IL-6 between infected and non-infected shoulder arthroplasties. They also showed that the sensitivity, specificity, positive predictive value, negative predictive value, and accuracy were 14%, 95%, 67%, 61%, and 62%, respectively [21]. This compares to sensitivity, specificity, positive predictive value, negative predictive value, and accuracy for serum WBC of 7%, 95%, 50%, 59%, and 59%; for ESR of 21%, 65%, 30%, 54%, and 47%; and for CRP of 0%, 95%, 0%, 57%, and 56%, in the same study. Similarly, in the study by Grosso et al., the sensitivity of serum IL-6 was 12%, and the specificity was 93%, making it less sensitive than ESR and CRP (42% and 46%, respectively) in their series [23]. While an elevated serum ESR, CRP, or WBC should raise concern for a potential PJI of the shoulder, a negative result does not rule out an infected arthroplasty. Based on the lack of additional benefit, serum IL-6 is not a recommended tool for the work-up of shoulder PJI.

A variety of imaging studies have been used to aid in the diagnosis of shoulder PJI. Plain radiographs are always obtained when evaluating a painful shoulder arthroplasty and can often be helpful in the diagnosis of shoulder PJI. In particular, it is important to examine the images for any signs of radiolucency around that implant or gross loosening of one or both components that could be attributable to infection. Of particular concern is implant radiolucencies or loosening that develops in the early years after the index procedure. Periosteal new bone formation can also be seen in the setting of shoulder PJI. CT can confirm evidence of implant radiolucencies or loosening seen on plain radiographs or detect more subtle signs of these findings that cannot be seen on plain radiographs, particularly when using metal artifact reduction techniques. Ultrasound and MRI have been used for detection of a fluid collection if there is clinical concern. Ultrasound may be a better test as the presence of a significant metal artifact may make MRI difficult to interpret [14]. PET scan has been shown to be helpful in diagnosis of PJI of the hip [14, 31], but no literature exists evaluating its use for detection of shoulder PJI. A technetium Tc-99 bone scan and indium In-111-labeled WBC scan have been used for diagnosis of hip and knee PJI and may be useful in a limited role for the shoulder if other testing is equivocal [26].

Aspiration can be attempted as another part of the diagnostic work-up of shoulder PJI. The volume of fluid aspirated, however, can often preclude performing multiple synovial fluid tests due to less synovial fluid production with indolent shoulder PJI when compared to the knee and hip. Successful shoulder aspiration rates have been reported from 38.8% to 56% [8, 32]. If aspiration is successful, it is critical that the patient is not currently on any antibiotics that may cause a false negative result and that the aspirate is cultured for an appropriate length of time. Patients should be off of antibiotics for a minimum of 2–3 weeks to obtain an accurate culture [26], and a culture should be held anaerobically for 14 days to increase the likelihood of detecting less virulent bacteria, like *P. acnes*, although incubation times of up to 21 days have been reported for *P. acnes* [14, 33–35]. Synovial fluid WBC with differential from the aspirate has been shown to be useful in the diagnosis of hip and knee PJI; however, no literature with regard to cut-off levels for shoulder PJI is currently available.

Several recent studies have evaluated the utility of synovial fluid biomarkers for diagnosing PJI of the shoulder. Synovial IL-6 was prospectively evaluated by Frangiamore et al. in a study of 35 painful shoulder arthroplasties undergoing revision surgery. Using receiver operating characteristic curve analysis, a cutoff value of 359.3 pg/mL led to sensitivity, specificity, and positive and negative likelihood ratios of 87%, 90%, 8.45, and 0.15, respectively. Seven patients with negative preoperative work-up were later diagnosed with infection based on multiple positive intraoperative cultures, and the synovial IL-6 level was elevated in five of them, with a mean level of 1400 pg/mL. Levels were also significantly elevated in patients with *P. acnes*-positive cultures [22]. In a similarly modeled study, Frangiamore et al. evaluated synovial α-defensin (Synovasure, CD Diagnostics) in 33 painful shoulder arthroplasties undergoing revision surgery. Sensitivity, specificity, and positive and negative likelihood ratios were 63%, 95%, 12.1, and 0.38, respectively, and α-defensin was significantly elevated in patients with *P. acnes*-positive cultures and moderately correlated with the number of positive intraoperative cultures [36]. Nearly all culture-positive cases in these two studies were *P. acnes*, coagulase-negative *Staphylococcus*, or another indolent organism. Following these single synovial biomarker studies, Frangiamore et al. prospectively evaluated a multiplex assay of 9 synovial fluid cytokines in 75 cases of revision shoulder arthroplasty. When evaluating the individual cytokines in this study, the authors found that synovial IL-1B, IL-6, IL-8, and IL-10 showed the best combined sensitivity and specificity for predicting infection (Table 12.1). However, cytokine combinations were also assessed for diagnostic performance, and a 3-cytokine statistical model using IL-6, TNF-alpha, and IL-2 was found to have better diagnostic test characteristics than any individual synovial cytokine alone (Table 12.1). A nomogram was developed from the model to predict likelihood of infection for a given patient based on their specific cytokine levels [24].

Table 12.1 Synovial fluid cytokine diagnostic test characteristics for infection

Cytokine	AUC[a]	Optimal cut-off[a] (pg/mL)	Sensitivity	Specificity	PPV	NPV	LR+	LR−
IL-6	0.87	453.6	0.82	0.87	0.79	0.89	6.4	0.20
GM-CSF	0.70	1.5	0.54	0.85	0.68	0.75	3.6	0.55
IFN-γ	0.69	4.9	0.60	0.80	0.62	0.78	3.0	0.50
IL-1β	0.80	3.6	0.71	0.87	0.77	0.84	5.6	0.33
IL-12	0.60	6.0	0.36	0.94	0.77	0.71	5.6	0.69
IL-2	0.70	1.6	0.54	0.87	0.71	0.76	4.2	0.53
IL-8	0.78	1502.4	0.71	0.79	0.67	0.82	3.4	0.36
IL-10	0.76	28.1	0.72	0.82	0.69	0.84	4.0	0.34
TNF-α	0.60	4.5	0.92	0.33	0.43	0.88	1.4	0.24
Combined[b]	0.87	0.4	0.80	0.93	0.87	0.89	12.0	0.21

Used with permission from Frangiamore et al. [24]

+ positive, − negative, *AUC* area under the curve, *GM-CSF* granulocyte-macrophage colony-stimulating factor, *IFN* interferon, *IL* interleukin, *LR* likelihood ratio, *NPV* negative predictive value, *PPV* positive predictive value, *TNF* tumor necrosis factor

[a]AUC and optimal cutoff were determined using receiver operating characteristics curves. Sensitivity, specificity, PPV, NPV, LR+, LR− were determined from the receiver operating characteristic curve analysis

[b]Represents the diagnostic test characteristics of the combined 3-cytokine (IL-6, TNF-α, IL-2) model found to have the optimal predictive power

Leukocyte esterase is another synovial fluid diagnostic test that has shown promising results in hip and knee PJI [37, 38]. However, Nelson et al. evaluated its utility in the shoulder and showed sensitivity, specificity, and positive and negative predictive values of only 30%, 67%, 43%, and 83%. In addition, aspirates that contain blood must be centrifuged prior to leukocyte esterase testing, and 29% of the time, even after centrifuging, the aspirate was too bloody for analysis [20]. The authors did not recommend routine use of this test in the shoulder.

If work-up of a painful shoulder arthroplasty is negative for infection but there is no other indication for revision surgery and the concern for PJI remains high, arthroscopic tissue biopsy may be considered. Multiple tissue samples can be taken from around the components, as well as from the joint capsule, for culture and other causes of pain can also be evaluated, including component loosening and rotator cuff deficiency. Dilisio et al. retrospectively evaluated 19 patients with painful shoulder arthroplasties who underwent arthroscopic biopsy prior to revision surgery, 7 (41%) of which grew *P. acnes*. The sensitivity, specificity, and positive and negative predictive values were all 100%, and all arthroscopic cultures matched with cultures taken during the revision surgery [39]

If a patient is taken to the operating room for revision surgery, intraoperative frozen sections and cultures should be obtained. It is important, as described previously, that the patient be off antibiotics for 2–3 weeks prior to surgery. Historically, an intraoperative gram stain was used to determine if bacteria were present at the time of revision; however, its value has been called into question [40–42], and its routine use is no longer recommended. Appropriate cultures should be sent and incubated for an adequate length of time, including aerobic and anaerobic cultures (incubate up to 21 days), fungal (4 weeks), and mycobacterium (8 weeks) [14]. As noted above, we recommend holding cultures anaerobically for 14 days to increase the likelihood of detecting less virulent bacteria, as the most commonly cultured organisms during revision shoulder arthroplasty are *P. acnes* and *coagulase-negative Staphylococcus* species in recent studies [22, 24, 36]. Intraoperative cultures have been reported to be negative in otherwise clinically confirmed cases of infected shoulder arthroplasty in some earlier studies [8, 15, 43], which is likely due to insufficient tissue samples, inadequate culture length, or remaining on or failing to discontinue antibiotics early enough before surgery. Recommendations from recent literature are to obtain 4–5 tissue specimens for culture at the time of revision surgery [35, 44]. Tissue samples should ideally be taken from the joint capsule, from the prosthesis-bone interface around both the humeral and glenoid components, and from the intramedullary canal of the humerus. Some of this tissue should also be sent for histology. Intraoperative frozen section is another important diagnostic test for infection, with a criterion of more than five polymorphonuclear leukocytes (PMNs) per high-power field (400x) typically considered positive for PJI in hip and knee arthroplasty [8, 14, 27, 28, 45]. However, this threshold may not be sensitive enough for detecting indolent bacteria in the shoulder, with a recent study investigating the use of alternate criteria. Grosso et al. evaluated 45 patients who underwent frozen section histology during revision shoulder arthroplasty, including 18 *P. acnes* infections and 12 infections from other organisms. Using a standard threshold of 5 PMNs per high-power field, the sensitivity was 50% for *P. acnes* infections and 67% for other infections, while the specificity was 100%. Using a new threshold of 10 PMNs total in the 5 densest high-power fields, the sensitivity for *P. acnes* infections improved to 72% and for other infections improved to 75%, while the specificity remained 100% [46].

Implant sonication fluid culture has also been evaluated with the hopes of improving diagnostic accuracy by culturing the biofilms from explanted prosthetic components [34]. Piper et al. showed that sonication fluid culture significantly improved sensitivity for diagnosis of shoulder PJI from 54.5% to 66.7%, when compared to periprosthetic tissue culture. However, this sensitivity still remained relatively low for culture, and a more recent study by Grosso et al. found no additional benefit to sonication cultures over standard intraoperative cultures for diagnosing shoulder PJI [47]. Based on the results of these two studies, and the increased laboratory support needed to perform this test, implant sonication is not used routinely for diagnosis of shoulder PJI at our institution.

Currently there is no clinical practice guideline available for the work-up and diagnosis and no agreed-upon diagnostic criteria for PJI of the shoulder. The Musculoskeletal Infection Society (MSIS) has defined consensus criteria for PJI of the hip and knee but acknowledged that in low-grade infections, which predominate in the shoulder, several of these criteria may not be routinely met [48, 49] (Table 12.2). In our practice, serum ESR and CRP are obtained in the painful shoulder arthroplasty, and joint aspiration is attempted. If the synovial fluid sample is a large enough volume to send for multiple tests, synovial alpha-defensin and synovial WBC with differential can also be obtained. At the time of surgery, intraoperative tissue specimens and another synovial fluid sample should be obtained and sent for culture and frozen section histology. Frozen sections may help guide decision-making on performing a one- versus two-stage revision, with positive frozen sections a potential indicator of a more aggressive infection that requires two-stage revision. We routinely obtain four to five tissue specimens for culture during revision shoulder arthroplasty from the joint capsule and periprosthetic humeral and glenoid tissue and hold each for aerobic and anaerobic culture for a period of 14 days.

Table 12.2 Definition of periprosthetic joint infection according to the 2013 International Consensus Group

PJI is present when one of the major criteria exists or three out of five minor criteria exist	
Major criteria	Two positive periprosthetic cultures with phenotypically identical organisms, *or*
	A sinus tract communicating with the joint, *or*
Minor criteria	1. Elevated serum C-reactive protein (CRP) *and* erythrocyte sedimentation rate (ESR)
	2. Elevated synovial fluid white blood cell (WBC) count *or* ++change on leukocyte esterase test strip
	3. Elevated synovial fluid polymorphonuclear neutrophil percentage (PMN%)
	4. Positive histological analysis of periprosthetic tissue
	5. A single positive culture

Used with permission from Parvizi and Gehrke [49]

Declaration: The consensus group wishes to state that PJI may be present without meeting these criteria, specifically in the case of less virulent organisms (e.g., *Propionibacterium acnes*). Thus, the clinicians are urged to exercise their judgment and clinical acumen in reaching the diagnosis of PJI

Diagnostic Considerations with *P. Acnes*

P. acnes is a relatively slow-growing organism that can be difficult to isolate in routine cultures with standard incubation periods and can remain in the soft tissues even after adequate antisepsis. Lee et al. showed that after skin preparation, punch biopsies of seven of ten male volunteers were culture positive for *P. acnes* [50]. Matsen et al. showed that three of ten male patients had *P. acnes* growth from deep tissues during primary arthroplasty after skin preparation and intravenous antibiotics [51].

Many have recognized the need to incubate cultures for longer than standard incubation times of 5 days and to utilize both aerobic and anaerobic culture techniques, in order to improve the ability to detect *P. acnes*. Butler-Wu et al. recommended holding cultures for 13 days, as those that grew after this point were considered to be contaminants. They also noted that holding only the anaerobic cultures for prolonged incubation periods would have missed 29.4% of *P. acnes* isolates and suggest holding both aerobic and anaerobic cultures for this time frame [52]. More recently, Matsen et al. found that a culture protocol of obtaining four deep tissue specimens and culturing them for a minimum of 17 days in three different media (aerobic, anaerobic, and broth) had a 95% chance of detecting all *P. acnes* cultures in a cohort of patients undergoing revision shoulder arthroplasty [44]. Other factors have also been shown to impact *P. acnes* recovery, including preoperative antibiotic hold at the time of revision shoulder arthroplasty (increases *P. acnes* recovery) and specimen type (intraoperative tissue specimens have higher *P. acnes* recovery than fluid) [17, 35, 44, 53]. Ahsan et al. also demonstrated the uneven distribution of *P. acnes* within culture-positive revision shoulder arthroplasty cases, emphasizing the importance of taking an adequate number of culture samples at the time of revision surgery to avoid missing detection of *P. acnes* that may be present [53].

P. acnes-positive cultures have been reported in patients undergoing first time open shoulder surgery in multiple recent studies. Levy et al. cultured aspirates and tissue specimens in 55 consecutive patients undergoing primary shoulder arthroplasty and noted that 41.8% of patients were culture-positive for *P. acnes*. No patient developed a postoperative infection, though the authors treated culture-positive patients with 4 weeks of oral antibiotics and also suggested that *P. acnes* may be implicated as a possible cause for glenohumeral osteoarthritis based on the high positive culture rate [54]. Other recent studies, however, using strict specimen collection protocols and/or control specimens suggest that *P. acnes*-positive cultures during first time shoulder surgery may be less common and at least a portion of them likely represent contaminants. Maccioni et al. utilized a strict specimen collection protocol in 32 patients undergoing primary shoulder arthroplasty in which 5 capsule/synovium specimens were sent for culture and a sixth was sent for histopathology and noted that only 3 patients (9.4%) grew *P. acnes*, with only 1 showing growth on more than 1 specimen. Histopathology was negative for infection in all positive culture cases [55]. Mook and Garrigues also recently reported a 17.1% (14/82) rate of positive *P. acnes* cultures in patients undergoing first time open shoulder surgery, with most cases representing an isolated result (three capsule specimens taken per case) that grew late. In addition, a sterile gauze sponge was sent as a control culture specimen in all of the prospectively enrolled patients in the study and had a 13.0% (7/54) rate of positive culture (5/7 positive cultures grew *P. acnes*). Taken together, these studies suggest a contamination rate with *P. acnes*-positive cultures, likely due to the increased incubation times for these specimens and the increased handling of samples as a result of the longer culture times [56].

In the setting of revision shoulder arthroplasty, interpretation of a positive *P. acnes* culture result should be made in the context of the overall clinical picture. This should take into account other positive preoperative and intraoperative markers for infection, including traditional serum markers (ESR and CRP) and intraoperative frozen section findings, as well as newer synovial fluid biomarkers, if available, and the characteristics of the positive culture result(s) themselves, such as the timing of the first positive culture and the number of positive culture results relative to the overall number of cultures taken. Such data taken together can help determine whether a positive culture is likely to represent a false-positive result consistent with contamination or a true positive finding that is concerning for infection. A recent study by Frangiamore et al. highlights this approach. In 46 patients who underwent revision shoulder arthroplasty and had at least one positive *P. acnes* culture, cases were classified into one of two groups based on culture results and other perioperative findings of infection: a probable true positive culture group and a probable contaminant group. Time to *P. acnes* growth in culture was found to be significantly shorter in the probable true positive culture group compared with the probable contaminant group (median of 5 days compared with 9 days). There were also significantly fewer days to *P. acnes* culture growth among cases with a higher number of positive cultures and a higher proportion of positive cultures, regardless of group classification [57].

Treatment

Treatment Options

There is no well-defined algorithm to guide treatment for PJI of the shoulder. Treatment should proceed with the goals of eradicating infection, improving shoulder function, and decreasing pain. A variety of patient-specific factors can help to guide the treating surgeon toward the appropriate treatment. These factors include the results of preoperative testing, chronicity of the infection, organism isolated, implant fixation, medical status of the patient, status of the soft tissues (rotator cuff, axillary nerve, and deltoid), and remaining bone stock. Treatment options for shoulder PJI include long-term antibiotic suppression, irrigation and debridement with implant retention, one-stage exchange arthroplasty with antibiotic-impregnated cement, two-stage exchange with antibiotic-impregnated cement spacer, resection arthroplasty with or without placement of a permanent antibiotic spacer, arthrodesis, and amputation [8, 15, 16, 19, 27, 28, 32, 35, 43, 45, 58–67].

In the hip and knee literature, a comprehensive periprosthetic infection (PJI) classification has been utilized to guide treatment. This classification is based on the time of onset of the infection following surgery and involves four types: Type 1 is the presence of positive cultures at the time of revision arthroplasty, type 2 is an acute infection detected within 30 days of arthroplasty, type 3 is an acute hematogenous infection that may occur at any time, and type 4 is a chronic infection [68]. Given the subtler appearance of shoulder PJI, it is sometimes difficult to apply this classification to shoulder PJI. For the ease of organization and to give a general framework, these criteria can be applied loosely to the shoulder.

Nonsurgical treatment of shoulder PJI is most often reserved for patients who are not candidates for surgery due to multiple medical comorbidities. There is also a group of patients who feel that their symptoms do not justify another surgery. For this subgroup of patients, long-term antibiotic suppression is an option. Long-term antibiotic suppression can be a reasonable option given the indolent nature of the infections and the lack of host immune response. There is no high-quality data regarding the outcomes of long-term suppressive antibiotics in the shoulder. Many antibiotics have been shown to be active against *P. acnes* isolated from orthopedic implants [69], and antibiotic selection and treatment should be co-managed along with an infectious disease specialist.

Surgery is the mainstay of treatment for those patients who are willing and able to undergo one or more additional operations. If an infection is diagnosed in the early postoperative period or develops as an acute hematogenous infection, treatment with irrigation and debridement along with component retention can be an appropriate treatment strategy. When chosen, it is important to perform a thorough and aggressive debridement of all tissues that appear to be involved in the disease process. If the humeral component is modular, separation of the head from the stem will yield improved exposure of the glenoid and the ability to culture at the modular interface. In cases where RSA is in place, exchange of the polyethylene liner and glenosphere will accomplish the same goals. Following surgery, the patient should be placed on culture-specific IV antibiotics through a peripherally inserted central catheter (PICC) for a period of 6 weeks [70]. This is often followed by oral antibiotic therapy with the guidance of infectious disease. In the case of culture-negative infection, an antibiotic covering *P. acnes* should be used. Dennison et al. retrospectively reviewed ten shoulders in nine patients who underwent irrigation and debridement with component retention for acute postoperative or acute delayed onset hematogenous shoulder PJI. The assumption was made that because the diagnosis occurred within 6 weeks of the development of infection, no biofilm would be present and irrigation and debridement would be sufficient. Seven of the ten shoulders in this study retained components after irrigation and debridement at a mean of 4.1 years' follow-up. Five of the seven shoulders with retained components were placed on long-term suppressive antibiotics. Function was maintained in the shoulders that retained their prosthesis with forward elevation greater than 110° and external rotation greater than 40° in all shoulders. Deep infection recurred in the other three shoulders, and resection arthroplasty was subsequently performed [71].

Unfortunately, the majority of infections after shoulder arthroplasty are subclinical or subtle for long periods of time before a diagnosis is made because of the indolent nature of the common infecting organisms. Patients with chronic, indolent infection may also present after failure of a more conservative treatment option. In these situations, removal of the prosthesis is required to eradicate the infection. One- or two-stage reimplantation of components is the goal when the clinical scenario allows; however, in special situations resection arthroplasty alone can be used as the definitive procedure. The goal of the initial implant removal should be removal of the implant, aggressive debridement of bone and soft tissue, and removal of all cement or other foreign material [32, 35, 45, 58, 64, 66, 67]. A variety of instrumentation should be available for cement removal as well as for removal of the implant. Specialized sonic devices and fine-tipped, high-speed burrs can be used along with instruments such as reamers, rongeurs, curettes, saws, and osteotomes to aid in removal. Identification of the prosthesis prior to surgery with the help of previous documentation or radiographs is helpful, as many companies have removal tools developed for their particular implant. Fluoroscopic guidance is helpful during cement and component removal to visualize surrounding bone to avoid cortical perforations or fractures. In some cases, a longitudinal unicortical osteotomy (episiotomy) or a cortical window is needed to aid in implant removal. The episiotomy cut should be made the length of the stem and lateral to the bicipital groove to minimize the risk of unintended humeral fracture during implant removal. The split can be gently hinged open to loosen the stem and remove cement, or if needed, the split can be converted to a cortical window and secured back at the end of the case with a monofilament cerclage [72]. Depending on the clinical picture, removal of the implant with irrigation and debridement could be the definitive procedure. The other options are placement of an antibiotic spacer or reimplantation at the time of removal or in staged fashion.

Resection arthroplasty is reserved for patients with recalcitrant infections after failed shoulder arthroplasties, patients who do not have enough bone stock remaining to support a prosthesis or with a severe neurologic deficit that precludes a functional prosthesis, or those with medical comorbidities that prevent further operations. This technique should be used as a salvage option only as functional results are very poor, although significant pain relief can be obtained [32, 59–61, 73, 74]. Muh and colleagues reviewed 26 patients who underwent resection arthroplasty for failed primary total shoulder arthroplasty and found significantly improved pain scores and no change in function. They noted that forward flexion tended to be better in patients who had an anatomic implant removed when compared with those who had a RSA removed [74]. Rispoli followed 18 patients with resection arthroplasty

(13 for infected arthroplasty) and reported significant pain relief in all, though 5 still had moderate to severe pain. Patients had significant functional limitations, with mean elevation of 70° and mean external rotation of 31°, Simple Shoulder Test (SST) score of 3.1, and American Shoulder and Elbow Surgeons (ASES) score of 36 [60]. Despite low functional scores, Stevens et al. found that patients tend to be satisfied after resection in salvage situations, with 86% saying that would undergo the procedure again [73].

Permanent placement of an antibiotic cement spacer can be performed for the same indications as resection arthroplasty. An additional subset of patients may be satisfied with the pain relief and function of a spacer initially placed as part of a two-stage protocol and may not wish to undergo the second-stage reimplantation. A study of nine patients with antibiotic spacers who elected not to undergo reimplantation because of satisfaction with the spacer reported satisfaction in all nine patients, no or mild pain, and adequate performance of ADLs. Mean abduction was 75°, mean external rotation was 25°, and QDASH scores were 37.5 [16].

While removal of the implant can provide pain relief, the most predictable means of achieving satisfactory functional outcomes is by reimplantation either in one or two stages. One-stage exchange involves placement of a new prosthesis at the time of irrigation and debridement. Patients who undergo one-stage exchange arthroplasty are also treated with approximately 6 weeks of culture-specific intravenous antibiotics through a PICC line. This treatment option is best for patients who are infected with less virulent organisms, such as *P. acnes* [35, 75], and also commonly occurs in the setting of unexpected positive culture results following one-stage revision shoulder arthroplasty [17, 27, 28, 76, 77]. In this clinical scenario, a one-stage revision shoulder arthroplasty is performed due to an aseptic indication, with a lack of overt clinical findings of infection and negative perioperative diagnostic tests, but postoperative growth of intraoperative cultures occurs. Growth of *P. acnes* or other indolent bacteria is common in the setting of unexpected positive culture results.

Two-stage exchange arthroplasty consists of implant removal with irrigation and debridement with antibiotic cement spacer placement followed by a course of intravenous antibiotics and delayed reimplantation (Fig. 12.1). Based upon the hip and knee literature, two-stage revision is the most commonly accepted treatment of PJI of the shoulder, particularly in a more virulent organism. Placement of the intra-articular cement spacer serves to maintain length to prevent soft tissue contracture, as well as provide high concentrations of antibiotics to the area of resection. If the spacer provides adequate stability to the joint, the patient may perform gentle range of motion exercises to further prevent contracture. The antibiotic-impregnated cement spacer can be molded by the surgeon at the time of surgery with or without custom molds, or newer prefabricated designs can be used (Fig. 12.1). Antibiotic concentrations have varied across studies, but recommended amounts have ranged from 1.2 to 4.8 grams of tobramycin, 40 milligrams to 4.8 grams of gentamicin, 1–6 grams of vancomycin, and 4.5–6 grams of cefazolin per 40 grams of polymethylmethacrylate powder [16, 59, 65, 78].

For a two-stage exchange, the treating surgeon must ensure that the infection has been eradicated. After completion of antibiotic therapy, the patient is usually given a 4–6-week period off of antibiotics prior to placement of a new prosthesis. Serum lab evaluation (ESR, CRP) is again undertaken, and joint aspiration is performed after this antibiotic-free period to confirm the laboratory studies have normalized and the joint aspirate is negative [66]. As in the initial resection surgery, intraoperative tissue samples should be obtained for culture and pathology, including frozen section, prior to reimplantation [66]. If there are concerning signs that an infection is still present, such as positive preoperative bloodwork or aspirate or positive intraoperative frozen section, a repeat debridement procedure with placement of a new antibiotic spacer should be performed.

If the infection has been cleared, the choice of prosthesis is made based on the status of the bone, rotator cuff, and deltoid. An anatomic TSA or hemiarthroplasty may be possible if glenoid bone

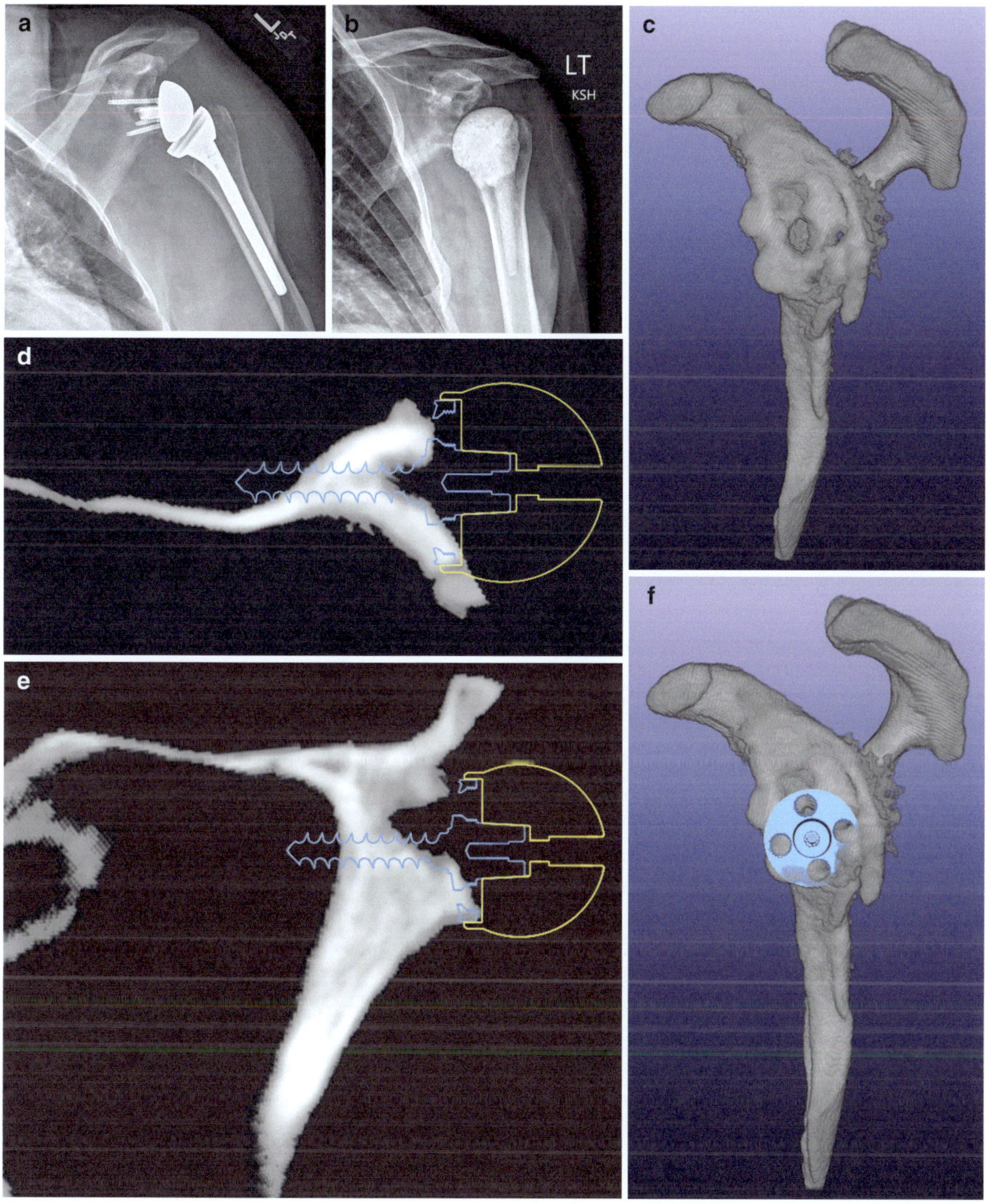

Fig. 12.1 (**a**) Anteroposterior (AP) radiograph of a left reverse total shoulder arthroplasty 1 year after surgery with signs of radiolucencies around both the glenoid and humeral component, worrisome for loosening. Preoperative work-up for infection showed elevated ESR and CRP, and the patient was taken for revision surgery with high suspicion for infection. Intraoperative frozen section tissue specimens demonstrated acute inflammation concerning for infection, and intraoperative cultures subsequently grew out *P. acnes* (7/9 cultures positive). The patient underwent two-stage exchange, with (**b**) placement of a temporary antibiotic-impregnated cement spacer and a 6-week course of IV antibiotics. (**c**) Preoperative three-dimensional CT scan was obtained prior to reimplantation surgery and demonstrated a central contained glenoid defect at the prior center peg site. (**d**–**f**) Preoperative planning software was utilized to plan the implant position prior to reimplantation surgery. (**g**) AP radiograph following reimplantation with a reverse total shoulder arthroplasty. Cancellous allograft bone chips were used to fill the central contained glenoid defect, and the humeral component was secured with antibiotic-containing cement

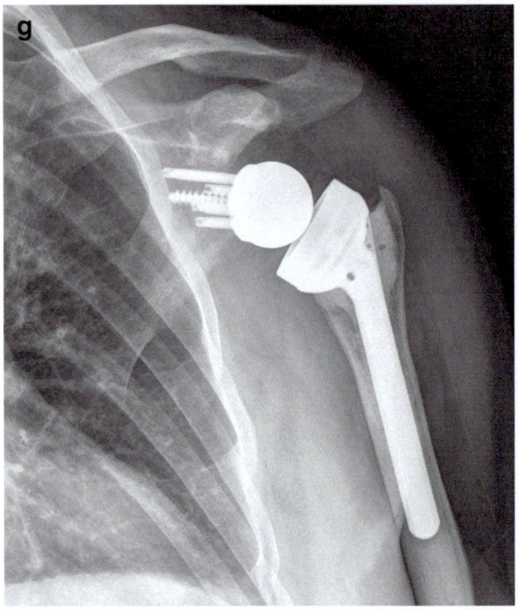

Fig. 12.1 (continued)

stock is sufficient and the rotator cuff and deltoid are functional and intact. Hemiarthroplasty or RSA should be utilized in cases where glenoid deficiency precludes placement of an anatomic glenoid component and/or soft tissue defects, particularly rotator cuff deficiency, are present. RSA may provide the most reliable functional outcome, particularly in the setting of rotator cuff deficiency and advanced glenoid bone loss. Preoperative computed tomography (CT) may be useful for surgical planning in order to better evaluate the degree of glenoid bone loss that is present (Fig. 12.1).

Arthrodesis, although rarely performed, is an option in those with axillary nerve or brachial plexus injuries or combined loss of the rotator cuff and deltoid. Functional outcome is typically better than resection arthroplasty as it provides a stable platform for distal function; however, it is a technically demanding procedure given the bone loss typically present after implant removal. Scalise and Iannotti reported on a series of seven patients who underwent arthrodeses after failed arthroplasty and noted the need for a vascularized fibula in three patients and subsequent operations to obtain union in four [79].

Treatment Outcomes of One- and Two-Stage Exchange

Evaluating treatment outcomes for shoulder PJI is somewhat difficult given the small amount of literature available and its heterogeneity. Most studies report on revision arthroplasty utilizing non-standardized treatment protocols with variable follow-up lengths. The evidence that is available is primarily retrospective case series, typically involving a small number of patients. A few comparative studies are available at this point, but there is yet to be any prospective data published. Comparing results of one- and two-stage revision approaches is difficult due to the lack of uniform criteria across studies in choosing each approach and in the definitions of PJI. Functional outcomes are also difficult to compare since the majority of the data available is based upon revision to hemiarthroplasty, with only more recent data including revision to RSA. Given the limited data, it is difficult to draw conclusions on specific treatment methods. Below we summarize outcomes for one- and two-stage exchange.

One-Stage Exchange

Hsu and colleagues recently compared outcomes of one-stage exchange in *P. acnes* culture-positive (>1 culture positive) revisions (27 cases) to a control group of one-stage revisions with no culture growth or an isolated positive *P. acnes* culture (28 cases). At the time of revision surgery, five sets of cultures were obtained prior to administration of antibiotics, irrigation and debridement, and exchange arthroplasty in all patients. In their treatment protocol, all patients with multiple positive *P. acnes* cultures were given a 6-week course of IV antibiotics followed by 6 months of oral antibiotics. The control group of patients discontinued antibiotics at 3 weeks after cultures were final. At a mean follow-up of 47.8 months, the Simple Shoulder Test (SST) scores improved in both groups with no significant difference in pain, stiffness, or component loosening between the two groups. There were no recurrent infections in the 27 culture-positive shoulders [35].

Ince et al. reported on their experience with one-stage exchange for the treatment of infected shoulder arthroplasty [63]. Sixteen cases were performed, and 15 were converted to a hemiarthroplasty and 1 to a RSA. All revision implants were cemented with antibiotic-impregnated cement. The two most common isolated organisms were a *Staphylococcus* species (8 shoulders) or a *Propionibacterium* species (4). Mean course of antibiotic therapy was only 8.6 days (range, 5–14) and was stopped once the CRP began to decline. Nine patients were available for follow-up at a mean of 5.8 years (range, 1.1–13.25). Six patients were satisfied with their outcome. Mean shoulder abduction was only 51.6°. The mean Constant score was 33.6 and the mean UCLA score was 18.3 (maximum score, 35). There were three cases not in the final follow-up that required revision surgery: one for a periprosthetic fracture, one for an acromial pseudarthrosis, and one for recurrent instability. There were no recurrent infections, and the authors concluded that eradication of infection is possible with a one-stage exchange [63].

More recently, Beekman et al. reported on a series of 11 cases of one-stage revisions performed for infected reverse TSA [62]. All patients were revised to a cemented RSA with antibiotic-impregnated cement. No primary reverse TSA was loose at the time of revision surgery. The isolated organisms were *P. acnes* (7 shoulders), coagulase-negative *Staphylococcus* (5), methicillin-resistant *Staphylococcus aureus* (1), and *Escherichia coli* (1), including two multibacterial infections. A minimum of 3 days of IV antibiotic therapy was given to all patients, and the minimum overall course of antibiotic treatment (combined IV and oral) was 3 months. Antibiotics were stopped when the ESR and CRP normalized for 6 weeks. Mean follow-up was 24 months (range, 12–36). There was one recurrent infection that persisted despite a subsequent two-stage exchange. The organism was *Propionibacterium* species, and the patient was ultimately cleared of the infection after placement of a long-term spacer. Overall, the mean Constant score was 55 at final follow-up [62]. Klatte et al. evaluated 35 patients treated with single-stage revision to various implants and a mean of 10.6 days of antibiotics. Two patients (5.7%) developed recurrent infection and were treated with resection arthroplasty. Mean Constant scores were 43.3 for hemiarthroplasties, 56.0 for bipolar hemiarthroplasties, and 61 for RSAs [75]

Two-Stage Exchange

Two-stage exchange is still the most commonly recommended treatment option available in shoulder PJI, though this is mostly extrapolated from the success of this treatment option in the hip and knee literature. With many cases of shoulder PJI due to chronic, indolent infections, a two-stage exchange may not be necessary in all instances, but further data is needed to determine the criteria for performing a one- versus a two-stage exchange.

Strickland et al. evaluated 19 shoulders that were treated with two-stage exchange for a deep shoulder prosthetic infection [8]. Four cases had previously been treated with either long-term antibiotic suppression (2) or irrigation and debridement with implant retention (2) and had failed to eradicate the infection. All patients underwent placement of an antibiotic-impregnated spacer after implant removal and received 4–6 weeks of organism-specific IV antibiotic therapy. The most common isolated organisms were either *P. acnes* or *coagulase-negative Staphylococcus* (10 shoulders) and *Staphylococcus aureus* (3). Mean time to reimplantation was 11 weeks (range, 6–31) after resection and was either with hemiarthroplasty (13) or TSA (5). Mean follow-up was 35 months (range, 24–80), with mean shoulder elevation to 89°, mean external rotation to 43°, and mean internal rotation to L5. Pain was significantly improved ($p = 0.0001$) postoperatively, but results were rated as unsatisfactory in 13/19 (68%) shoulders. There were 14 complications and 5 further operations following reimplantation, including 2 irrigation and debridements and a resection arthroplasty in a patient with continued infection. The infection was considered cleared in 12/19 (63%) shoulders. Seven recurrent infections were defined based on six patients requiring long-term antibiotics due to continued concern for infection and the one patient who required a resection arthroplasty [8].

Coffey et al. reported on their experience with two-stage exchange for infected shoulder arthroplasty and native septic arthritis using a commercially produced antibiotic-impregnated spacer [65]. The series consisted of 16 shoulders, 11 of which were infected shoulder prostheses. This included six hemiarthroplasties, three RSA, and two standard TSA. An organism was isolated in 12 of 16 cases, including 3 with methicillin-resistant *Staphylococcus aureus*, 3 with *Staphylococcus epidermidis*, and 1 with *P. acnes*. All patients underwent placement of a commercially manufactured gentamycin-impregnated spacer after implant removal and received culture-specific IV antibiotic therapy postoperatively. Mean IV antibiotic treatment was 5.6 weeks (range, 2–6). Reimplantation occurred when the patient's serum IL-6 level was decreasing or had normalized at a mean of 11.2 weeks (range, 6–30) after implant removal and spacer placement. Nine shoulders were reimplanted with a RSA and two with a standard TSA, and one shoulder underwent arthrodesis because of deltoid deficiency. Four patients refused revision and retained their antibiotic spacer. Mean follow-up was 20.5 months (range, 12–30) after spacer placement. Pain was improved, with mean active forward flexion increased from 65° before spacer placement to 110° at final follow-up and mean active external rotation increased from −5° to 20°. The mean UCLA score was 26, the mean Simple Shoulder Test (SST) score was 6.6, the mean ASES score was 74, and the mean Constant score was 57 at final follow-up. None of the postoperative outcome measures were separated out by preoperative etiology (infected shoulder arthroplasty versus native septic arthritis) or final revision implant. There were no recurrent infections [65].

Sabesan et al. evaluated the outcomes of two-stage exchange in the treatment of infected shoulder arthroplasty, in which reimplantation was with a reverse TSA [64]. Twenty-seven shoulders were identified that had undergone two-stage reimplantation for a shoulder PJI, with 17 revised to a RSA. The most common isolated bacteria were a *Staphylococcus* species (7 shoulders) and *P. acnes* (5). Patients received organism-specific IV antibiotic therapy for a mean of 6.3 weeks (range, 4–54) postoperatively and had a median of 4.0 months (range, 1.8–61) between explant and reimplantation. Mean follow-up was 46.2 months (range, 22–80). There was one recurrent infection from *P. acnes* that was ultimately cleared with a second two-stage exchange. Mean Penn shoulder score was significantly improved from preoperative levels at final follow-up (24.9–66.4), with mean forward flexion of 123° and mean external rotation of 26°. Seven complications developed postoperatively, requiring seven additional surgeries. One postoperative hematoma developed that required irrigation and debridement. Five surgeries were performed for instability with polyethylene exchange or revision of the glenosphere. The other additional surgery was the repeat two-stage exchange for recurrent infection [64].

Recently, two more retrospective studies have evaluated two-stage exchange for shoulder PJI. Buchalter and colleagues reviewed 19 patients with a mean time from index procedure to revision of 40 months. Diagnosis was made based upon serum lab studies, clinical presentation, and aspiration. A standard two-stage protocol was undertaken with resection and antibiotic spacer placement. All patients were given 6 weeks of intravenous antibiotics, and infectious disease was consulted. Reimplantation was undertaken when the patient had been found to have cleared the infection based upon lab studies and aspiration. A deep infection recurred in 26% of the 19 patients. Overall complication rate was 42% with two patients having aseptic loosening, one with fracture, and five developing recurrent infections. Forward elevation significantly improved after two-stage revision, but external rotation did not improve. The authors found that patients infected with *P. acnes* had poorer outcomes than those who did not isolate *P. acnes* [67]. In another retrospective review, Assenmacher et al. reviewed 35 shoulders with PJI treated with two-stage exchange. The organisms isolated from the shoulder were *P. acnes* in 13 cases, *Staphylococcus epidermidis* in 12, and methicillin-resistant *Staphylococcus aureus* in 2. No growth was obtained in four of the cases. VAS pain scores were significantly improved from a mean of 4.4 to 2 out of 5. Mean forward elevation improved from 64° to 118°. Mean ER improved from 14° to 41°. Outcome was excellent in 10, satisfactory in 12, and unsatisfactory in 13 on the Neer modified rating scale. Function and pain did not change depending on prosthesis implanted. There were six reinfections, three due to *P. acnes*, two from *Staphylococcus epidermidis*, and one from polymicrobial with methicillin-resistant *Staphylococcus aureus* and *Enterococcus*. While infection was eradicated in 85% of patients using two-stage revision, the rate of unsatisfactory results was nearly 40% [58].

Comparative Studies

Several studies have directly compared treatment methods. Verhelst et al. evaluated 11 patients treated with resection arthroplasty and 10 patients with permanent spacers and noted no difference in recurrence rate or functional outcomes [59]. Codd et al. compared resection arthroplasty in 5 patients to reimplantation in 13 patients. Pain relief was similar in the two groups, though elevation was 66° compared to 117°, external rotation was 27° compared to 38°, and internal rotation was to the sacrum compared to L2 [32]. Stine compared permanent spacers to two-stage exchange in 30 patients. There were no recurrent infections and no differences in functional outcomes [66]. Cuff et al. compared one-stage exchange in 10 patients to two-stage exchange in 12 patients. There were no recurrent infections and no differences in functional outcomes between groups; however, there were 11 complications in 7 shoulders [45]. More recently, Stone et al. retrospectively compared one- and two-stage exchange in 79 patients with shoulder PJI but evaluated patients in 3 groups, those that underwent an incomplete one-stage exchange with some component retention (15 patients), those that underwent a complete one-stage exchange (45 patients), and those that underwent a two-stage exchange (19 patients). There was no difference in noninfectious complications, pain, and functional improvement between groups; but one-stage incomplete exchange and growth of either *S. aureus* or coagulase-negative staph species were found to be significantly associated with reoperation for infection [80]. Nelson et al. also recently performed a systematic review of outcomes in the treatment of shoulder PJI, evaluating a total of 669 patients across 30 studies. *P. acnes* was the most commonly reported bacteria in the included studies. They found no significant differences in eradication rates of PJI in one- and two-stage exchange surgeries and resection arthroplasties (all >90%), while antibiotic suppression (50%) and irrigation and debridement with implant retention (68.6%) had significantly worse PJI eradication rates (Table 12.3) [81].

Studies with Unexpected Positive Culture Results

Several studies have evaluated outcomes in case with unexpected positive culture results. Topolski et al. reported on 75 cases of revision arthroplasty with unexpected positive cultures. Fifty-four of 75 were treated with standard postoperative antibiotics. Ten patients underwent a second revision surgery, only one of which was for a documented recurrent infection, though seven of

Table 12.3 Infection outcomes by treatment regimen

	Antibiotics only	Resection or arthrodesis	I&D, implant retention	Antibiotic spacer	One-stage revision (+UPC)	One-stage revision (−UPC)	Two-stage revision
Total	8	90	35	31	282	72	97
Successful treatment	4	84	24	28	254	66	91
% Cured	50%	93.3%	68.6%	90.3%	90.1%	91.7%	93.8%
Failed treatment	4	6	11	3	28	6	6
% Failed	50%	6.7%	31.4%	9.7%	9.9%	8.3%	6.2%

Used with permission from Nelson et. al. [81]
Data pooled from the following references: [1, 3, 5–7, 9, 10, 17, 22–24, 28, 29, 34, 41, 43–45, 50–57]
I&D irrigation and débridement, *+UPC* included unexpected positive cultures as one-stage revisions, *−UPC* excluding unexpected positive cultures

the ten had positive cultures at the time of the second revision [27]. Kelly and Hobgood evaluated eight patients with unexpected positive cultures and noted that two of eight developed a late infection. They recommended placing all revisions on oral antibiotics until cultures are negative and that culture-positive patients should be treated with 6 weeks of IV antibiotics [28]. Grosso et al. similarly reviewed 17 patients with unexpected positive cultures who were not treated with prolonged antibiotic therapy and noted recurrent infection in 1 of 17. There was no difference in recurrence rate or functional outcomes in these patients compared to one- and two-stage revisions for infection [82]. In the largest series to date, Foruria et al. evaluated the results of 107 consecutive cases of revision shoulder arthroplasty without preoperative or intraoperative signs of infection that were found to have at least one positive intraoperative culture. Sixty-eight (64%) of the cases grew *P. acnes*. Following one-stage revision, 53 cases were treated with an extended course of antibiotics, while 54 were not. At mean follow-up of 5.6 years, 11/107 (10%) cases had a subsequent positive culture result either by aspirate or during a second revision surgery that matched the culture result of the original revision surgery. Ten of the cases were *P. acnes* positive. Treatment with antibiotics did not appear to lower the risk of having a second positive culture result [77].

Authors Preferred Management

Currently, our preferred management approach for a chronic PJI of the shoulder is a two-stage reimplantation when one or more perioperative signs of infection are present, particularly positive serum ESR and CRP, positive preoperative synovial aspirate, positive intraoperative gross findings of infection, and positive intraoperative frozen sections. However, many patients with a chronic indolent infection may have none of these positive perioperative signs of infection and, therefore, undergo a one-stage revision shoulder arthroplasty for an aseptic indication. We, therefore, routinely maintain all presumed aseptic revision shoulder arthroplasty cases on oral antibiotics postoperatively until all cultures are negative, due to the possibility of postoperative growth of intraoperative cultures. In this scenario, cases found to have multiple positive intraoperative cultures are treated with 6 weeks of IV antibiotic therapy, with transition to a more extended course of oral antibiotics based on the clinical presentation. If only one intraoperative culture turns positive, no further antibiotic therapy may be needed if the clinical picture is suggestive of a probable contaminant result. This is particularly true if the culture growth is late and all prior components were removed at revision surgery; however, retention of some of the prior components may still be an indication for postoperative antibiotic treatment.

Conclusions

Diagnosis and treatment of infection after shoulder arthroplasty is a complex and challenging problem. Evaluation of a persistently painful shoulder arthroplasty should start with a thorough history and physical examination and a high index of suspicion for infection by the treating surgeon. Serum laboratory studies and other standard diagnostic tests have been shown to be less sensitive in the shoulder than in the hip and knee but can still play a role in diagnosis if a positive result is obtained. Newer synovial biomarker tests have shown promise for diagnosing shoulder PJI. Most studies on outcomes of treatment for infected shoulder arthroplasty report results on only a small number of patients, often with varying treatment protocols. This lack of uniformity in treatment approach, as well as in reported outcome measures, makes it difficult to draw definitive conclusions on specific treatment methods. As the most common clinical scenario in shoulder PJI is a chronic infection involving an indolent organism, further data is particularly needed to better define the indications and outcomes in cases of one- and two-stage exchange. Improved diagnostic testing to better identify *P. acnes* and other less virulent organisms preoperatively or intraoperatively may help to more clearly define indications for one- versus two-stage exchange, as well as the need for postoperative antibiotic therapy in the setting of a presumed aseptic one-stage revision with unexpected positive culture results.

This chapter highlights the lack of precise algorithms for both diagnosis and treatment of shoulder PJI. Essential to development of such algorithms is arriving at a consensus definition for shoulder PJI, based on a combination of preoperative and intraoperative findings and intraoperative culture results. The evaluation and management of the painful shoulder arthroplasty remains highly variable and needs to be standardized in such areas as preoperative surgical site preparation, choice and timing of intraoperative antibiotics during revision surgery, number and type of intraoperative cultures obtained during revision surgery, culture methods and length of time for culture incubation, and choice and length of postoperative antibiotic therapy. A consensus definition of PJI and a standardized approach to evaluation and management will aid in developing and interpreting future research studies and will ultimately lead to more refined diagnostic algorithms and clinical treatment pathways. Currently, decision-making for each patient should be based on the results of preoperative testing, time since the index arthroplasty, the infecting organism, patient comorbidities, the status of implant fixation, glenoid and humeral bone stock, and the status of the deltoid and rotator cuff.

References

1. Kim SH, Wise BL, Zhang Y, Szabo RM. Increasing incidence of shoulder arthroplasty in the United States. https://doi.org/10.2106/JBJS.J.01994.
2. Padegimas EM, Maltenfort M, Ramsey ML, Williams GR, Parvizi J, Namdari S. Periprosthetic shoulder infection in the United States: incidence and economic burden. J Shoulder Elb Surg. 2015. https://doi.org/10.1016/j.jse.2014.11.044.
3. Kamal Bohsali BI, Wirth MA, Rockwood CA Jr. Complications of total shoulder arthroplasty. J Bone Joint Surg. 2006;88:2279–92.
4. Gonzalez JF, Alami GB, Baque F, Walch G, Boileau P. Complications of unconstrained shoulder prostheses. J Shoulder Elb Surg. 2011. https://doi.org/10.1016/j.jse.2010.11.017.
5. Zumstein MA, Pinedo M, Old J, Boileau P. Problems, complications, reoperations, and revisions in reverse total shoulder arthroplasty: a systematic review. J Shoulder Elb Surg. 2011. https://doi.org/10.1016/j.jse.2010.08.001.
6. Trappey GJ, O'Connor DP, Bradley Edwards T. What are the instability and infection rates after reverse shoulder arthroplasty? Clin Orthop Relat Res. 2011. https://doi.org/10.1007/s11999-010-1686-9.
7. Walch G, Bacle G, Nove-Josserand L, John Smithers C. Do the indications, results, and complications of reverse shoulder arthroplasty change with surgeons experience? J Shoulder Elb Surg. 2012;21:1470–7.
8. Strickland JP, Sperling JW, Cofield RH, Sperling RJW. The results of two-stage re-implantation for infected shoulder replacement. J Bone Joint Surg Br. 2008;90:460–5.

9. Cheung EV, Sperling JW, Cofield RH. Infection associated with hematoma formation after shoulder arthroplasty. Clin Orthop Relat Res. 2008;466:1363. https://doi.org/10.1007/s11999-008-0226-3.
10. Hatta T, Werthel J-D, Wagner ER, Itoi E, Steinmann SP, Cofield RH, Sperling JW. Effect of smoking on complications following primary shoulder arthroplasty. 2017. https://doi.org/10.1016/j.jse.2016.09.011.
11. Werthel JD, Hatta T, Schoch B, Cofield R, Sperling JW, Elhassan BT. Is previous nonarthroplasty surgery a risk factor for periprosthetic infection in primary shoulder arthroplasty? J Shoulder Elb Surg. 2017;26:635. https://doi.org/10.1016/j.jse.2016.10.020.
12. Bala A, Penrose CT, Visgauss JD, Seyler TM, Randell TR, Bolognesi MP, Garrigues GE. Total shoulder arthroplasty in patients with HIV infection: complications, comorbidities, and trends. J Shoulder Elb Surg. 2016;25:1971. https://doi.org/10.1016/j.jse.2016.02.033.
13. Singh JA, Sperling JW, Schleck C, Harmsen WS, Cofield RH. Periprosthetic infections after total shoulder arthroplasty: a 33-year perspective. J Shoulder Elb Surg. 2012;21:1534. https://doi.org/10.1016/j.jse.2012.01.006.
14. Saltzman MD, Marecek GS, Edwards SL, Kalainov DM. Infection after shoulder surgery. J Am Acad Orthop Surg. 2011;19:208.
15. Coste JS, Reig S, Trojani C, Berg M, Walch G, Boileau P, Surgeon O. Shoulder the management of infection in arthroplasty of the shoulder. J Bone Joint Surg Br. 2004;86:65–9.
16. Themistocleous G, Zalavras C, Stine I, Zachos V, Itamura J. Prolonged implantation of an antibiotic cement spacer for management of shoulder sepsis in compromised patients. J Shoulder Elb Surg. 2007;16:701. https://doi.org/10.1016/j.jse.2007.02.118.
17. Pottinger P, Butler-Wu S, Neradilek MB, Merritt A, Bertelsen A, Jette JL, Warme WJ, Matsen FA. Prognostic factors for bacterial cultures positive for Propionibacterium acnes and other organisms in a large series of revision shoulder arthroplasties performed for stiffness, pain, or loosening. J Bone Joint Surg Am Vol. 2012;94:2075. https://doi.org/10.2106/JBJS.K.00861.
18. Millett PJ, Yen YM, Price CS, Horan MP, Van Der Meijden OA, Elser F. Propionobacter acnes infection as an occult cause of postoperative shoulder pain: a case series. Clin Orthop Relat Res. 2011;469:2824. https://doi.org/10.1007/s11999-011-1767-4.
19. Dodson CC, Craig E V, Cordasco FA, Dines DM, Dines JS, Dicarlo E, Brause BD, Warren RF. Propionibacterium acnes infection after shoulder arthroplasty: a diagnostic challenge. https://doi.org/10.1016/j.jse.2009.07.065.
20. Nelson GN, Paxton ES, Narzikul A, Williams G, Lazarus MD, Abboud JA. Leukocyte esterase in the diagnosis of shoulder periprosthetic joint infection. J Shoulder Elb Surg. 2015;24:1421. https://doi.org/10.1016/j.jse.2015.05.034.
21. Villacis D, Merriman JA, Yalamanchili R, Omid R, Itamura J, Hatch III GFR. Serum interleukin-6 as a marker of periprosthetic shoulder infection. https://doi.org/10.2106/JBJS.L.01634.
22. Frangiamore SJ, Saleh A, Kovac MF, Grosso MJ, Zhang X, Bauer TW, Daly TM, Ricchetti ET, Iannotti JP. Synovial interleukin-6 as a predictor of periprosthetic shoulder infection. J Bone Joint Surg. 2015;97:63–70.
23. Grosso MJ, Frangiamore SJ, Saleh A, Kovac MF, Hayashi R, Ricchetti ET, Bauer TW, Iannotti JP. Poor utility of serum interleukin-6 levels to predict indolent periprosthetic shoulder infections. J Shoulder Elb Surg. 2014;23:1277. https://doi.org/10.1016/j.jse.2013.12.023.
24. Frangiamore SJ, Saleh A, Grosso MJ, Farias Kovac M, Zhang X, Daly TM, Bauer TW, Derwin KA, Iannotti JP, Ricchetti ET. Neer Award 2015: analysis of cytokine profiles in the diagnosis of periprosthetic joint infections of the shoulder. J Shoulder Elb Surg. 2017;26:186–96.
25. White J, Kelly M, Dunsmuir R. C-reactive protein level after total hip and total knee replacement. J Bone Joint Surg Br. 1998;80–B:909–11.
26. Della Valle C, Parvizi J, Bauer TW, et al. Diagnosis of periprosthetic joint infections of the hip and knee overview and rationale. J Am Acad Orthop Surg. 2010;18:760–70.
27. Topolski MS, Chin PYK, Sperling JW, Cofield RH. Revision shoulder arthroplasty with positive intraoperative cultures: the value of preoperative studies and intraoperative histology. J Shoulder Elb Surg. 2006;15:402. https://doi.org/10.1016/j.jse.2005.10.001.
28. Kelly JD, Hobgood ER. Positive culture rate in revision shoulder arthroplasty. Clin Orthop Relat Res. 2009;467:2343. https://doi.org/10.1007/s11999-009-0875-x.
29. Nodzo SR, Boyle KK, Bhimani S, Duquin TR, Miller AO, Westrich GH. Propionibacterium acnes host inflammatory response during periprosthetic infection is joint specific. HSS J. 2017;13:159. https://doi.org/10.1007/s11420-016-9528-2.
30. Di Cesare PE, Chang E, Preston CF, Liu C. Serum interleukin-6 as a marker of periprosthetic infection following total hip and knee arthroplasty. J Bone Joint Surg Am. 2005;87:1921–7.
31. Chryssikos T, Parvizi J, Ghanem E, Newberg A, Zhuang H, Alavi A. FDG-PET imaging can diagnose periprosthetic infection of the hip. Clin Orthop Relat Res. 2008;466:1338. https://doi.org/10.1007/s11999-008-0237-0.
32. Codd T, Yamaguchi K, Pollock R, Flatow E, Bigliani L. Infected shoulder arthroplasties: treatment with staged reimplantations vs. resection arthroplasty. J Shoulder Elb Surg. 1996;5:2.
33. Patel A, Calfee RP, Plante M, Fischer SA, Green A. Propionibacterium acnes colonization of the human shoulder. J Shoulder Elb Surg. 2009;18:897–902.
34. Piper KE, Jacobson MJ, Cofield RH, et al. Microbiologic diagnosis of prosthetic shoul-

der infection by use of implant sonication. J Clin Microbiol. 2009;47:1878. https://doi.org/10.1128/JCM.01686-08.
35. Hsu JE, Gorbaty JD, Whitney IJ, Matsen FA III. Single-stage revision is effective for failed shoulder arthroplasty with positive cultures for Propionibacterium. J Bone Joint Surg. 2016;98:2047–51.
36. Frangiamore SJ, Saleh A, Grosso MJ, Farias Kovac M, Higuera CA, Iannotti JP, Ricchetti ET. α-Defensin as a predictor of periprosthetic shoulder infection. J Shoulder Elb Surg. 2015;24:1021–7.
37. Tischler EH, Cavanaugh PK, Parvizi J. Leukocyte esterase strip test: matched for musculoskeletal infection society criteria. J Bone Joint Surg Am Vol. 2014;96:1917. https://doi.org/10.2106/JBJS.M.01591.
38. Wetters NG, Berend KR, Lombardi AV, Morris MJ, Tucker TL, Della Valle CJ. Leukocyte esterase reagent strips for the rapid diagnosis of periprosthetic joint infection. J Arthroplast. 2012;27:8–11.
39. Dilisio MF, Miller LR, Warner JJ, Higgins LD. Arthroscopic tissue culture for the evaluation of periprosthetic shoulder infection. J Bone Joint Surg Am Vol. 2014;96:1952. https://doi.org/10.2106/JBJS.M.01512.
40. Della Valle CJ, Scher DM, Kim YH, Oxley CM, Desai P, Zuckerman JD, Di Cesare PE. The role of intraoperative Gram stain in revision total joint arthroplasty. J Arthroplast. 1999;14:500–4.
41. Oethinger M, Warner DK, Schindler SA, Kobayashi H, Bauer TW. Diagnosing periprosthetic infection false-positive intraoperative Gram stains. 2010. https://doi.org/10.1007/s11999-010-1589-9.
42. Morgan PM, Sharkey P, Ghanem E, Parvizi J, Clohisy JC, Burnett RSJ, Barrack RL. The value of intraoperative gram stain in revision total knee arthroplasty. J Bone Joint Surg Am Vol. 2009;91:2124. https://doi.org/10.2106/JBJS.H.00853.
43. Sperling JW, Tomasz KW, Hanssen AD, Cofield RH. Infection after shoulder arthroplasty. Clin Orthop Relat Res. 2001;382:206–211б.
44. Matsen FA III, Butler-Wu S, Carofino BC, Jette JL, Bertelsen A, Bumgarner R. Origin of Propionibacterium in surgical wounds and evidence-based approach for culturing Propionibacterium from surgical sites. J Bone Joint Surg. 2013;95–A:e1811–7.
45. Cuff DJ, Virani NA, Levy J, Frankle MA, Derasari A, Hines B, Pupello DR, Cancio M, Mighell M. The treatment of deep shoulder infection and glenohumeral instability with debridement, reverse shoulder arthroplasty and post- operative antibiotics. J Bone Joint Surg Br. 2008;90:336–42.
46. Grosso MJ, Frangiamore SJ, Ricchetti ET, Bauer TW, Iannotti JP. Sensitivity of frozen section histology for identifying Propionibacterium acnes infections in revision shoulder arthroplasty. J Bone Joint Surg. 2014;96:442. https://doi.org/10.2106/JBJS.M.00258.
47. Grosso MJ, Frangiamore SJ, Yakubek G, Bauer TW, Iannotti JP, Ricchetti ET. Performance of implant sonication culture for the diagnosis of periprosthetic shoulder infection. J Shoulder Elb Surg. 2018;27:211. https://doi.org/10.1016/j.jse.2017.08.008.
48. Parvizi J, Jacovides C, Zmistowski B, Kwang Am Jung. Definition of periprosthetic joint infection is there a consensus? 2011. https://doi.org/10.1007/s11999-011-1971-2.
49. Parvizi J, Gehrke T. Definition of periprosthetic joint infection. J Arthroplast. 2014;29:1331.
50. Lee MJ, Pottinger PS, Butler-Wu S, Bumgarner RE, Russ SM, Matsen FA. Propionibacterium persists in the skin despite standard surgical preparation. J Bone Joint Surg Am Vol. 2014;96:1447–50.
51. Matsen FA, Russ SM, Bertelsen A, Butler-Wu S, Pottinger PS. Propionibacterium can be isolated from deep cultures obtained at primary arthroplasty despite intravenous antimicrobial prophylaxis. J Shoulder Elb Surg. 2015;24:844. https://doi.org/10.1016/j.jse.2014.10.016.
52. Butler-Wu SM, Burns EM, Pottinger PS, Magaret AS, Rakeman JL, Matsen FA, Cookson BT. Optimization of periprosthetic culture for diagnosis of Propionibacterium acnes prosthetic joint infection. J Clin Microbiol. 2011;49:2490. https://doi.org/10.1128/JCM.00450-11.
53. Ahsan ZS, Somerson JS, Matsen Iii FA. Characterizing the Propionibacterium load in revision shoulder arthroplasty a study of 137 culture-positive cases. J Bone Joint Surg. 2017;99–A:150–4.
54. Levy O, Iyer S, Atoun E, Peter N, Hous N, Cash D, Musa F, Narvani AA. Propionibacterium acnes: an underestimated etiology in the pathogenesis of osteoarthritis? J Shoulder Elb Surg. 2013;22:505. https://doi.org/10.1016/j.jse.2012.07.007.
55. Maccioni CB, Woodbridge AB, Balestro J-CY, Figtree MC, Hudson BJ, Cass B, Young AA. Low rate of Propionibacterium acnes in arthritic shoulders undergoing primary total shoulder replacement surgery using a strict specimen collection technique. 2015. https://doi.org/10.1016/j.jse.2014.12.026.
56. Mook WR, Klement MR, Green CL, Hazen KC, Garrigues GE. The incidence of Propionibacterium acnes in open shoulder surgery a controlled diagnostic study. https://doi.org/10.2106/JBJS.N.00784.
57. Frangiamore SJ, Saleh A, Grosso MJ, Alolabi B, Bauer TW, Iannotti JP, Ricchetti ET. Early versus late culture growth of Propionibacterium acnes in revision shoulder arthroplasty. https://doi.org/10.2106/JBJS.N.00881.
58. Assenmacher AT, Alentorn-Geli E, Dennison T, Baghdadi YMK, Cofield RH, Sánchez-Sotelo J, Sperling JW. Two-stage reimplantation for the treatment of deep infection after shoulder arthroplasty. J Shoulder Elb Surg. 2017;26:1978. https://doi.org/10.1016/j.jse.2017.05.005.
59. Verhelst L, Stuyck J, Bellemans J, Debeer P. Resection arthroplasty of the shoulder as a salvage procedure for deep shoulder infection: does the use of a cement spacer improve outcome? J Shoulder Elb Surg. 2011;20:1224. https://doi.org/10.1016/j.jse.2011.02.003.

60. Rispoli DM, Sperling JW, Athwal GS, Schleck CD, Cofield RH. Pain relief and functional results after resection arthroplasty of the shoulder. J Bone Joint Surg Br. 2007;89:1184–7.
61. Braman JP, Sprague M, Bishop J, Lo IK, Lee EW, Flatow EL. The outcome of resection shoulder arthroplasty for recalcitrant shoulder infections. J Shoulder Elb Surg. 2006;15:549. https://doi.org/10.1016/j.jse.2005.11.001.
62. Beekman PDA, Katusic D, Berghs BM, et al. One-stage revision for patients with a chronically infected reverse total shoulder replacement. J Bone Joint Surg Br. 2010;92:817–22.
63. Ince A, Seemann K, Frommelt L, Katzer A, Loehr JF. One-stage exchange shoulder arthroplasty for peri-prosthetic infection. J Bone Joint Surg Br. 2005;87:814–8.
64. Sabesan VJ, Ho JC, Kovacevic D, Iannotti JP. Two-stage reimplantation for treating prosthetic shoulder infections. Clin Orthop Relat Res. 2011;469:2538. https://doi.org/10.1007/s11999-011-1774-5.
65. Coffey MJ, Ely EE, Crosby LA. Treatment of glenohumeral sepsis with a commercially produced antibiotic-impregnated cement spacer. J Shoulder Elb Surg. 2010;19:868. https://doi.org/10.1016/j.jse.2010.01.012.
66. Stine IA, Lee B, Zalavras CG, Hatch G, Itamura JM. Management of chronic shoulder infections utilizing a fixed articulating antibiotic-loaded spacer. J Shoulder Elb Surg. 2010;19:739. https://doi.org/10.1016/j.jse.2009.10.002.
67. Buchalter DB, Mahure SA, Mollon B, Yu S, Kwon YW, Zuckerman JD. Two-stage revision for infected shoulder arthroplasty. J Shoulder Elb Surg. 2017;26:939. https://doi.org/10.1016/j.jse.2016.09.056.
68. Segawa H, Tsukayama DT, Kyle RF, Becker DA, Gustilo RB. Infection after total knee arthroplasty a retrospective study of the treatment of eighty-one infections*. J Bone Joint Surg Am. 1999;81:1434–45.
69. Khassebaf J, Hellmark B, Davidsson S, Unemo M, Nilsdotter-Augustinsson Å, Söderquist B. Antibiotic susceptibility of Propionibacterium acnes isolated from orthopaedic implant-associated infections. Anaerobe. 2015;32:57–62.
70. Ricchetti ET, Frangiamore SJ, Grosso MJ, Alolabi B, Saleh A, Bauer TW, Iannotti JP. Diagnosis of Periprosthetic infection after shoulder arthroplasty: a critical analysis review. JBJS Rev. 2013;1:1–9.
71. Dennison T, Alentorn-Geli E, Assenmacher AT, Sperling JW, Sánchez-Sotelo J, Cofield RH. Management of acute or late hematogenous infection after shoulder arthroplasty with irrigation, débridement, and component retention. J Shoulder Elb Surg. 2017;26:73. https://doi.org/10.1016/j.jse.2016.05.018.
72. Sperling JW, Cofield RH. Humeral windows in revision shoulder arthroplasty. J Shoulder Elb Surg. 2005;14:258. https://doi.org/10.1016/j.jse.2004.09.004.
73. Stevens NM, Kim HM, Armstrong AD. Functional outcomes after shoulder resection: the patient's perspective. J Shoulder Elb Surg. 2015;24:e247–54.
74. Muh SJ, Streit JJ, Lenarz CJ, et al. Resection arthroplasty for failed shoulder arthroplasty. J Shoulder Elb Surg. 2013;22:247. https://doi.org/10.1016/j.jse.2012.05.025.
75. Klatte TO, Junghans K, Al-Khateeb H, et al. Single-stage revision for peri-prosthetic shoulder infection outcomes and results. Bone Joint J. 2013;9595:391–5.
76. McGoldrick E, McElvany MD, Butler-Wu S, Pottinger PS, Matsen FA. Substantial cultures of Propionibacterium can be found in apparently aseptic shoulders revised three years or more after the index arthroplasty. J Shoulder Elb Surg. 2015;24:31. https://doi.org/10.1016/j.jse.2014.05.008.
77. Foruria AM, Fox TJ, Sperling JW, Cofield RH. Clinical meaning of unexpected positive cultures (UPC) in revision shoulder arthroplasty. J Shoulder Elb Surg. 2013;22:620. https://doi.org/10.1016/j.jse.2012.07.017.
78. Jaeblon T. Polymethylmethacrylate: properties and contemporary uses in orthopaedics. J Am Acad Orthop Surg. 2010;18:297–305.
79. Scalise JJ, Iannotti JP. Glenohumeral arthrodesis after failed prosthetic shoulder arthroplasty. https://doi.org/10.2106/JBJS.G.00203.
80. Stone GP, Clark RE, O'Brien KC, Vaccaro L, Simon P, Lorenzetti AJ, Stephens BC, Frankle MA. Surgical management of periprosthetic shoulder infections. J Shoulder Elb Surg. 2017;26:1222. https://doi.org/10.1016/j.jse.2016.11.054.
81. Nelson GN, Davis DE, Namdari S. Outcomes in the treatment of periprosthetic joint infection after shoulder arthroplasty: a systematic review. J Shoulder Elb Surg. 2016;25:1337–45.
82. Grosso MJ, Sabesan VJ, Ho JC, Ricchetti ET, Iannotti JP. Reinfection rates after 1-stage revision shoulder arthroplasty for patients with unexpected positive intraoperative cultures. J Shoulder Elb Surg. 2012;21:754. https://doi.org/10.1016/j.jse.2011.08.052.

13 Diagnosis, Management, and Prevention of the Unstable Shoulder Arthroplasty

Alexander Martusiewicz and Aaron Chamberlain

Background

The native shoulder has various structures that contribute to joint stability depending on the magnitude of load [1]. Shoulder arthroplasty alters many of these restraints, so careful attention must be directed to implant size, position, and balancing of soft tissues during replacement surgery. Maintaining stability can be difficult, and instability remains the number one combined complication after total and reverse shoulder arthroplasty. Total shoulder arthroplasty (TSA) has reported rates of instability ranging from 1.0% to 31% [2–4]. Reverse shoulder arthroplasty (RSA) has a 2.7–4.7% incidence of instability despite its more constrained design [5, 6].

An unstable shoulder arthroplasty is one of the most difficult complications to manage as noted from the high rate of recurrent instability. Even after revision surgery for instability, over two-thirds of patients can have recurrent symptoms [7]. When revision surgery is limited to a soft tissue repair, only 24% have excellent or satisfactory results [7]. After component revision, the rate of satisfactory results only improves to 48% [8].

The goal of this chapter is to discuss risk factors for instability and how to prevent the complication with appropriate preoperative planning and intraoperative decision-making during shoulder arthroplasty. The chapter will also review how to accurately diagnose instability after arthroplasty, determine its etiology, and institute appropriate management.

Diagnosis of Instability

A recent review of studies in the past decade showed the overall incidence of instability after arthroplasty has decreased, but it is still common [4]. Subtype analysis revealed that instability was the most common complication after RSA and the third most common after anatomic TSA (followed by glenoid loosening and glenoid wear) [4]. Most authors acknowledge that the most important factor in prevention of instability during the index procedure is to utilize meticulous technique. However, when symptoms present, a thorough history and physical exam with appropriate imaging is necessary to diagnose and understand the etiology of instability.

Several different factors may contribute to an unstable arthroplasty. Soft tissue imbalance is a major cause of instability after anatomic TSA and present in most cases, but component malposition also plays a role [5, 7, 9]. Superior and inferior instability can be due to cuff deficiency (in TSA) or inappropriate restoration of humeral length and soft tissue tension after RSA.

A. Martusiewicz, MD · A. Chamberlain, MD, MSc (✉)
Department of Orthopedic Surgery, Washington University, St. Louis, MO, USA
e-mail: amchamberlain@wustl.edu

R. Z. Tashjian (ed.), *Complex and Revision Shoulder Arthroplasty*,
https://doi.org/10.1007/978-3-030-02756-8_13

Factors associated with anterior and posterior instability are less well established. Capsular disruption and subscapularis insufficiency can contribute to anterior instability after anatomic TSA. Humeral component version and head offset can also affect sagittal plane stability. Although there is an overlap in factors contributing to instability in anatomic and reverse shoulder arthroplasty, there are additional implant-specific factors that contribute to instability in reverse shoulder arthroplasty such as adduction impingement and acromiohumeral impingement leading to leveraging of the humeral component away from the glenosphere.

Identifying risk factors for instability preoperatively is one of the most important steps in prevention. In 2016 Boileau et al. found that humeral or glenoid bone loss and soft tissue deficiency were risk factors for instability after RSA [10]. A shortened humerus due to fracture or deformity could lead to failure in restoring humeral length. Excessive medialization in the setting of a glenoid bone defect can also lead to instability. Soft tissue pathology such as subscapularis or rotator cuff deficiency and deltoid atrophy were also contributing factors [10]. The rate of instability is three times higher for reverse shoulder arthroplasty performed in the revision setting compared to primary reverse shoulder arthroplasty [11].

Clinical signs and symptoms of instability may be obvious such as in the case of a locked dislocation, but instability can also present with less obvious findings. There may be subtle mechanical symptoms with pain or exam findings consistent with decreased range of motion and strength [7, 12]. Several authors also stress the importance of physical exam maneuvers to assess translation or dislocation with directional force [7, 12]. An exaggerated sulcus, anterior apprehension, or a positive load and shift can help make the diagnosis.

Radiographic evaluation of the shoulder should include AP, true AP (Grashey), axillary, and scapular-Y views to assess the overall position of the prosthetic components. An axillary view is essential in evaluating glenoid wear and subluxation tendencies of the humerus relative to the glenoid. This information can inform the surgeon as to whether there is sufficient glenoid bone stock to accommodate an anatomic glenoid prosthesis. Understanding preoperative subluxation provides context as to the relative risk of subluxation tendency after anatomic TSA. In cases of severe glenoid wear and/or subluxation, a reverse shoulder arthroplasty should be considered. Contralateral measured humerus x-rays can be helpful with inferior instability to confirm arm lengths in the setting of RSA as failure to restore humeral length is a known risk for recurrent instability [13].

Advanced imaging such as CT arthrogram or ultrasound can be used to evaluate the integrity of the rotator cuff after anatomic TSA. These modalities can quantify tear size, quality of soft tissues, and atrophy of rotator cuff muscle bellies. Ultrasound, which is not affected by metallic artifact, can also assess biceps tendon abnormalities, subacromial or subdeltoid bursitis after shoulder arthroplasty [14]. CT scans provide additional detail when analyzing bony deformity and heterotopic ossification which may lead to impingement and component wear.

Management of Instability in Anatomic Total Shoulder Arthroplasty

After accurately diagnosing the type of shoulder instability, management is based on its direction and etiology. Classifying the direction of instability guides the treatment algorithm. Most common directions of instability are anterior, posterior, and superior (anterosuperior escape). Inferior instability has also been described after a hemiarthroplasty was implanted inferiorly [15]. As previously described, most cases of instability have factors relating to improper soft tissue balancing and component malposition. Both these factors should be scrutinized and corrected as necessary.

Anterior Instability

Anterior instability occurs in 0.9% of cases after TSA and often occurs as a result of an acute event

[3]. Subscapularis rupture or insufficiency often plays a role and can be due to several factors. Overstuffing the joint with an inappropriately large humeral head can cause excessive tension on the subscapularis repair leading to failure. Excessive anteversion (less than 20° of retroversion) or anteriorly directed offset of the humeral head can also increase tension on the subscapularis [1]. Miller reported that previous z-lengthening or medialization of the subscsapularis repair is also a risk factor for rupture [16]. The choice of subscapularis management technique performed at the index procedure may affect risk of subscapularis deficiency. Most commonly the subscapularis is managed with a tenotomy, peel technique, or lesser tuberosity osteotomy. While there is no Level I evidence that conclusively demonstrates superior clinical outcomes of any of these techniques, biomechanical studies have shown a lesser tuberosity osteotomy to have a higher load to failure compared to tenotomy. Variable rates of subscapularis tenotomy repair failures have been reported in the literature ranging up to 40%. However, this did not correlate with clinical exam. Lower rates of tenotomy repair failure have been published using transosseous repair techniques (30% failure) at 4 years' follow-up. In a Level I study, Lapner et al. found no difference in subscapularis strength in the Western Ontario Osteoarthritis of the Shoulder Index (WOOS) or American Shoulder and Elbow Surgeons (ASES) scores at 24 months postoperatively. More recent studies have found a higher rate of a normal lift-off test after LTO (90%) compared to subscapularis peel (70%).

Less commonly, anterior deltoid dysfunction can be a contributing factor to anterior instability. This can be due to muscle-tendon injury or injury to the axillary nerve [1]. Failure to correct excessive anterior glenoid erosion or polyethylene wear may also play a role, especially in cases of post-instability arthropathy.

Early described techniques to manage anterior instability after TSA utilized MERSILENE tape or an allograft Achilles tendon augmentation [12]. A static restraint is created by securing a bone-tendon allograft from the glenoid neck to the humeral head; however, outcome data is limited. Ianotti et al. subsequently described capsular reconstruction using ITB with successful outcomes in seven patients [17]. Sanchez-Sotelo reported on a combination of component revision, cuff repair, capsular plication, and interval closure [17]. Three of seven shoulders with anterior instability required a reoperation for recurrence of the problem. Anterior instability was also associated with a higher failure rate compared to posterior instability. Of the 19 shoulders considered failures (56%), 14 were treated for anterior instability [17].

Dynamic tendon transfers have been described to manage anterior stability. One tendon transfer that has been well described is that of the pectoralis major tendon. Variations of a pectoralis major transfer include transfers superficial or deep to the conjoint tendon as well as complete or split transfers (including only one head of the insertion). Konrad et al. performed a biomechanical analysis comparing transfer of the pectoralis major either above or below the conjoint tendon [18]. The tendon transfer deep to the conjoint tendon restored glenohumeral kinematics that more closely resembled a subscapularis intact shoulder [18]. Ahrens et al. repaired the subscapularis and transferred the pectoralis in the setting of an unstable TSA [19]. More than half of the 33 unstable shoulders had recurrent instability. However the three shoulders converted to a reverse shoulder arthroplasty did not have recurrent symptoms. Similarly Elhassan et al. reported poor results with pectoralis major transfer for anterior instability in TSA, thus advocating for a reliable and predictable solution: reverse shoulder arthroplasty [20].

Authors' Recommendation: Anterior Instability After Anatomic TSA

One of the most common reasons for anterior instability after anatomic TSA is related to subscapularis insufficiency. The decision regarding revision subscapularis repair vs revision to reverse shoulder arthroplasty should be based on the etiology of instability, patient's age, and comorbidities. In the case of an acute subscapularis repair disruption in the setting of viable subscapularis tissue within 6 weeks of the index procedure, revision repair should be considered. The recommendation for revision repair is strengthened if there is anterior subluxation noted on axillary radiographs. Humeral head exchange or component revision should also be optimized at the time of revision repair especially if an oversized humeral head prosthesis was placed originally. In an elderly patient or in anterior instability related to chronic subscapularis deficiency, a reverse shoulder arthroplasty provides a reliable outcome and would be the primary recommendation.

Given the lack of convincing data supporting capsular reconstruction, capsular plication, and pectoralis major tendon transfer, these procedures should be reserved for an increasingly young population where revision subscapularis repair is not possible but the patient is a poor candidate for a reverse shoulder arthroplasty. However, given its increased durability and predictable outcomes, the reverse shoulder arthroplasty should be considered even in appropriately indicated younger populations.

Posterior Instability

Posterior instability occurs at about the same frequency as anterior instability (1% incidence) [3]. Posterior instability after anatomic TSA most commonly occurs early in the postoperative period. However, it may also occur chronically in shoulders that exhibit preoperative posterior subluxation. B-type glenoid wear patterns are associated with an increased risk of posterior instability after TSA. Patients with osteoarthritis often have posterior glenoid erosion with contracture and tightening of the anterior capsule and subscapularis. The combination of increased glenoid retroversion and posterior humeral head translation can predispose patients to posterior instability [13]. Sanchez-Sotelo reported on a cohort of 14 patients with posterior instability. A combination of posterior cuff dysfunction, component malposition, posterior bone loss, and capsular laxity were identified as risk factors predisposing to posterior instability in this group [7].

In terms of component positioning, excessive humeral retroversion (greater than 45°) and/or glenoid retroversion (greater than 20°) has been associated with posterior instability [1]. Subscapularis contracture or lateral malunion of the lesser tuberosity can also cause a posteriorly directed force on the humeral head. This highlights the importance of releases around the subscapularis for mobilization and anatomic reduction of the lesser tuberosity.

To address posterior instability, soft tissue tension and component position must again be evaluated. If implant version is outside the parameters above, component revision should be performed. In the setting of minor humeral version differences, compensatory relative humeral anteversion has been shown to be ineffective at significantly altering the center of rotation or address posterior instability [17]. Anteriorly offsetting the eccentric humeral head centers the prosthetic humeral head on the prosthetic glenoid and has been shown to increase the force and energy required to displace the prosthesis posteriorly [21]. Hsu et al. reported on a small cohort of patients who were noted to have posterior decentering of the humeral head by placing the eccentricity of the humeral head prosthesis in an anterior position rather than in the normal posterior offset.

Posterior capsular plication is a beneficial technique to address persistent posterior instability. When noted intraoperatively, removal of the prosthetic humeral head with lateral translation of the humerus will expose the posterior capsule. Multiple nonabsorbable sutures can then be placed with a figure-of-eight technique while the humerus is translated. The lateral translation is then released, and the sutures are tied to allow adequate tensioning of the posterior capsule. Alentorn-Geli showed restoration of soft tissue balance in 71% of shoulders with persistent intraoperative posterior instability [22]. Gee also describes arthroscopic capsular plication using two suture anchors as a sole treatment of posterior instability [23]. The technique restored soft tissue balance in 27 of the 38 shoulders (71%). The remaining 11 shoulders had evidence of residual posterior subluxation, two of which dislocated [23].

With respect to the glenoid, there are several techniques to correct version and improve stability. A high-side (anterior) ream, bone graft, or an augmented glenoid can all be used to restore anatomic or near-anatomic glenoid retroversion. Published data describing outcomes using these techniques is limited in quantity and follow-up. Techniques have also been described in which an arthroscopic technique is used to place a bone block posteriorly to improve stability [24]. Again, clinical outcomes data using this technique is very limited.

If a subscapularis contracture is present, mobilization can be improved by performing a thorough 360° release of all scar tissue and glenohumeral ligaments around the tendon [25]. There is also an option for a z-lengthening of the tendon, although this can predispose injury to the tissue [26]. When severe internal anterior contracture is noted, medializatino of the repaired insertion of the subscapularis (in the setting of a subscapularis peel) will decrease the posteriorly directed force on the humeral head.

Prior to closure, humeral translation relative to the glenoid should be evaluated. If there is greater than 50% translation without "bounce back," the rotator interval can be closed with a lateral suture to increase stability.

Despite treatment with stem revision, glenoid grafting, and posterior plication, Sanchez-Sotelo reported persistent instability in 36% of patients [7]. Although these outcomes are improved compared to anterior instability, it reiterates the difficulty in treating this complication. Postoperative immobilization in external rotation can also help the posterior soft tissues heal in appropriate tension [27].

Author's Recommendation: Posterior Instability After Anatomic TSA

It is important to follow a consistent algorithm in cases with posterior instability. Intraoperatively, component positioning should be optimized. Partial or complete correction of glenoid retroversion with a high-side reaming or glenoid implant technique (bone graft or augmented prosthesis) should be performed first.

The humeral components should then be optimized with appropriate head size selection. Stability can then be tested with trial components in place. If needed, the height of the humeral head can be increased slightly; however, care should be taken to avoid "overstuffing" as this will cause excessive strain on the rotator cuff. If persistent posterior instability persists, the authors will then dial the eccentricity of the humeral head prosthesis anteriorly (opposite the normal posterior anatomic offset) in order to translate the center of rotation anteriorly and center the humeral head prosthesis on the glenoid prosthesis.

If posterior instability is persistent after glenoid and humeral head parameters are optimized, posterior capsular plication stiches are then placed as described above. Stability is trialed once more, and if there is subtle posterior translation, this can be addressed with rotator interval closure. If there remains some concern for instability, one should consider immobilizing the shoulder in a relatively externally rotated position and may consider altering postoperative rehabilitation to avoid forward elevation for a period of up to 6 weeks. If there is excessive posterior translation without "bounce back" noted at the time of surgery, a reverse shoulder arthroplasty is a reliable and predictable option in the appropriately indicated patient.

Superior Instability (Anterosuperior Escape)

Superior (anterosuperior escape) is the most common direction of shoulder instability after total shoulder arthroplasty, occurring with a 3% incidence [27]. Rotator cuff deficiency is the primary factor that affects superior instability. Although significant rotator cuff tears are the most common cause, Young et al. found that fatty infiltration of the infraspinatus was associated with proximal migration of the humeral implant in TSA [28]. There is also a correlation with tear size and the risk of proximal migration [29].

Other factors that contribute to anterosuperior escape include coracoacromial arch insufficiency, anterior deltoid dysfunction, and failure of tuberosity union after fracture. Superior humeral head malposition or "overstuffing" with a large humeral head can also increase stress on the rotator cuff and cause eventual tearing.

Managing superior instability involves soft tissue reconstruction and component modification. Achilles allograft reconstruction of the coracoacromial (CA) arch is a reported technique, but outcome data is limited [13]. Galatz reported good success with subcoracoid pectoralis major transfer in the setting of anterosuperior escape [30]. However, the most predictable revision is to reverse shoulder arthroplasty with 78% excellent or good results and consistent improvements with forward elevation from 50° to 130° [31].

Since the introduction of the reverse shoulder arthroplasty (RSA) in the United States after FDA approval in 2003, it has been demonstrated to be a reliable solution for instability secondary to cuff deficiency after TSA. The increased constraint of the implant and the option to increase length and offset make it an especially attractive option [32]. Abdel initially reported good short-term results [33]. Of 33 unstable anatomic shoulder arthroplasties, 31 maintained stability after conversion to reverse at 3.5 years. The other two dislocated at 2.5 weeks and 3 months postoperatively. They also demonstrated consistent improvements in forward elevation, averaging over 50°. Hernandez showed similar results with 87% and 79% survivorship free from dislocation at 2 and 5 years, respectively [32]. Patients with a BMI > 35 and a prior hemiarthroplasty were also found to be at increased risk for persistent instability [32].

Conversion to RSA is an excellent tool to address cuff deficiency after TSA and its associated instability. However, attention must be directed to ensure correct implant placement, as instability is the most common complication after reverse shoulder arthroplasty [4].

Authors' Recommendation: Anterosuperior Instability After Anatomic TSA

Anterosuperior instability after TSA is most commonly due to rotator cuff failure. This may include failure of the subscapularis repair and/or a disruption of the posterosuperior cuff. In the setting of significant posterosuperior cuff failure with or without subscapularis deficiency, there are not many surgical options that provide reliable and predictable management for anterosuperior escape. In this setting, the authors recommend a reverse shoulder arthroplasty as it is most likely to produce a reliable, predictable outcome given its inherent stabilizing constraint and distalization of the humerus as described above.

Inferior Instability

Inferior instability most frequently occurs as a complication of acute fracture treatment [1]. Excessive shortening of the humeral shaft and low placement of the humeral component result in inappropriate deltoid tensioning. This leads to relative dysfunction of the deltoid in maintaining axial stability of the implant. Less commonly an axillary nerve palsy or rotator interval defect may also contribute.

To address inferior instability, revising the humeral stem to the proper height is critical.

Intraoperatively the pectoralis major tendon can serve as a landmark for humeral height. The superior border of this tendon lies on average 5.64 cm from the top of the humeral head [34]. Lo also advises the use of intraoperative fluoroscopy to confirm appropriate height and positioning of the humeral component. The Gothic arch technique can be useful in assessing the anatomic relationship of the humeral neck to the scapular neck [27]. The relative height of the greater tuberosity to the humeral head can also be used as an intraoperative landmark (8 mm +/− 3 mm) [35]. Ideally, after implant placement, the humeral head should translate with traction to a point in the upper one-third of the glenoid [13].

Management of Instability in Reverse Shoulder Arthroplasty

Although published dislocation rates after reverse total shoulder arthroplasty have decreased from 15% to 3% over the past decade, various factors can still be modified to avoid the complication [4, 36–38]. Appropriate implant version and offset and arm length are critical for implant stability. Kohan et al. reported the two main etiologies for instability were inappropriate soft tissue balancing and instability due to impingement or liner failure. After 3 months, 80% of dislocated RSAs dislocated due to adduction impingement with evidence of either heterotopic ossification or asymmetric polyethylene wear [5].

Padegimas reported revision reverse total shoulder arthroplasty (odds ratio of 7.5) and a higher body mass index (odds ratio of 1.09) to be independent risk factors for RSA dislocations [38]. Their results were also consistent with previous studies that male sex, revision surgery, and subscapularis insufficiency were risks factors for instability after RSA [38].

Initial closed reduction in the setting of early instability has modest success rates of 44–62% and can be initially attempted, but if instability persists, it should be addressed operatively [37, 39].

Impingement

Impingement after RSA can occur in several locations including posterior, anterior, and inferior, all of which should be thoroughly evaluated during revision for an unstable RSA. Incomplete resection of osteophytes, especially posteriorly where access can be more difficult, may cause the implant to lever. Non-united tuberosity fragments posteriorly can also be a source of impingement as well. Acromial impingement may also occur in high-offset implants with minimal lengthening. Implants with a valgus neck shaft angle, particularly in thin patients, can cause adduction impingement. Inferior impingement with adduction can lead to instability and is commonly a result of inferior heterotopic ossification along the axillary border of the scapula and glenoid neck as well as inferior scar tissue.

In any arthroplasty, impingement can be addressed by increasing the angle at which bone or implant contact occurs to cause levering. Appropriate excision of osteophytes or heterotopic ossification should be the initial focus. Component positioning should then be evaluated. Inferior placement and/or lateralization of the glenosphere center of rotation can prevent adduction impingement along the inferior glenoid neck. Inferior placement can also increase the distance from the acromion to avoid proximal impingement. Care should be taken with significantly reducing the neck-shaft angle of the humerus as this will limit impingement but will also increase instability due to the biomechanics of the implant.

Glenospheres with increased diameter can also provide improved stability and range of motion as long as the humeral cup depth-diameter ratio is favorable [40]. Differences in glenosphere offset and polyethylene component morphology have also been shown to effect notching (adduction impingement) [41]. A lateral-based prosthesis will decrease the rate of notching compared to a Grammont style design [42]. Depending on whether the impingement is proximal or in adduction, choosing a humeral implant with an appropriate neck-shaft angle can prevent the implant from engaging the area of concern.

Deltoid Dysfunction

A reverse shoulder arthroplasty functions through optimizing the deltoid moment arm. Implant malposition that negates this principle or any insult to the deltoid can lead to instability in RSA.

Suboptimal deltoid tensioning is often a result of incorrect surgical technique. Insufficient lengthening, superior baseplate tilt, or excessive glenoid medialization may all be contributing factors [4]. Addressing these issues involves revising component position.

Deltoid dysfunction can also occur from intraoperative injury to the axillary nerve or iatrogenic trauma that causes the deltoid to rupture. A displaced acromial fracture and subsequently displaced os acromiale are variations. Depending on the magnitude of injury, repair can be considered; however, given the unpredictable results of surgical management of these fractures, these injuries are typically treated conservatively.

An axillary nerve injury is an infrequent but devastating complication. Appropriate retractor placement at every stage of the operation is critical to protect the nerve. Checking the tension of the nerve, especially during glenoid exposure and after implant placement, is crucial. Prevention is key in avoiding this complication.

Subscapularis Status

Management of the subscapularis remains controversial as it relates to anterior instability in RSA. Some data suggests that dislocations are more common with prior surgery or an irreparable subscapularis [43]. Other data suggests that the state of the subscapularis does not contribute to stability in the setting of a RSA [44]. Further studies are needed to truly discern if a subscapularis repair would minimize instability after RSA.

Alternative Revision Options

Although suboptimal, resection arthroplasty can be used as a salvage operation for refractory instability after RSA. A constrained fixed-fulcrum RSA is also an option [45]. This type of implant causes concern for increased strain at bone/cement/implant interfaces, as well as suboptimal function and range of motion. Evidence is limited, but initial results show reasonable function in patients with epilepsy and recurrent instability after RSA [45].

Postoperative Rehabiliation

In order to optimize soft tissue healing and prevent recurrent instability, postoperative rehabilitation should be modified after revision RSA for instability. Depending on the direction of instability, the arm may be positioned in relative internal or external rotation utilizing a customized brace or sling [28]. An intraoperative range of motion assessment (as permitted by repair) can provide information on adjustment of the postoperative rehabilitation program. This can guide range of motion limitations to allow appropriate soft tissue healing [2]. Delaying motion and strengthening exercises may also be appropriate depending on the stability of the final implant.

Prevention of Instability in Shoulder Arthroplasty

As previously discussed, managing instability can be a difficult task due to the incidence of recurrence. In shoulder arthroplasty, foresight is key. In anatomic total shoulder arthroplasty, meticulous dissection should be the initial focus. Protecting the rotator cuff during the humeral head osteotomy and subsequently during glenoid exposure is also critical.

When placing implants, appropriate version and size should be verified. Excessive humeral anteversion can lead to anterior instability and place excess tension on the subscapularis repair. Extreme retroversion can also lead to posterior instability. Placing an oversized humeral head can strain the rotator cuff and lead to an unstable shoulder arthroplasty if rotator cuff deficiency results. If excess translation is present while trialing implants, corrective version may be helpful to maintain a stable construct [13]. Adjusting the direction of humeral head offset is also useful to help improve stability [21].

Appropriate humeral head height can be confirmed by using various soft tissue landmarks during trialing implants. The greater tuberosity and pectoralis major can be used as intraoperative landmarks. The superior border of the pectoralis major tendon lies on average 5.64 cm from the top of the humeral head [34].

Appropriate correction of glenoid deformity should also be evaluated. Preoperative planning with two-dimensional corrected CT scans or three-dimensional templating software can help improve glenoid component positioning and deformity correction [46]. These modern tools are invaluable in assessing bone loss and wear patterns that would otherwise be underestimated at the time of surgery. Depending on the deformity present, previously discussed techniques such as a corrective glenoid reaming, bone grafts, or augments may be utilized. CT-guided planning can help execute superior-inferior placement of the glenoid prosthesis as well by differentiating osteophytes from native glenoid anatomy.

After humeral and glenoid component placement, translation and range of motion should be evaluated. The rotator interval can be closed with a lateral suture if there is excessive (greater than 50%) translation. If there is persistent instability or implant gapping, capsular plication of the posterior capsule can be helpful in addition to verifying component position.

In reverse shoulder arthroplasty, many of the same principles apply. Complete osteophyte excision and correct component version are keys to avoid impingement and premature implant gapping. Balancing length and offset on both the glenoid and humeral sides are important to establish appropriate deltoid tension. Prior to closure, trialing implants through the planes of motion should be performed at the end of every surgery. There should be reasonable tension in the short head of the biceps and coracobrachialis. There should be minimal gapping with axial traction. There should be no instability with direct lateral translation of the proximal humeral implant by placing a finger on the medial calcar and trying to dislocate the humerus laterally. If instability is present, spacers or constrained liners can be utilized. If instability persists prior to completing the RSA, the aforementioned principles should be re-evaluated.

Conclusion

The incidence of instability after shoulder arthroplasty has decreased over time but is still a potential complication. A thorough history and physical exam can help diagnose the direction and etiology. Advanced imaging may also be helpful in diagnosis and planning for revision surgery. Several techniques have been developed to address failed anatomic total shoulder arthroplasty due to instability, but a properly positioned RSA has the most predictable results in restoring function. Most surgeons agree that meticulous technique and implant positioning during index surgery is the most important factor in preventing the complication. Adjusting the implant position and correcting soft tissue imbalance after trialing implants can help avoid an unstable shoulder arthroplasty.

References

1. Wirth M, Rockwood C. Complications of total shoulder-replacement arthroplasty. J Bone Joint Surg. 1996;78-A(4):603–16.
2. Cofield RH, Edgerton BC. Total shoulder arthroplasty: complications and revision surgery. Instr Course Lect. 1990;39:449–62.
3. Bohsali I, Wirth A, Rockwood C. Complications of total shoulder arthroplasty. J Bone Joint Surg. 2006;88:2279–92.
4. Bohsali K, Bois A, Wirth M. Complications of shoulder arthroplasty. J Bone Joint Surg. 2017;99:256–69.
5. Kohan EM, Chalmers PN, Salazar D, Keener JD, Yamaguchi K, Chamberlain AM. Dislocation following reverse total shoulder arthroplasty. J Shoulder Elb Surg. 2017;26:1238–45.
6. Zumstein MA, Pinedo M, Old J, Boileau P. Problems, complications, reoperations, and revisions in reverse total shoulder arthroplasty: a systematic review. J Shoulder Elb Surg. 2011;20:146–57.
7. Sanchez-Sotello J, Sperling J, Rowland C, Cofield R. Instability after shoulder arthoplasty: results of surgical treatment. J Bone Joint Surg. 2003;85A(4):622–31.
8. Cofield RH, Chang W, Sperling JW. Complications of shoulder arthroplasty. In: Iannotti JP, Williams GR, editors. Disorders of the shoulder. Philadelphia: Lippincott; 1999.
9. Kany J, Jose J, Katz D, Werthel J, Sekaran P, Amaravathi R, Valenti P. The main cause of instability after unconstrained shoulder prosthesis is soft tissue deficiency. J Shoulder Elb Surg. 2017;26:e243–51.
10. Boileau P. Complications and revision of reverse total shoulder arthroplasty. Orthop Traumatol Surg Res. 2016;102:S33–43.
11. Walch G, Wall B, Mottier F. Complications and revision of the reverse pros-thesis: a multicenter study of 457 cases. Reverse shoulder arthroplasty. Montpellier: Sauramps Médical; 2006. p. 35–52.
12. Moeckel B, Altchek D, Warren R, Wickiewicz T, Dines D. Instability of the shoulder after arthroplasty. J Bone Joint Surg. 1993;75-A(4):492–7.
13. Warren R, Coleman S, Dines J. Instability after arthroplasty: the shoulder. J Arthroplast. 2002;17(4-1):28–31.
14. Sofka CM, Adler RS. Original report. Sonographic evaluation of shoulder arthroplasty. AJR Am J Roentgenol. 2003;180:1117–20.
15. Wiater BP, Moravek JE, Wiater JM. The evaluation of the failed shoulder arthroplasty. J Shoulder Elb Surg. 2014;23:745–58.

16. Miller BS, Joseph TA, Noonan TJ, Horan MP, Hawkins RJ. Rupture of the subscapularis tendon after shoulder arthroplasty: diagnosis, treatment, and outcome. J Shoulder Elb Surg. 2005;14:492–6.
17. Iannotti JP, Antoniou J, Williams GR, Ramsey ML. Iliotibial band reconstruction for treatment of glenohumeral instability associated with irreparable capsular deficiency. J Shoulder Elb Surg. 2002;11(6):618–23.
18. Konrad G, Sudkamp N, Kreuz P, Jolly J, McMahon P, Debski R. Pectoralis major tendon transfers above or underneath the conjoint tendon in subscapularis-deficient shoulder. J Bone Joint Surg Am. 2007;89:2477–84.
19. Ahrens P, Boileau P, Walch G. Anterior and posterior instability after unconstrained shoulder arthroplasty. In: Walch G, Boileau P, Molé D, editors. 2000 shoulder prostheses: two to ten year follow-up. Montpellier: Sauramps Medical; 2001. p. 359–93.
20. Elhassan B, Ozbaydar M, Massimini D, Diller D, Higgins L, Warner JJP. Transfer of pectoralis major for the treatment of irreparable tears of subscapularis: does it work? J Bone Joint Surg Br. 2008;90(8):1059–65.
21. Kim H, Chacon A, Andrews S, Roush E, Cho E, Conaway W, Kunselman A, Lewis G. Biomechanical benefits of anterior offsetting humeral head component in posteriorly unstable total shoulder arthroplasty. J Orthop Res. 2016;34:666–74.
22. Alentorn-Geli E, Assenmacher AT, Sperling JW, Cofield RH, Sanchez-Sotelo J. Plication of the posterior capsule for intraoperative posterior instability during anatomic total shoulder arthroplasty. J Shoulder Elb Surg. 2017;26:982–9.
23. Gee A, Angeline M, Dines J, Dines D. Shoulder instability after total shoulder arthroplasty: a case of arthroscopic repair. Hosp Spec Surg J. 2014;10:88–91.
24. Galvin J, Eichinger J, Boykin R, Szollosy G, Lafosse L. Posterior shoulder instability following anatomic total shoulder arthroplasty: a case report and review of management. Int J Should Surg. 2015;9(4):131–4.
25. Keener JD. Subscapularis management in total shoulder arthroplasty. World Clin Orthoped. 2014;1(1):1–15.
26. Williams G, Yamaguchi K, Ramsey M, Galatz L. Complication of shoulder arthroplasty. Shoulder and elbow arthroplasty, vol. 16. 1st ed. Philadelphia: Lippincott Williams & Wilkins; 2005. p. 235–42.
27. Lo E, Moen T, Burkhead W. Instability failure in total shoulder arthroplasty. Semin Arthroplast. 2013;24:28–32.
28. Young A, Walch G, Pape G, Gohlke F, Favard L. Secondary rotator cuff dysfunction following total shoulder arthroplasty for primary glenohumeral osteoarthritis: results of a multicenter study with more than five years of follow-up. The J Bone Joint Surg Am. 2012;94:685–93.
29. Haines F, Trail IA, Nuttall D, Birch A, Barrow A. The results of arthroplasty in osteoarthritis of the shoulder. J Bone Joint Surg Br. 2006;88:496–501.
30. Galatz LM, Connor PM, Calfee RP, Hsu JC, Yamaguchi K. Pectoralis major transfer for anterior-superior subluxation in massive rotator cuff insufficiency. J Shoulder Elb Surg. 2003;12(1):1–5.
31. Walker M, Willis MP, Brooks JP, Pupello D, Mulieri P, Frankle MA. The use of reverse shoulder arthroplasty for treatment of failed total shoulder arthroplasty. J Shoulder Elb Surg. 2012;21(4):514–22.
32. Hernandez NM, Chalmers BP, Wagner ER, Sperling JW, Cofield RH, Sanchez-Sotelo J. Revision to reverse total shoulder arthroplasty restores stability for patients with unstable shoulder prostheses. Clin Orthop Relat Res. 2017;475(11):2716–22.
33. Abdel MP, Hattrup SJ, Sperling JW, Cofield RH, Kreofsky CR, Sanchez-Sotelo J. Revision of an unstable hemiarthroplasty or anatomical total shoulder replacement using a reverse design prosthesis. J Bone Joint Surg Am. 2013;95-B:668–72.
34. Torrens C, Corrales M, Melendo E, Solano A, Rodríguez-Baeza A, Cáceres E. The pectoralis major tendon as a reference for restoring humeral length and retroversion with hemiarthroplasty for fracture. J Shoulder Elb Surg. 2008;17:947–50.
35. Iannotti JP, Gabriel JP, Schneck SL, Evans BG, Misra S. The normal glenohumeral relationships. An anatomical study of one hundred and forty shoulders. J Bone Joint Surg Am. 1992;74:491–500.
36. Gallo R, Gamradt S, Mattern C, et al.; Sports Medicine and Shoulder Service at the Hospital for Special Surgery, New York, NY. Instability after reverse total shoulder replacement. J Shoulder Elb Surg. 2011;20(4):584–90.
37. Chalmers P, Rahman Z, Romeo A, Nicholson G. Early dislocation after reverse total shoulder arthroplasty. J Shoulder Elb Surg. 2014;23(5):737–44.
38. Padegimas E, Zmistowski B, Restrepo C, Abboud J, Lazarus M, Ramsey M, Williams G, Namdari S. Instability after reverse total shoulder arthoplasty: which patients dislocate? Am J Orthop. 2016;45(7):E444–50.
39. Teusink M, Pappou I, Schwartz D, Cottrell B, Frankle M. Results of closed management of acute dislocation after reverse shoulder arthroplasty. J Shoulder Elb Surg. 2015;24(4):621–7.
40. Favard L, Levigne C, Nerot C, Gerber C, De Wilde L, Mole D. Reverse prostheses in arthropathies with cuff tear: are survivorship and function maintained over time? Clin Orthop Relat Res. 2011;469(9):2469–75.
41. Kowalsky MS, Galatz LM, Shia DS, Steger-May K, Keener JD. The relationship between scapular notching and reverse shoulder arthroplasty prosthesis design. J Shoulder Elb Surg. 2012;21:1430–41.

42. Huri G, Familiari F, Salari N, Petersen S, Doral M, McFarland E. Prosthetic design of reverse shoulder arthroplasty contributes to scapular notching and instability. World J Orthop. 2016;7(11):738–45.
43. Edwards TB, Williams MD, Labriola JE, Elkousy HA, Gartsman GM, O'Connor DP. Subscapularis insufficiency and the risk of shoulder dislocation after reverse shoulder arthroplasty. J Shoulder Elb Surg. 2009;18(6):892–6. Epub 2009 Mar 17.
44. Clark JC, Ritchie J, Song FS, Kissenberth MJ, Tolan SJ, Hart ND, Hawkins RJ. Complication rates, dislocation, pain, and postoperative range of motion after reverse shoulder arthroplasty in patients with and without repair of the subscapularis. J Shoulder Elb Surg. 2012;21(1):36–41. Epub 2011 July 31.
45. Thangarajah T, Higgs D, Bayley J, Lambert S. Constrained fixed-fulcrum reverse shoulder arthroplasty improves functional outcome in epileptic patients with recurrent shoulder instability. World J Orthop. 2016;7(7):434–41.
46. Chalmers PN, Salazar D, Chamberlain A, Keener JD. Radiographic characterization of the B2 glenoid: the effect of computed tomographic axis orientation. J Shoulder Elb Surg. 2017;26(2):258–64.

14 Treatment of Periprosthetic Fractures of the Shoulder

Benjamin J. Lindbloom, Michael C. Cusick, and Mark A. Mighell

Introduction

Periprosthetic fractures of the humerus can be a devastating complication following shoulder arthroplasty. Although they occur relatively infrequently, with an incidence of 0.6–3%, they are often challenging to treat. [1, 2] Most fractures occur intraoperatively and are more commonly seen in total shoulder arthroplasty than hemiarthroplasty due to maneuvering for glenoid exposure. Risk factors for periprosthetic fractures include osteopenia, advanced age, female sex, and rheumatoid arthritis [2, 3]. As the indications for arthroplasty continue to expand and frequency of shoulder arthroplasty increases, an understanding of periprosthetic shoulder fractures and how to treat them becomes critical. Good clinical outcomes and osseous healing can be accomplished following appropriate treatment of periprosthetic humeral fractures.

B. J. Lindbloom · M. A. Mighell (✉)
Shoulder and Elbow Service, Florida Orthopaedic Institute, Tampa, FL, USA
e-mail: mmighell@floridaortho.com

M. C. Cusick
Department of Orthopedic Surgery, McGovern Medical School, The University of Texas Health Science Center, Houston, TX, USA

Classification

Several classification systems have been introduced in the description of periprosthetic humerus fractures. Perhaps the most widely utilized classification system was introduced in 1995 by Wright and Cofield [4]. This classification primarily describes the fracture based on its location relative to the humeral stem. Type A fractures begin around the humeral stem and extend proximally. Type B fractures begin around the stem and extend distal to the tip. Type C fractures both begin and remain distal to the stem tip. One study demonstrated poor interobserver reliability (kappa coefficients of 0.24 for first attempts and 0.50) but good intraobserver reliability (kappa coefficient 0.69) [5]. Another common concern with the Wright and Cofield classification raised by clinicians is its lack of description of how well-fixed the stem is and the quality and quantity of the remaining bone.

Campbell et al. categorized periprosthetic proximal humerus fractures based on fracture location in four specific regions. Region 1 were fractures involving the greater or lesser tuberosity. Region 2 were fractures occurring in the humeral metaphysis and surgical neck. Region 3 involved the proximal humeral diaphysis and region 4 the mid- and distal diaphysis. Fracture location was classified by the most distal extent of the fracture line.

R. Z. Tashjian (ed.), *Complex and Revision Shoulder Arthroplasty*,
https://doi.org/10.1007/978-3-030-02756-8_14

The morphology and features of the fracture are also important considerations for treatment and prognosis. Transverse and short oblique fractures have less intrinsic fracture stability and less surface area available for healing, resulting in a higher incidence of non-union than long oblique or spiral fractures. A fracture gap larger than 2 mm is also associated with higher incidence of non-union in periprosthetic humerus fractures.

It is important to consider the bone stock remaining when a periprosthetic humerus fracture occurs. Campbell et al. described their system of evaluating the presence of osteopenia on the preoperative plain radiographs [6]. The authors calculated the ratio of the combined width of the mid-diaphyseal cortices to the diameter of the diaphysis. The bone is described as normal if the ratio was greater than 50%, mild osteopenia if ratio was 25% to 50%, and severe osteopenia if the ratio was less than 25%. Remaining bone quality is important in considering the final construct. For example, locking screws, orthogonal plating constructs, and allograft bone plates may be considered in patients with osteopenic bone as they provide greater rigidity and support.

Another critical consideration is the stability of the implant. While the ultimate determination of whether the implant remains well-fixed is made intraoperatively, several radiographic features have been described to help the surgeon anticipate the stability based off the preoperative radiographs. Sperling et al. described eight radiographic zones surrounding a press-fit humeral implant and determined the humeral component was "at risk" for clinical component loosening when a lucent line 2 mm or greater was present in three or more of the eight zones [7]. Humeral components are also considered loose when there is tilt or subsidence of the component [8]. Sanchez-Sotelo et al. demonstrated these same parameters can be used in cemented humeral components as well with good accuracy [9].

At our institution, we feel that although fracture location is the focus of the two main classifications discussed, the most important clinical parameters to consider remain implant stability and quality of bone stock. These two considerations have a great impact on implant consideration, operative approach, and fixation construct, as will be discussed in the next section.

Treatment

Treatment of periprosthetic humerus fractures involves careful consideration of the fracture characteristics, bone stock, implant stability, and patient factors. Non-operative treatment with a fracture brace or orthosis may be used to treat periprosthetic fractures that are minimally displaced or nondisplaced in the setting of a well-fixed prosthesis [6, 10]. Satisfactory alignment of humerus fractures is defined as within 20° of flexion/extension, 30° of varus/valgus, and 20° of rotational alignment [11].

Operative treatment strategies can be stratified generally by considering the regions involved in the fracture. Campbell et al. described four fracture regions [6]. Region 1 are isolated fractures of the greater and/or lesser tuberosities. These fractures are fixed with cerclage sutures or wires to securely fix the tuberosities back to a standard "fracture-type" humeral stem. Region 2 are fractures that occur in the metaphyseal flare below the tuberosities. Region 2 fractures are treated with intramedullary fixation with a standard or long humeral stem implant that extends at least three cortical widths distal to the fracture. Region 3 occurs in the proximal diaphyseal region. These can be treated with intramedullary fixation with a long humeral stem implant. Bone stock must also be considered in these fractures, and often times these fractures may require allograft bone proximally in the form of an allograft prosthetic composite or an allograft bone strut with supplemental plate and cerclage fixation. Region 4 fractures occur in the mid- or distal humeral diaphysis. In region 4 fractures, which are often distal to the stem of the humeral component, the stability of the implant is the primary consideration. In the setting of a loose prosthetic, revision with a long stem implant plus the potential for allograft bone and plate supplementation similar to the treatment described for region 3 is required. If the prosthetic remains well-fixed in a region 4 fracture, then the fracture may be reconstructed using plate osteosynthesis with periprosthetic "stem skiving" cortical screws, unicortical locking screws, and/or cerclage wires which may be used to obtain fixation in the proximal fragment [5]. (Reference the Anderson paper)

Operative approach must be determined by the surgeon upon considering the fracture characteristics and planned fixation construct. The anterolateral approach is extensile, allows the patient to be positioned supine with some elevation of the head, and allows for access to the shoulder joint to revise a potentially loose prosthetic. The posterior approach to the proximal humerus allows for direct visualization of the radial nerve, facilitates the possible use of a sterile tourniquet, and is well suited for fixing region 4 fractures that occur distal to a well-fixed stem. The main drawback of the posterior approach is difficulties and risks associated with prone or lateral positioning and the lack of ability to perform a revision of the arthroplasty and access the shoulder joint.

Fixation constructs also have many considerations when applied to the treatment of periprosthetic humerus fractures. The question of whether to use a single plate or using smaller plates applied orthogonally to allow for more options for points of fixation should be considered, especially in patients with poor bone stock or patients with a large diameter stem in place. Allograft cortical bone plates may also be a useful adjuvant with screws or cerclage fixation to restore or reinforce poor bone stock. Although allograft bone is useful in settings of bone loss, it does carry a slightly increased risk of infection. As a result, if there is not substantial bone loss and optimizing the fracture healing biology is the goal, we prefer autograft bone grafting. When placing cerclage fixation around the humerus, always pass from lateral to medial and be conscious of the course of the radial nerve in the surgical field to avoid injury. There are certain "safe zones" for placing cerclage fixation around the humerus: (1) above the level of the surgical neck near the tuberosities, as one is above the axillary nerve, and (2) at the level of the latissimus dorsi tendon, as it is between the axillary and radial nerves. At other levels, care and consideration must be given to elevate the periosteum and not entrap soft tissues with cerclage fixation to minimize the risk of injury to neurovascular structures. Retractors must also be placed carefully, and long-levered retractors such as Homans should not be placed laterally distal to the deltoid tuberosity on the humerus due to the course of the radial nerve.

In cases where the prosthetic is also loose, there are many considerations for revision arthroplasty to treat periprosthetic humerus fractures. A cemented allograft prosthetic composite may be constructed on the back table in cases of extensive proximal bone loss. To decrease the effects of rotational forces, step cuts are made in the native diaphyseal humerus and allograft. Interdigitation of the host and allograft segments will improve the stability of the allograft prosthetic construct.

Conclusion

Periprosthetic fractures about total shoulder arthroplasty are an infrequent but difficult scenario encountered by the shoulder surgeon. Many occur intraoperatively and can be addressed during the index operation, but an increasing number of traumatic periprosthetic fractures are occurring as the prevalence of shoulder arthroplasty increases. It is crucial to the treating surgeon to understand and appropriately classify the fracture, evaluate the bone quality, and estimate implant stability in order to appropriately plan their operative strategy and approach. The treatment for these fractures includes non-operative treatment, open reduction internal fixation, and revision arthroplasty. With the appropriate treatments, satisfactory outcomes and reliable healing can be achieved in the majority of these fractures (Figs. 14.1, 14.2, and 14.3).

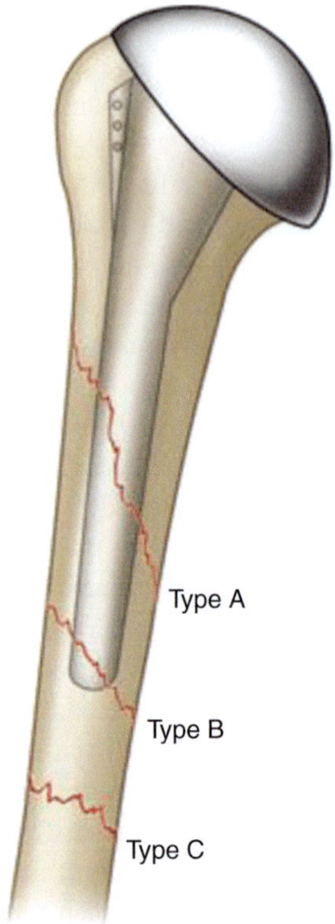

Fig. 14.1 Wright and Cofield classification of periprosthetic humerus fractures

Author's Preferred Methods

Fracture of Tuberosity Occurring During Revision or Primary Arthroplasty

When periprosthetic tuberosity fractures occur intraoperatively, they must be identified, and the fracture fragments must be controlled and well-fixed to the final construct. At our institution, we will switch to a fracture-type stemmed reverse humeral prosthetic. Three large structural sutures (we use Arthrex FiberTape) are placed in the posterior rotator cuff (infraspinatus and teres minor) at the tendon-osseous junction in a simple configuration. A fourth suture is placed in the anterior supraspinatus to use as a traction stitch to assist with reduction. Prior to placing the final stem, an anterior to posterior 2.0 mm drill hole is placed just lateral to the biceps groove and inferior to the surgical neck. Using a Hewson suture passer, FiberTape and FiberWire sutures are placed through the humerus to serve as vertical limb fixation sutures. The stem and humeral component are then impacted. The prosthesis is reduced, and then the tuberosity is

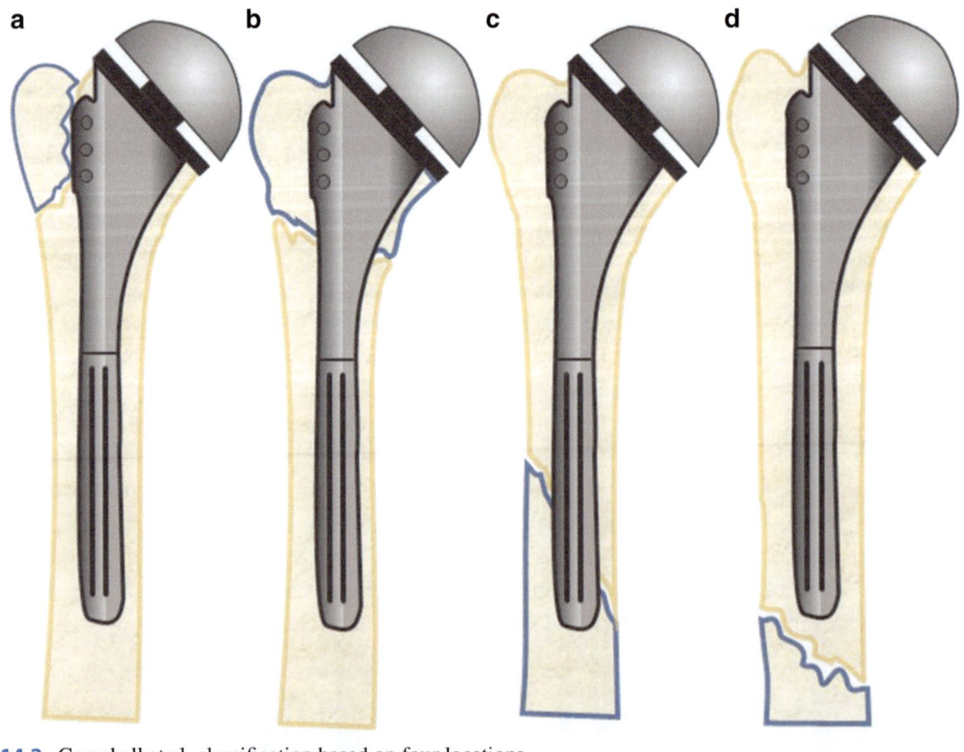

Fig. 14.2 Campbell et al. classification based on four locations

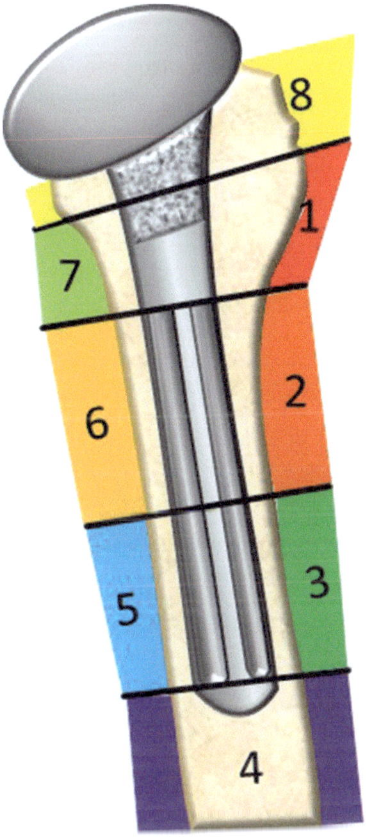

Fig. 14.3 Eight radiographic zones to evaluate humeral ingrowth

reduced to the prosthesis and fixed with the three sutures. The vertical limb two sutures are then passed anterior to posterior for one and posterior to anterior for the other, creating a "figure of eight" tension band fixation laterally with the vertical limb sutures. These are tightly tied with the arm positioned in shoulder abduction. This abduction position is critical, because when the arm is then lowered, the sutures become even tighter and compress the greater tuberosity fragment, further securing it. We will use our typical shoulder immobilizer for 4 weeks following this and avoid any pendulum range of motion exercises.

Midshaft Fracture Requiring Revision to Long-Stemmed Component

In fractures that occur in the midshaft and require revision to a long-stemmed component, there can be challenges with maintaining an adequate fracture reduction while placing the long-stemmed implant. For these fractures at our institution, we position the patient supine and elevate the radiolucent portion of the bed 30°. The C-arm is positioned to come in from the head of the patient. We utilize a deltopectoral approach and extend it into an anterolateral approach to the humerus. In these situations, we prefer to get a provisional reduction and stability at the fracture site prior to placing the long stem. Often times this stability can be achieved with tibial cortical strut allografts, which can be utilized as "bone plates" and affixed with cortical screws to the proximal and distal fracture fragments. In addition to stabilizing the fracture, this technique can help by providing additional bone stock in poor quality bone or bone loss situations. Another technique involves bridge plating the fracture with unicortical locking fixation. This can be performed with either large fragment 4.5 mm plates or orthogonal small fragment 3.5 mm plates. Following final long-stemmed placement, stem skiving cortical screws may be employed within the plate to increase the rigidity of the final construct.

Supracondylar Fracture Occurring Distal to a Well-fixed Stem

For supracondylar or distal humerus shaft fractures occurring below a well fixed stem, we will typically position the patient lateral with a beanbag and the arm over a post to perform a posterior paratricipital or triceps splitting approach. We prefer the added rigidity of parallel plating for these fractures, especially if there is intra-articular extension into the distal humerus. The limitation of this approach is that it does not allow for any revision of the prosthesis, if it turns out to not be well-fixed.

1. Case examples from Dr Mighell/Dr Frankle (Monahos, Shiela Schumacker)

Bibliography

1. Williams GR, Iannotti JP. Management of periprosthetic fractures: the shoulder. J Arthroplast. 2002;17(4):14–6. https://doi.org/10.1054/arth.2002.32683.

2. Steinmann SP, Cheung EV. Treatment of periprosthetic humerus fractures associated with shoulder arthroplasty. J Am Acad Orthop Surg. 2008;16(4):199–207. http://www.ncbi.nlm.nih.gov/pubmed/18390482
3. Wagner ER, Houdek MT, Elhassan BT, Sanchez-Sotelo J, Cofield RH, Sperling JW. What are risk factors for intraoperative Humerus fractures during revision reverse shoulder arthroplasty and do they influence outcomes? Clin Orthop Relat Res. 2015;473(10):3228–34.https://doi.org/10.1007/s11999-015-4448-x.
4. Wright TW, Cofield RH. Humeral fractures after shoulder arthroplasty. J Bone Joint Surg Am. 1995;77(9): 1340–6.https://doi.org/10.2106/00004623-199509000-00008.
5. Andersen JR, Williams CD, Cain R, Mighell M, Frankle M. Surgically treated humeral shaft fractures following shoulder arthroplasty. J Bone Joint Surg Am. 2013;95(1):9–18. https://doi.org/10.2106/JBJS.K.00863.
6. Campbell JT, Moore RS, Iannotti JP, Norris TR, Williams GR. Periprosthetic humeral fractures: mechanisms of fracture and treatment options. J Shoulder Elb Surg. 1998;7(4):406–13. http://www.ncbi.nlm.nih.gov/pubmed/9752653
7. Sperling JW, Cofield RH, O'Driscoll SW, Torchia ME, Rowland CM. Radiographic assessment of ingrowth total shoulder arthroplasty. J Shoulder Elb Surg. 2000;9(6):507–13. https://doi.org/10.1067/mse.2000.109384.
8. Sanchez-Sotelo J, Wright TW, O'Driscoll SW, Cofield RH, Rowland CM. Radiographic assessment of uncemented humeral components in total shoulder arthroplasty. J Arthroplast. 2001;16(2):180–7. https://doi.org/10.1054/arth.2001.20905.
9. Sanchez-Sotelo J, O'Driscoll SW, Torchia ME, Cofield RH, Rowland CM. Radiographic assessment of cemented humeral components in shoulder arthroplasty. J Shoulder Elb Surg. 2001;10(6):526–31. https://doi.org/10.1067/mse.2001.118482.
10. Kim DH, Clavert P, Warner JJP. Displaced periprosthetic humeral fracture treated with functional bracing: a report of two cases. J Shoulder Elb Surg. 2005;14(2):221–3. https://doi.org/10.1016/j.jse.2004.05.006.
11. Kumar S, Sperling JW, Haidukewych GH, Cofield RH. Periprosthetic humeral fractures after shoulder arthroplasty. J Bone Joint Surg Am. 2004;86-A(4):680–9. https://doi.org/10.2106/00004623-199509000-00008.

Salvage Options for Failed Arthroplasty: Arthrodesis and Resection

15

Jason Scalise

Introduction

Shoulder arthroplasty, including hemiarthroplasty, anatomic total shoulder arthroplasty (TSA), and reverse total shoulder arthroplasty (RSA) have been proven to be effective treatment options for glenohumeral arthritis. There has been rapid adoption of these techniques over the last 15 years such that the incidence of these procedures worldwide has risen substantially [1, 2]. As a result the incidence of failed arthroplasty has also risen and will continue to rise in the future.

In many cases, the reason or reasons for the failed arthroplasty can be addressed during revision surgery at which time new prosthetic components are inserted. In the setting of a failed shoulder arthroplasty, every consideration should be made to maintain the functionality of the glenohumeral joint; however, in cases with severe glenohumeral bone loss, loss of the deltoid muscle and rotator cuff, or the presence of recalcitrant infection, the likelihood of a successful outcome with a revision arthroplasty may be unacceptably low. In these circumstances, glenohumeral arthrodesis or resection arthroplasty may become the only other surgical option.

J. Scalise (✉)
The CORE Institute, Phoenix, AZ, USA
e-mail: jason.scalise@thecoreinstitute.com

Arthrodesis

Failure of a shoulder arthroplasty often leads to poor functional outcomes if not addressed. Pain and loss of sufficient motion to allow for some activities of daily living can occur. With the advent of reverse shoulder arthroplasty, many patients have been successfully revised to this style of construct that has resulted in acceptable outcomes in several series [3–8].

However, in some circumstances, revision to a new arthroplasty construct may not be a viable alternative. Such circumstances can include complete deltoid dysfunction, inability to eradicate infection, insufficient bone stock to allow stable implantation of a shoulder arthroplasty, or other concomitant neuromuscular disorders that would prevent durable shoulder stability or function. Although glenohumeral arthrodesis remains a proven and durable technique to restore function in select patients with a native shoulder, those outcomes are not comparable to arthrodesis in the setting of failed arthroplasty [9]. Poor quality bone stock, sometimes massive bone loss, and poor soft tissue envelopes all make successful salvage with arthrodesis more challenging when in the setting of a failed arthroplasty.

The primary indication for an arthrodesis in the setting of failed arthroplasty is for the alleviation of pain while still allowing for some waist-to-shoulder level elevation. A successful arthrodesis can result in durable pain relief and

R. Z. Tashjian (ed.), *Complex and Revision Shoulder Arthroplasty*,
https://doi.org/10.1007/978-3-030-02756-8_15

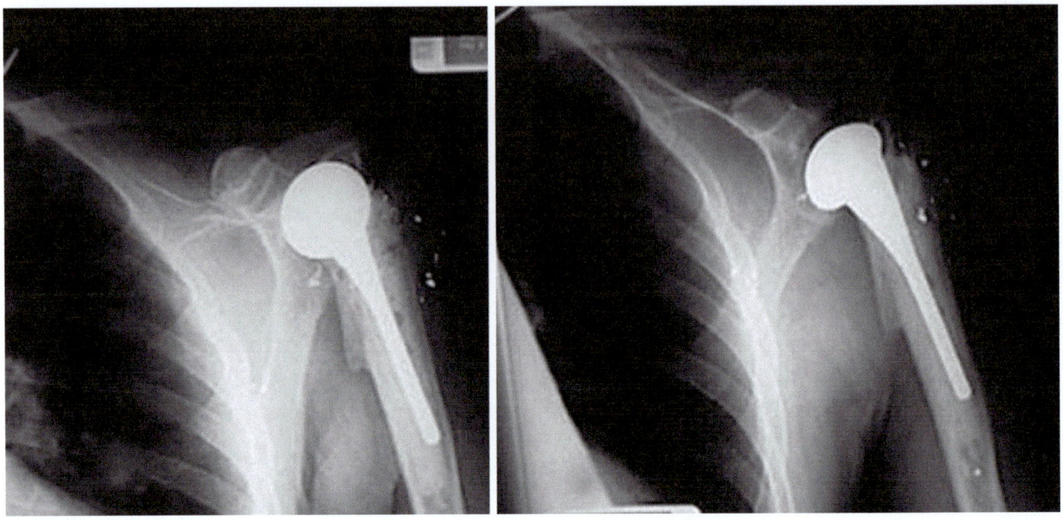

Fig. 15.1 Radiographs of a failed, painful prosthetic replacement in a 53-year-old police officer. Complete deltoid deficiency was present following multiple surgeries and an initial shotgun injury

provide a stable platform for upper extremity use [10–12]. Younger patients that are wishing to perform additional but moderately laborious activities with the involved extremity may therefore be candidates for arthrodesis consideration.

The decision to consider arthrodesis after failed arthroplasty is usually coupled with the presence of severe deltoid dysfunction given that the option of revision to RSA is compromised. Complete deltoid dysfunction may be seen in injury to the axillary nerve, brachial plexopathies, primary muscle dysfunction, or dehiscence from its origin. It should be noted, however, that in the presence of partial deltoid function, acceptable outcomes for RSA have been reported [13, 14] and that the decision to consider arthrodesis or resection would be consigned to situations where complete or near-complete deltoid functional loss is present.

Persistent prosthetic sepsis in some patients is a contraindication for implantation of prosthetic components. In this setting and typically after multiple failed attempts at infection treatment, arthrodesis remains a salvage option assuming the infection is treated and no longer active. Recalcitrant prosthetic instability following unconstrained or reverse total shoulder arthroplasty is a very challenging problem. When soft tissue stabilization procedures or revision arthroplasty have been exhausted, arthrodesis may be indicated (Fig. 15.1).

Factors relevant to the decision to proceed with arthrodesis will include the health status of the patient, postoperative expectations of the patient, the feasibility that a fusion can be obtained, and the ability of the patient to cooperate with the postoperative rehabilitation program. The most important contraindication to glenohumeral arthrodesis following failed total shoulder arthroplasty is when other reasonable reconstructive options exist. This underscores the salvage nature of arthrodesis in the treatment of failed glenohumeral arthroplasty and that all practical reconstructive options should be first considered. Patients with progressive neurological disorders that may result in paralysis of the trapezius, serratus anterior, or levator scapulae muscles represent a contraindication to arthrodesis as the fused shoulder relies upon these muscles to move the extremity through the scapulothoracic articulation.

Patients whose overall health status would preclude them from the substantial operative procedure are also discouraged from arthrodesis. In many cases arthrodesis for failed prosthetic arthroplasty requires more than one procedure to achieve bony fusion [3, 10, 12].

Technique

The surgeon and patient should recognize that glenohumeral arthrodesis for failed prosthetic replacement is a technically demanding procedure. Prosthesis and cement extraction along with proper bone grafting techniques and correct arm positioning all are pertinent. A complete set of radiographs of shoulder and humerus to the elbow must be obtained. One should also evaluate the soft tissues surrounding the shoulder for the need for flap coverage when the soft tissue envelope is compromised.

The need for and type of bone graft should be determined preoperatively. In cases with intact proximal humerus tuberosities, non-vascularized bone graft can be sufficient so long as the native humeral bone can be placed into direct contact with the decorticated glenoid fossa. In these cases there is still a need for bulk structural graft substrate that cannot typically be accommodated from the patient's iliac crest alone. Often, one large femoral head is sufficient for this purpose. Cancellous autograft can be obtained from the iliac crest. In some severe cases, where the tuberosities are missing or not attached to the humeral shaft and a large portion of the proximal humerus is deficient, a vascularized fibular autograft is required and can provide a reconstructive solution for this level of bone loss. In many respects, these situations resemble the reconstructive challenges found in tumor cases about the shoulder.

The patient is positioned in a beach-chair configuration, while the operative shoulder is brought over the edge of the table allowing full range of motion of the shoulder and global surgical access. If iliac crest bone graft is to be obtained, the hip area must also be appropriately draped. If vascularized fibula is needed, both legs are prepped from the groin to the toes. Saphenous vein graft harvest may be required in some cases.

The incision is made over the spine of the scapula, curving anteriorly over the acromion. Often, the scar from previous deltopectoral incisions can be incorporated as the distal extent of the incision. After the deltopectoral interval is developed to the clavicle, the anterior and middle portions of the deltoid are detached subperiosteally from the clavicle and acromion and then reflected distally, thus exposing the entire proximal humerus. The prosthetic components are now removed and the remaining bone stock and soft tissue defects evaluated. Scar in the surgical bed is resected to expose the bone surfaces and allow apposition of those surfaces. The entire glenoid fossa, rim, and vault walls need be exposed to define the best placement of the graft material.

Position of Extremity

The optimal position of the arthrodesed extremity is debated. In fusion for failed arthroplasty, the position that will allow proper function needs to be balanced with the position of the remaining humeral and glenoid bone to optimize bone contact, stability, and ultimately union of the fusion. Given this balance of objectives, the position of fusion is a range of 10–20° of abduction, 10–20° flexion, and 35–45° internal rotation. This position will generally allow the patient to reach their mouth, waist, back pocket, and contralateral shoulder, facilitating activities of daily living. In patients with a larger body habitus, larger degrees of forward flexion or abduction will still allow for the patient to comfortably bring the arm to the side of their body and will allow for greater degrees of active forward elevation. When there is sufficient humeral bone remaining (intact tuberosities) provisional fixation using large 3 mm crossed Steinmann pins through the acromion, proximal humerus and glenoid can allow for a gentle range of motion trial to ensure that the arm can come to the side, to the groin, and to the mouth or forehead. When the optimal position is achieved, definitive fixation can be placed.

If the tuberosities are intact, they can be shaped with minimal bone removal to fit the glenoid. The presence of intact tuberosities and their blood supply enhances the potential for fusion. Fixation of the tuberosities to the glenoid should be with separate fixation using large cancellous screws. 4.5 mm screws with washers provide

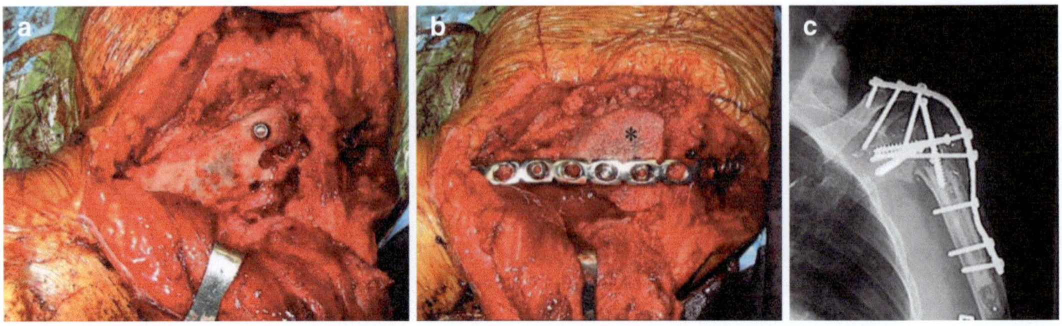

Fig. 15.2 (**a**) Intraoperative photograph demonstrating initial fixation of the humerus to the glenoid. (**b**) Large fragment reconstruction plate is shown fixing the humeral shaft to the acromion and scapula spine. The bulk allograft (asterisk) is shown between the plate and proximal humeral shaft. (**c**) Postoperative radiograph demonstrating the arthrodesis construct

interfragmentary stability and compression of the tuberosities to the glenoid. Larger screws for the tuberosity fixation may risk fragmentation. Soft tissue from the underside of the acromion should be removed and its undersurface gently planed to provide a flat surface for fusion. After initial fixation with screws, the structural allograft may be cut to fit between the tuberosities and the acromion and the humeral shaft. 6.5 mm terminally threaded screws with washers can then be used to provide strong, independent fixation of the humerus graft composite to the glenoid. A large fragment pelvic reconstruction plate may be contoured to the spine of the scapula, the acromion, bone graft, and the humeral shaft distally (Fig. 15.2). A 12- or 14-hole plate is commonly used given the extent of contouring required and length needed to span the fusion mass. Although a minimum of three screws on either side of the fusion site should be used for stability, the interfragmentary compression screws are critical to the integrity of this construct as the plate functions largely in a neutralization role. Therefore, a wide distribution of screws enhances the strength of the construct. Where feasible, screws engaging the plate can also engage the humerus, graft, and glenoid. Use of intraoperative fluoroscopy is important to confirm screw position as well as the final construct.

The use of bone graft supplements such as demineralized bone matrix and/or recombinant bone morphogenic protein to enhance the fusion mass can be considered when the quantity or quality of native, viable bone is minimal (as can be encountered in such salvage scenarios). However, these should not be considered substitutes to robust compression and stability that is obtained with adherence to proper fixation techniques.

Vascularized Fibula Graft

When a vascularized fibula autograft is necessary, it is ideal to utilize two surgical teams. During the harvesting of the graft, the reconstructive team may focus on the prosthesis extraction and preparing the bone bed. The bone gap is measured with traction on the arm to achieve normal or near-normal arm length. The fibula graft is harvested giving at least 6 centimeters more bone length than the measured bone deficiency (top of the glenoid fossa to the proximal end of the humeral shaft). The humeral canal is prepared so that the fibula can be placed within the medullary canal and at least two cortical (4.5 mm) screws are placed into the humeral shaft transfixing the fibula. The optimal arm position is determined, and the angle that of the proximal fibula is used to carve a tunnel in the glenoid so that it is doweled into the glenoid vault or has close side-to-side contact with the glenoid vault. Two 4.5 mm cortical screws are placed into the proximal fibula and then into the glenoid vault in lag fashion. Smaller-diameter screws (e.g., 3.5 mm) should be considered if the size of the fibula is small so as to minimize the risk of fracturing the fibula. A large fragment pelvic reconstruction plate is contoured to fit the spine of the acromion and humerus distally and then fixed with screws. The fibula is then vascularized by the microvascular team. After vascularization, cancellous bone graft is used at both the proximal and distal osteosynthesis sites.

Postoperatively, the shoulder is immobilized in a brace that will hold the new arm position or spica cast for 12–16 weeks or until radiographic evidence of fusion is present. After the fusion has been established, scapular range of motion and strengthening exercises are initiated. If there is lack of bony healing at 3–4 months after surgery, there should be regrafting before there is failure of the hardware and loss of fixation.

Results

Given the salvage nature of an arthrodesis after failed shoulder arthroplasty, results of this procedure should be viewed as having limited goals. Providing pain relief and a stable platform for elbow and hand function are the primary goals of glenohumeral arthrodesis, as well as allowing some active elevation of the shoulder through scapula motion.

Arthrodesis has been recommended in settings when revision prosthetic arthroplasty is not indicated. However, peer-reviewed data specific to arthrodesis following failed prosthetic arthroplasty are limited. As this procedure is performed with relative infrequency, many of the results of this procedure are contained in reports of fusions performed for variable indications within heterogenous populations.

In 1 series of 43 shoulder arthrodeses, 2 were performed following removal of failed shoulder prostheses [15]. In one of these patients, deltoid dysfunction from axillary nerve palsy and subsequent glenoid component dislocation represented the indication for arthrodesis. Pseudarthrosis was observed in one patient in whom bone graft was not used. The authors suggest that the use of bone graft in the setting of such substantial bone loss can help avoid nonunion. In another report of 15 fusion cases, 2 were for failed prosthetic arthroplasty with the only nonunion in the series resulting in 1 of these 2 patients.[16]. The results of 57 glenohumeral arthrodesis were reviewed in another series in which two procedures were performed for failed TSA [17]. One of these patients experienced a nonunion and required revision surgery and bone grafting before fusion was obtained.

In one of the few dedicated series of patients that reported the results of arthrodesis for failed arthroplasty, eight shoulder fusion procedures were performed [10]. All patients had undergone multiple surgeries before their arthrodesis surgery. Three patients included vascularized fibular bone graft procedures due to massive bone loss with the other five patients needing structural allograft or iliac crest autograft or both. Two nonunions were seen in this group with four patients requiring two or more procedures to obtain fusion. Functional outcome improvement was reported in 7/8 patients.

Both surgeon and patient need be aware that multiple surgeries may be necessary to obtain fusion after prosthetic removal but that functional improvements can be achieved when compared to their pre-arthrodesis state.

Resection Arthroplasty

Removal of a failed shoulder arthroplasty without further reconstruction can be considered a viable option in some select patients. Functional outcomes of a resection arthroplasty may be less predictable [18–22]. However, patients with a relatively poor health status or with sufficiently low functional demands may represent candidates for this procedure. In some cases, these patients who have undergone multiple prior surgeries are wishing to avoid further procedures that have extended rehabilitation times and still may have relatively high risks of poor outcomes. This option is an alternative which is technically more approachable and avoids the prospect of complications such as nonunion or hardware failure.

Chronic infection that has been resistant to previous attempts at eradication can also represent an opportunity for select patients to consider resection arthroplasty [18, 22]. In those patients in whom deltoid function still exists yet the ability or desire to revise the shoulder with another arthroplasty option such as hemiarthroplasty or RSA is deemed unwarranted, the results of some series have demonstrated acceptable results with resection arthroplasty when proper deltoid strengthening programs are instituted and coupled with appropriate patient selection and expectations.

As in arthrodesis, the primary goal for resection arthroplasty is pain relief. These patients typically have low functional demands and, in some cases, cognitive deficits. Deep infections around the shoulder that have been recalcitrant to all reasonable treatments are often an indication for resection arthroplasty, and like arthrodesis, resection arthroplasty should be considered a salvage procedure. The objective is therefore to provide a straightforward procedure that results in the improvement of pain and allows the patient to avoid complex treatments or rehabilitation regimens postoperatively.

Technique

Patients are placed in a beach-chair position. Previous incision planes are used if possible. If a draining sinus is present, the incision is crafted so as to allow excision of the sinus tract and skin. The previous implants are removed including all cement and other foreign materials if infection is present so as to minimize the chance of infection recurrence. Devitalized or infected bone is also removed. The glenoid vault is similarly debrided, and exposure is typically generous in these situations. After thorough debridement and irrigation, any remnants of the anterior capsule or subscapularis can be secured to the anterior humerus in order to help promote anterior stability.

Patients are placed in a simple sling, and pendulum exercises may begin in 2 weeks. If a functional deltoid is present, gentle but progressive deltoid strengthening can begin once comfort allows. Improvements in deltoid strength and control may in time result in modest functional gains for patients.

Results

Several series have been reported for resection arthroplasty in this setting. Pain was reduced in one series 10 of 11 patients having a resection arthroplasty for failed shoulder arthroplasty despite also having very limited shoulder function [23]. In a different investigation, six of seven patients resulted in substantial or near-complete pain relief after resection arthroplasty despite limited functional results of that shoulder (average preoperative pain score decreased from 7.8 to 3.3 on a10-point visual analog scale) [21]. In yet another study, seven patients were reviewed in which all of the patients had sufficient function to perform basic activities of daily living and also had improvements in comfort allowing them to conclude that resection arthroplasty was an option in select patients who are otherwise poor candidates for other reconstructive efforts [18]. At follow-up, average forward flexion was 28° (range, 0–80), and average external rotation was 8° (range, −20 to −40); mean ASES scores after resection were 49.75 ± 26.1 (Fig. 15.3).

Conclusion

Both arthrodesis and resection arthroplasty in the setting of failed arthroplasty are considered salvage procedures for those patients in whom other reasonable reconstructive efforts are unwarranted. Appropriate patient selection and expectations combined with adherence to technical details are critical to the success of these surgical options. Arthrodesis is a technically challenging procedure and is complicated by relatively high rates of nonunion of the fusion site especially with increasing degrees of humeral bone loss. A successful arthrodesis, however, can provide durable pain relief, sufficient chest-level function, and a stable platform for patients to maintain some activity with their arm along with acceptable clinical outcomes. Resection arthroplasty is often indicated for a different population of patients in whom low functional demands combined with a desire to limit additional procedural and rehabilitation needs can result in adequate pain relief following implant extraction.

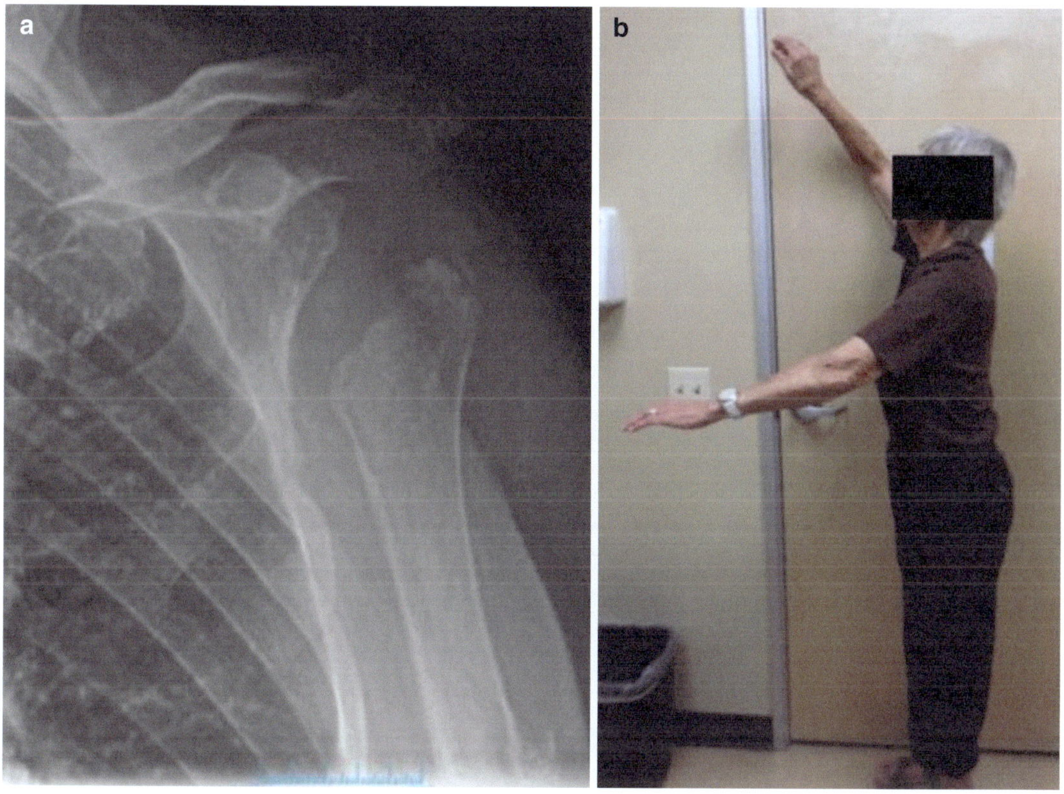

Fig. 15.3 (**a**) X-ray of the left shoulder of an 82-year-old female after resection of failed reverse shoulder arthroplasty for intractable deep infection and (**b**) clinical photo of the left shoulder after resection demonstrating waist-level elevation but with improved comfort

References

1. Issa K, Pierce CM, Pierce TP, Boylan MR, Zikria BA, Naziri Q, et al. Total shoulder arthroplasty demographics, incidence, and complications-a Nationwide inpatient sample database study. Surg Technol Int. 2016;39:240–6.
2. Trofa D, Rajaee SS, Smith EL. Nationwide trends in total shoulder arthroplasty and hemiarthroplasty for osteoarthritis. Am J Orthop (Belle Mead NJ). 2014;43(4):166–72.
3. McLendon PB, Cox JL, Frankle MA. Large diaphyseal-incorporating allograft prosthetic composites: when, how, and why: treatment of advanced proximal humeral bone loss. Orthopade. 2017;46(12):1022–7.
4. Merolla G, Wagner E, Sperling JW, Paladini P, Fabbri E, Porcellini G. Revision of failed shoulder hemiarthroplasty to reverse total arthroplasty: analysis of 157 revision implants. J Shoulder Elb Surg. 2018;27(1):75–81.
5. Stephens BC, Simon P, Clark RE, Christmas KN, Stone GP, Lorenzetti AJ, et al. Revision for a failed reverse: a 12-year review of a lateralized implant. J Shoulder Elb Surg. 2016;25(5):e115–24.
6. Alentorn-Geli E, Clark NJ, Assenmacher AT, Samuelsen BT, Sanchez-Sotelo J, Cofield RH, et al. What are the complications, survival, and outcomes after revision to reverse shoulder arthroplasty in patients older than 80 years? Clin Orthop Relat Res. 2017;475(11):2744–51.
7. Hernandez NM, Chalmers BP, Wagner ER, Sperling JW, Cofield RH, Sanchez-Sotelo J. Revision to reverse total shoulder arthroplasty restores stability for patients with unstable shoulder prostheses. Clin Orthop Relat Res. 2017;475(11):2716–22.
8. Porcellini G, Combi A, Merolla G, Bordini B, Stea S, Zanoli G, et al. The experience of the RIPO, a shoulder prosthesis registry with 6-year follow-up. Musculoskeletal Surg. 2017;(Dec):1–10.
9. Scalise JJ, Iannotti JP. Glenohumeral arthrodesis after failed prosthetic shoulder arthroplasty. Surgical technique. J Bone Joint Surg Am. 2009;91(Suppl 2):30–7.
10. Scalise JJ, Iannotti JP. Glenohumeral arthrodesis after failed prosthetic shoulder arthroplasty. J Bone Joint Surg Am. 2008;90(1):70–7.
11. Dubina A, Shiu B, Gilotra M, Hasan SA, Lerman D, Ng VY. What is the optimal reconstruction option

after the resection of proximal humeral tumors? a systematic review. Open Orthop J. 2017;11:203–11.
12. Viehweger E, Gonzalez J-F, Launay F, Legre R, Jouve J-L, Bollini G. Shoulder arthrodesis with vascularized fibular graft after tumor resection of the proximal humerus. Rev Chir Orthop Reparatrice Appar Mot. 2005;91(6):523–9.
13. Ladermann A, Walch G, Denard PJ, Collin P, Sirveaux F, Favard L, et al. Reverse shoulder arthroplasty in patients with pre-operative impairment of the deltoid muscle. Bone Joint J. 2013;95–B(8):1106–13.
14. Schneeberger AG, Muller TM, Steens W, Thur C. Reverse total shoulder arthroplasty after failed deltoid flap reconstruction. Arch Orthop Trauma Surg. 2014;134(3):317–23.
15. Ruhmann O, Schmolke S, Bohnsack M, Flamme C, Wirth CJ. Shoulder arthrodesis: indications, technique, results, and complications. J Shoulder Elb Surg. 2005;14(1):38–50.
16. Stark DM, Bennett JB, Tullos HS. Rigid internal fixation for shoulder arthrodesis. Orthopedics. 1991;14(8):849–55.
17. Richards RR, Beaton D, Hudson AR. Shoulder arthrodesis with plate fixation: functional outcome analysis. J Shoulder Elb Surg. 1993;2(5):225–39.
18. Braman JP, Sprague M, Bishop J, Lo IK, Lee EW, Flatow EL. The outcome of resection shoulder arthroplasty for recalcitrant shoulder infections. J Shoulder Elb Surg. 2006;15(5):549–53.
19. Debeer P, Plasschaert H, Stuyck J. Resection arthroplasty of the infected shoulder: a salvage procedure for the elderly patient. Acta Orthop Belg. 2006;72(2):126–30.
20. Muh SJ, Streit JJ, Lenarz CJ, McCrum C, Wanner JP, Shishani Y, et al. Resection arthroplasty for failed shoulder arthroplasty. J Shoulder Elb Surg. 2013;22(2):247–52.
21. Stevens NM, Kim HM, Armstrong AD. Functional outcomes after shoulder resection: the patient's perspective. J Shoulder Elb Surg. 2015;24(9):e247–54.
22. Verhelst L, Stuyck J, Bellemans J, Debeer P. Resection arthroplasty of the shoulder as a salvage procedure for deep shoulder infection: does the use of a cement spacer improve outcome? J Shoulder Elb Surg. 2011;20(8):1224–33.
23. Sperling JW, Kozak TK, Hanssen AD, Cofield RH. Infection after shoulder arthroplasty. Clin Orthop Relat Res [Internet]. 2001;382:206–16. Available from: http://www.ncbi.nlm.nih.gov/pubmed/11153989.

Part III

Revision Shoulder Arthroplasty Techniques

Surgical Exposure in Revision Shoulder Arthroplasty

16

Jason S. Klein and Charles L. Getz

Introduction

The first documented shoulder arthroplasty was completed for treatment of tuberculous arthritis in 1893 [1]. Since that time, advances in knowledge, surgical technique, shoulder implant technology, implant availability, and increasingly favorable outcomes have improved the surgeon's ability to care for a wide variety of shoulder pathologies. Moreover, the total number of shoulder arthroplasties performed has grown (11% increase from 2000 to 2008) to meet the demand of an aging population that is living longer with increasing incidence of advanced shoulder arthritis [2–4]. Additionally, the increased utilization of shoulder arthroplasty has been fueled by increased availability and expanding indications for reverse shoulder arthroplasty following its 2003 FDA approval for use in the United States [3].

Similar to other areas of joint reconstruction, shoulder replacements do not last forever. With revision as an endpoint, long-term implant survival rates for total shoulder arthroplasty are around 95% at 5 years, 90–95% at 10 years, and 79–92% at 15 years [5–7]. While recent implant survival data has been encouraging, the overall increase in shoulder arthroplasty utilization has resulted in an increased total number of complications requiring revision surgery. Five- and 10-year revision rates previously have been reported as 2–20% and 3–27%, respectively [8–13]. In a review of the National Hospital Discharge Survey database from 2001–2010, Schwartz et al. noted a fourfold increase in revision shoulder arthroplasty during that decade [14]. The demand for revision shoulder arthroplasty is expected to continue to rise in the coming years [15]. Therefore, we must be ready to take on the challenges of revision surgery.

The indications for reoperation often are multifactorial and include soft tissue-related failures (rotator cuff tears or instability, stiffness or adhesions), bone failures (fractures, malunion, nonunion), prosthetic failures (loosening, malposition, polyethylene wear), and infection [16–21]. Revision arthroplasty is technically more demanding and inherently fraught with more complications than primary arthroplasty [22–26]. Revision arthroplasty also has less predictable outcomes [27, 28] and results in inferior outcomes compared to primary arthroplasty [11, 24, 26, 29–34]. This is due in part to altered anatomy, muscle contractures, scar tissue and adhesions, bone loss, soft tissue deficiency, patient comorbidities, increased age at the time of revision surgery, and increased blood loss/transfusion requirements [11, 24, 26, 29–34].

The ability to recognize the causes of failure unique to each case is essential to successful treatment of these patients. Moreover, a thorough

J. S. Klein · C. L. Getz (✉)
Department of Orthopaedic Surgery, Thomas Jefferson University, Philadelphia, PA, USA
e-mail: Charlie.getz@rothmaninstitute.com

R. Z. Tashjian (ed.), *Complex and Revision Shoulder Arthroplasty*,
https://doi.org/10.1007/978-3-030-02756-8_16

understanding of surgical exposures and operative techniques to address a given cause of failure is critical in order to optimize patient outcomes. The focus of this chapter will be on the preoperative work-up of a failed arthroplasty and how this directs the technique of operative exposure.

Preoperative Assessment

Revision shoulder arthroplasty should be considered only after a comprehensive preoperative evaluation is completed. A thorough history should include an understanding of the original diagnosis and indication for the index procedure. Additionally, a review of previous operative notes and the postoperative course of care is mandatory. Documentation of the previous surgical approaches, implants used, rehabilitation regimen, response to therapy, and patient compliance should be performed as well in order to understand what techniques were used and the response to treatment. Early postoperative wound healing problems should be noted. The current physical status of the shoulder should be evaluated including the healing status of the prior incisions, overall skin problems of the shoulder (acne, erythema, swelling), range of motion, strength, stability, and neurovascular status. Complaints regarding function, pain, instability, and weakness are documented. A discussion about the patient's goals and expectations for the revision surgery should be performed. Finally, comprehensive examination of the entire upper extremity including cervical spine, scapulothoracic articulation, and ipsilateral chest is required.

The laboratory work-up should include an evaluation of inflammatory markers (sedimentation rate, C-reactive protein) even if there is not a concern for underlying infection (such as fevers, chills, erythema, warmth, or history of previous infection), as well as a complete metabolic panel to identify metabolic bone disease. If concern for infection persists, aspiration should be considered with synovial fluid held for at least 14 days to identify *Propionibacterium acnes* [35, 36]. A complete set of shoulder radiographs including an axillary view should be obtained and compared to previous radiographs looking for component malposition, subsidence, osteolysis and loosening, and fracture. Advanced imaging including ultrasounds and CT scans may be considered to evaluate the rotator cuff and to assess for the presence of soft tissue deficiencies and bone loss. Typically, MRI is of little use due to metal artifact although metal suppression techniques are being developed to improve the utility of MRI post-arthroplasty. The results of these studies will guide one's operative plan if surgery is indicated. In the case of suspected nerve injury, an EMG/nerve conduction study should be completed to document existing neurologic lesions and to plan for possible nerve or tendon transfers. Finally, a medical evaluation and clearance should be performed to optimize patient comorbidities prior to surgical intervention.

Revision Arthroplasty Surgical Technique

As with any surgery, preparation for the operating room begins prior to incision. Confirmation is required that revision instruments and implants are available. Typical instruments and equipment include implant extraction tools, flexible and rigid osteotomes, small microsagittal saws, burrs, drills, cables or cable systems, and allografts (struts and bulk) (Table 16.1). Fluoroscopy

Table 16.1 Planning for the OR

Pick list
System-specific trays (for primary and revision implants)
Revision implants
Universal extraction kits
Osteotomes (rigid and flexible)
Drill and drill bit rack
High-speed burr
Sagittal saw
Cables
Allografts
Fluoroscopy
Heavy permanent suture
Bovie and/or bipolar cautery
Hewson suture passer
Cement extraction instrumentation
Cement and cement restrictors
Culture swabs and specimen tubes

should be available. If vascular or soft tissue deficiencies may be encountered, consultation and coordination with appropriate services should be performed so that they are available and ready to intervene at the time surgery is required. Revision surgery is associated with a higher complication rate, including neurologic injury. Therefore, nerve monitoring can be utilized at the time of surgery as well as based upon surgeon preference.

The author's preferred patient position is a 45-degree beach chair position with appropriate padding of bony prominences and flexion about the knees to protect the sciatic nerve (Fig. 16.1a). The skin is prepared with an alcohol or Betadine wash and then with a chlorhexidine gluconate-based solution. The extremity is draped with the use of Ioban antimicrobial adhesive drapes (3 M, St. Paul, MN) to seal off the sterile field.

Old incisions should be utilized if possible, but the skin of the shoulder region is well vascularized, and adjacent incisions can be made with low risk for wound healing problems. The old incision can be extended for improved exposure and to aid dissection in native tissue where the anatomy has not been distorted. If the previous approach was not through the deltopectoral interval, a new anterior incision just proximal to the coracoid extending distally along the anterior portion of the deltoid to its insertion on the humerus should be utilized. Most of the goals of revision arthroplasty can be accomplished through the deltopectoral interval alone. Once through the skin, old suture may direct your path to the deltopectoral interval. Careful dissection of the soft tissues is of critically important to decrease the risk of wound breakdown or deltoid denervation/dysfunction, both of which are critical to the success of revision surgery maximizing function and stability.

The coracoid is the lighthouse of the shoulder and can be used as a guide to orient the surgeon to the proximal extent of the deltopectoral interval, particularly if the cephalic vein is absent or difficult to identify (Fig. 16.1b). If the cephalic vein cannot be safely dissected from surrounding scar, ligate the vein to maintain hemostasis and a dry operative field. The exposure is carried the full length of the incision to the base of the wound. Proximally, the clavicle should be easily palpable, and distally, the insertion of the deltoid is exposed. Initial dissection medial to the coracoid is minimized. The tissue plane between the deltoid and pectoralis is often scarred. The muscle bellies can be differentiated by contraction of the muscles using the bovie. Often the proximal extent of the interval has been left untouched by prior surgeons and can be a region to initiate dissection. Using cautery, the interval can be dissected from proximal to distal using a rake or Senn retractor on the deltoid to maintain tension in the tissue. The conjoined tendon should be the structure that is next approached during the dissection understanding that it is commonly scarred laterally so lateral dissection through the interval is important to avoid inadvertent injury to the conjoined tendon and nearby neurovascular structures.

Upon developing the deltopectoral interval, one should focus on developing the subdeltoid and subacromial spaces. The clavipectoral fascia lateral to the conjoined tendon is incised from the pectoralis major tendon to the coracoacromial ligament (Fig. 16.1c). The subscapularis is deep to the clavipectoral fascia and should not be injured when incising the clavipectoral fascia. A Mayo scissor is spread under the CA ligament in the subacromial space to start the adhesion release in the subacromial space (Fig. 16.1d). A Browne deltoid retractor is placed into the subacromial space between the acromion and supraspinatus if one is still intact. Care is taken to not place the retractor through the rotator interval potentially injuring the posterosuperior rotator cuff.

At this point, the arm may be placed in slight abduction and internal rotation, which helps identify the anterior deltoid. While some have found it easiest to first develop the subdeltoid space distally, adhesion release from proximal to distal by starting in the subacromial space and sweeping down distally to the deltoid insertion with blunt dissection or a Cobb elevator can also be performed and is our preference. If the leading edge of the deltoid is tightly adhered to the humerus, a knife or bovie is used parallel and in contact with the humerus to start the elevation of

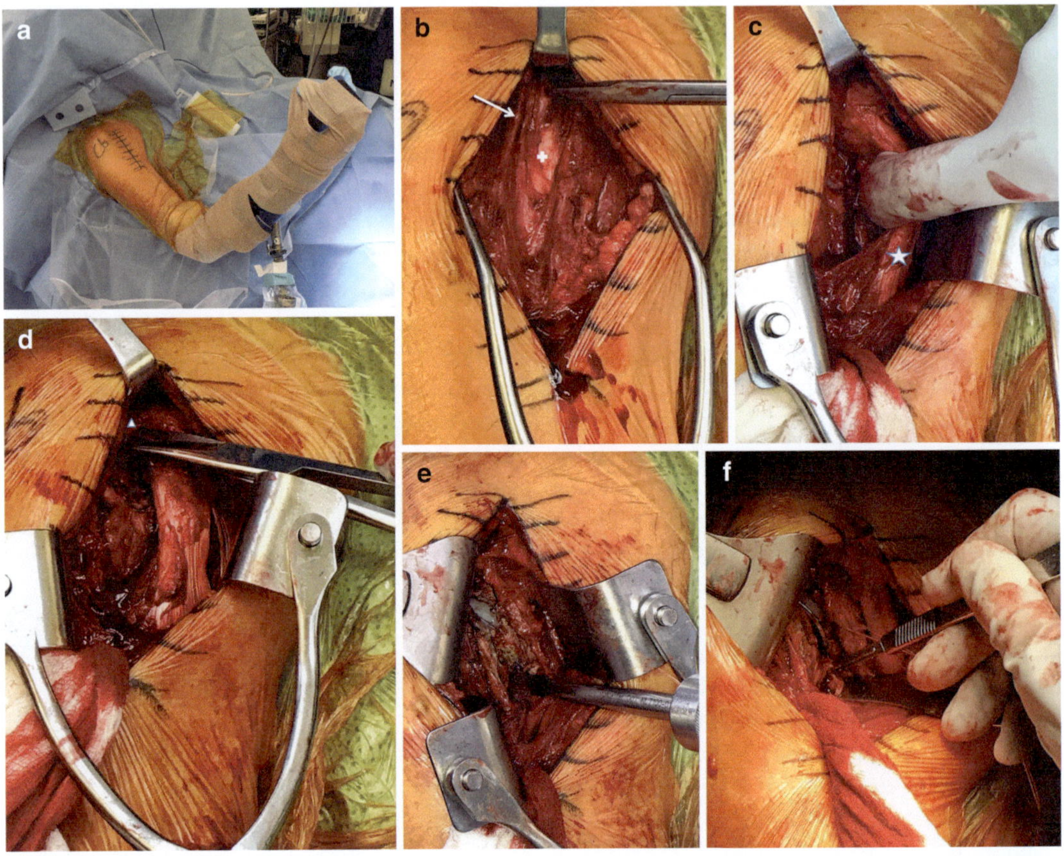

Fig. 16.1 (**a**) Patient is positioned 45° from horizontal in the lazy beach chair position. The arm may be secured with an arm positioner or rested on a Mayo stand. The anticipated incision is marked out, in this case over the previous incision. The end of the previous incision is marked to identify the extent of previous incision in case it needs to be extended for improved exposure and/or releases. (**b**) After incision and dissection through subcutaneous tissues, an army navy retractor placed just superficial to the coracoid. In this image, the scissor is pointing at the coracoid, which guides development of the deltopectoral interval distally as you carefully dissect through scar. The scarred cephalic vein (arrow) was retracted laterally. The + sign identifies the conjoined tendon in this image. (**c**) After taking down remaining clavipectoral fascia and scar tissue lateral to the conjoined tendon, blunt dissection of the subcoracoid space is performed. The axillary nerve should be identified in this space between the conjoined tendon (star) superficially and the subscapularis musculotendinous unit deep if it is still intact. (**d**) The subacromial space is developed by inserting scissors beneath the coracoacromial ligament (triangle) and by spreading into the subacromial space. Once this space is developed, the dissection can be continued distally into the subdeltoid space, taking down adhesions to the posterior aspect of the proximal humerus to allow for placement of a deltoid retractor. (**e, f**) After the rotator interval is opened and subscapularis taken down, a Cobb elevator is placed along the inferior humeral neck to assist with humeral releases and dislocation. (**g**) The axillary nerve seen here at the tip of the clamp should again be identified before proceeding with glenoid exposure and synovium/scar removal. The nerve is being identified posterior to the conjoined tendon and inferior to the subscapularis as it is passing posteriorly. (**h**) The subscapularis is grasped in this picture to allow for dissection of the subscapularis from the underlying capsule, beginning the releases and debridement around the glenoid. (**i**) After the space between the capsule and subscapularis has been developed and with a blunt Hohmann retractor placed between the subscapularis posteriorly and the axillary nerve anteriorly to protect the nerve, the capsule is released down to the glenoid vault. This accomplishes an inferior release often allowing the humerus to fall posteriorly thereby improving glenoid visualization. (**j**) To improve subscapularis excursion and exposure of glenoid, a Cobb elevator is carefully placed along the anterior glenoid to facilitate release of adhesions. The subscapularis is marked with the arrow. The capsule is marked with the star

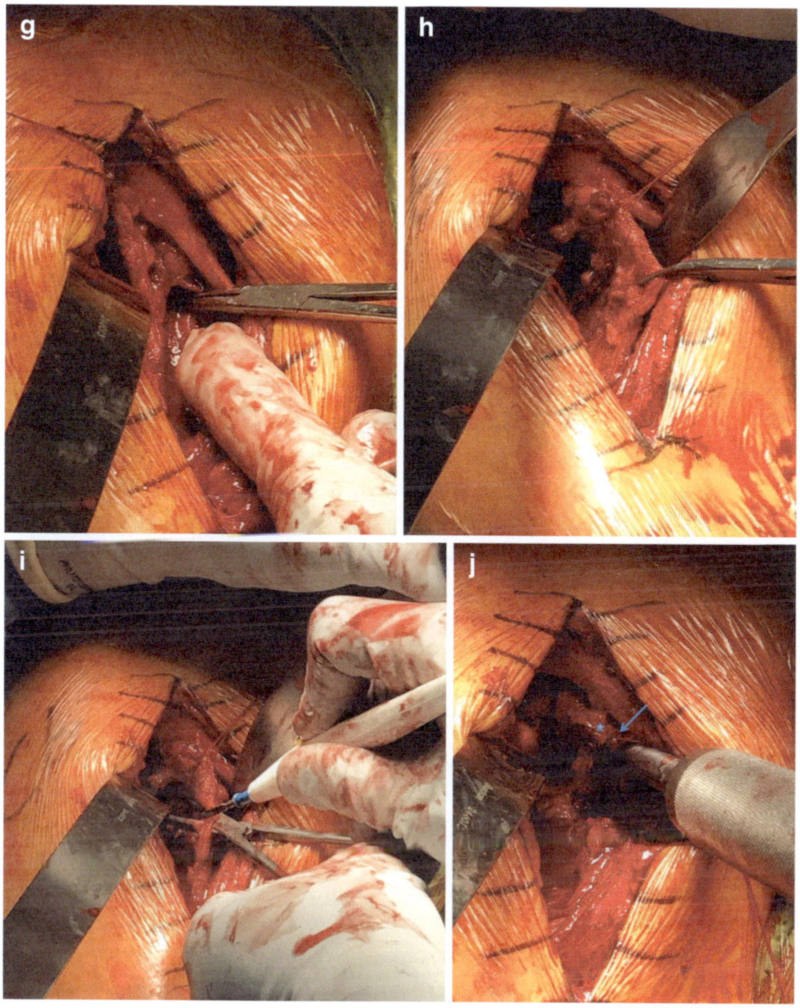

Fig. 16.1 (continued)

the deltoid taking care to avoid cutting the deltoid, the axillary nerve, or the rotator cuff. The anterior insertion of the deltoid can be released to facilitate exposure if needed. However, deltoid release should be done as a last resort and should be repaired at the end of the case to maximize deltoid function. The deltoid can be released from the clavicle, acromioclavicular joint, and acromion (and repaired again at the end of the procedure) to facilitate exposure in extreme cases although this has not been required in the authors' practice. In cases in which the rotator cuff is intact, the coracoacromial (CA) ligament can be partially incised to improve exposure; however complete release should be avoided in unconstrained arthroplasty to avoid anterosuperior escape [17, 37, 38]. The CA ligament can be sectioned without consequence in the setting of reverse total shoulder arthroplasty.

The subcoracoid space should be developed next. First, the coracoid and the conjoined tendon are identified. The pectoralis major is often scarred to the conjoined tendon; therefore careful dissection between these structures should be performed to facilitate improved exposure and motion. Next, the plane between the conjoined tendon and subscapularis muscle-tendon unit is developed allowing the axillary nerve to be identified and protected. Adduction and internal rotation of the shoulder as well as elbow flexion can facilitate exposure between the subscapularis and the conjoined tendon by relieving tension on the conjoined. Caution should be taken with this dissection due to the presence of significant scar, adhesions, and suture material from prior subscapularis repairs that often complicate these revision cases.

When the subscapularis is intact, the deep surface of the conjoined tendon can be freed with careful dissection taking care not to dissect medial to avoid neurovascular injury. When the subscapularis is ruptured, the dissection of the deep surface of the conjoined is more difficult. The authors like to start at the base of the coracoid to identify any residual capsule or tendon. If possible, a traction stitch or Kocher is placed to allow for lateral traction of the subscapularis. If no plane is identifiable, consideration is made for brachial plexus dissection to identify the axillary nerve at Erb's point medial to conjoined tendon to allow safe releases and scar/capsular excision. Alternative strategies besides going to a plexus exploration include (1) identifying the lower border of the subscapularis and working proximally as the lower border can often be healed despite superior border failure or (2) not identifying the nerve anterior the subscapularis but identifying it inferiorly during glenoid exposure. There is usually scar at the inferior border, but remnant of the circumflex vessels can guide the dissection medially if lower border dissection is performed. Care should be used to not enter the conjoined tendon as the musculocutaneous nerve is a risk at this level. If the nerve is only identified inferior to the glenoid, dissection should be carried lateral to medial from the released capsule from the humerus to the inferior edge of the glenoid separating capsule superficially from the axillary nerve.

Release and/or lengthening of the conjoined tendon is sometimes necessary to improve visualization, particularly in chronic anterior dislocated shoulders. Release of the conjoined tendon also is performed for emergency access to the axillary artery in the case of a vascular injury. Surgeons performing revision arthroplasty should be familiar with this exposure. The easiest method of release is to remove from the coracoid either with fleck of bone at the tip or cutting directly off the coracoid sharply with a bovie. The tendons can then be repaired using #5 high-strength suture in a Krackow fashion in the proximal 1.5 cm of the tendons and repair through a drill hole in the remaining coracoid tied over a bone bridge.

With the all three spaces developed, it is time to address the intra-articular pathology. The author's preferred technique is to identify the bicipital groove and open the rotator interval to the level of the glenoid while inspecting the surrounding structures. Identification of the rotator interval can be challenging in revisions as the anterior and superior cuff blend as a single sheet of tissue. Knowing the subscapularis upper border exits inferior to the coracoid will assist in identifying the interval and avoid violation of the supraspinatus or subscapularis muscles or tendons. The subscapularis is then taken down in the surgeon's preferred manner. A plane should be developed between any residual capsule and the subscapularis tendon and muscle belly either before or after subscapularis mobilization.

Aggressive humeral-sided releases are needed for exposure and postoperative range of motion. The muscular insertion of the subscapularis and the inferior capsule need to be released past 6 o'clock inferiorly on the humerus. In addition to releasing the upper border of the pectoralis major tendon, one can release the latissimus dorsi tendon release to aid exposure. Humeral releases are aided by external rotation, adduction, and forward flexion of the humerus and by placing a retractor (Darrach) along the humeral neck. Any residual rotator interval is released at this time as the medial rotator cuff interval tissue can tether the supraspinatus to the subscapularis limited posterior displacement of the humeral head (Fig. 16.1e, f).

With a retractor in the subacromial space, along the humeral neck, and in the glenohumeral joint, the arm is externally rotated and extended to perform a surgical dislocation. Care should be taken during this maneuver to not fracture the greater tuberosity or tear the posterosuperior rotator cuff. If there is significant difficulty, further releases should be performed. At this stage, the humeral implants can be removed with several techniques, which will be discussed in later sections of this book. However, if humeral osteotomies or bone windows are required, one may need to release the pectoralis major and deltoid insertions to improve visualization and to plan the osteotomies.

After the humerus is removed, glenoid exposure is performed. A Fukuda or double-pronged Bankart retractor is placed posterior to the glenoid to help move the proximal humerus lateral and posterior thereby improving one's visualization of the anterior and inferior capsule. The arm is placed into neutral rotation for the initial glenoid-sided releases. A blunt Hohmann can also be placed between the axillary nerve and any residual capsule/subscapularis to protect the nerve after it has been identified as seen in Fig. 16.1g. The plane between the capsule and overlying subscapularis is developed. While protecting the axillary nerve, the capsule can be split to the inferior glenoid to complete the inferior release. Once complete, the blunt Hohmann can be repositioned into the joint along the inferior glenoid. The anterior capsule can then be released from the overlying subscapularis and the anterior glenoid to complete the anterior releases as seen in Fig. 16.1h. A double-pronged Bankart retractor can then be placed along the anterior glenoid neck for optimal exposure. At this point all four surfaces of the subscapularis have been released, and excursion is checked. Repeating the rotator interval, superficial and deep dissections, and releases may be required to ensure maximal excursion.

Arm abduction and external rotation will allow the retractors to push the humeral head posteriorly in order to improve glenoid visualization. Excessive arm abduction should be avoided as this can place the brachial plexus on stretch leading to a palsy. Synovium and hypertrophic tissue should be excised to facilitate glenoid exposure. Removal of inferior scar tissues while protecting the axillary nerve will improve postoperative restoration of arm elevation (Fig. 16.1i).

Any residual adhesion along the capsule and anterior glenoid neck can be carefully released with Cobb elevators to improve subscapularis excursion, mobility, and glenoid exposure (Fig. 16.1j). Releasing the subscapularis from its fossa along the anterior neck of the glenoid is safe with a low risk for neurovascular injury. Posterior capsule can be released to improve posterior humeral excursion if needed to improve visualization of the glenoid. We caution against release of any structures such as insertion of intact teres minor or posterior capsule if it is not interfering with exposure in order to maintain and optimize function and stability postoperatively.

In revision arthroplasty, it is often necessary to extend the incision distally along the anterolateral approach to the humerus to facilitate exposure. As such, care should be taken preoperatively to prep and drape the entire arm so that access to the mid to distal arm is available. Earlier, we discussed the potential need for pectoralis major release for improved exposure and/or exposure of the neurovascular structures in the event of injury. However, one may also need to release the pectoralis major in preparation of humeral osteotomies for implant removal. Using bovie cautery, the pectoralis major can be released from the bone leaving a 5 mm stump of insertion on the humerus to facilitate soft tissue repair upon closure with ethibond or other nonabsorbable suture. The extension along the anterolateral approach to the humerus may also be necessary in the event of periprosthetic fracture and revision to a long-stem prosthesis with plate, screws, strut grafts, and/or cables.

There are several other approaches to the shoulder that can be used for revision shoulder arthroplasty, either by choice or because of previous incisions. These include a deltoid splitting, posterior Judet, or an extended superior deltopectoral approach with clavicular osteotomy. However, the authors have not found them to be easier or necessary to expose the shoulder completely for the purposes of revision shoulder arthroplasty, resection arthroplasty, or fusion. In the setting of failed proximal humerus fracture treated with lateral locking plates or hemiarthroplasty through a deltoid splitting technique, we have found it more difficult to identify and protect the axillary nerve as well as expose the glenohumeral joint for preparation and completion of revision shoulder arthroplasty if the prior deltoid split is used. Ultimately, it has been the authors' experience that meticulous dissection and exposure through the deltopectoral approach in a stepwise fashion as described above allow for safe and adequate exposure to perform revision arthroplasty based on the reason for failure identified in the preoperative work-up.

Summary

The demand for revision arthroplasty will rise over the next decade with increased utilization of shoulder arthroplasty. Recent experiences with revision shoulder arthroplasty illustrate less predictable and inferior outcomes with these challenging procedures. Identifying the cause of arthroplasty failure and developing a surgical plan are critical for success in these cases. Application of a systematic approach to the surgical exposure is critical in the complex cases in order to optimize results and avoid complications.

References

1. Lugli T. Artificial shoulder joint by Pean (1893): the facts of an exceptional intervention and the prosthetic method. Clin Orthop Relat Res. 1978;133:215–8.
2. Jain NB, Higgins LD, Guller U, et al. Trends in the epidemiology of total shoulder arthroplasty in the United States from 1990–2000. Arthritis Rheum. 2006;55:591–7.
3. Kim SH, Wise BW, Zhang Y, Szabo RM. Increasing incidence of shoulder arthroplasty in the United States. JBJS. 2011;93:2249–54.
4. Trofa D, Rajaee SS, Smith EL. Nationwide trends in total shoulder arthroplasty and hemiarthroplasty for osteoarthritis. Am J Orthop (Belle Mead NJ). 2014;43:166–72.
5. Fox TJ, Cil A, Sperling JW, et al. Survival of the glenoid component in shoulder arthroplasty. J Shoulder Elb Surg. 2009;18:859–63.
6. Singh JA, Sperling JW, Cofield RH. Revision surgery following total shoulder arthroplasty. J Bone Joint Surg (Br). 2001;93-B:1513–7.
7. Young A, Walch G, Boileau P, et al. A multicentre study of the long-term results of using a flat-back polyethylene glenoid component in shoulder replacement for primary osteoarthritis. J Bone Joint Surg (Br). 2011;93:210–6.
8. Fevang BT, Lie SA, Havelin LI, Skredderstuen A, Fumes O. Risk factors for revision after shoulder arthroplasty: 1825 shoulder arthroplasties from the Norwegian Arthroplasty Register. Acta Orthop. 2009;80:83–91.
9. Khan A, Bunker TD, Kitson JB. Clinical and radiological follow-up of the Aequalis third-generation cemented total shoulder replacement: a minimum ten-year study. J Bone Joint Surg (Br). 2009;91-B:1594–600.
10. Martin SD, Zurakowski D, Thornhill TS. Uncemented glenoid component in total shoulder arthroplasty: survivorship and outcomes. J Bone Joint Surg Am. 2005;87-A:1284–92.
11. Sperling JW, Cofield RH, Rowland CM. Neer hemiarthroplasty and Neer total shoulder arthroplasty in patients fifty years old or less: long-term results. J Bone Joint Surg Am. 1998;80-A:464–73.
12. Tammachote N, Sperling JW, Vathana T, et al. Long-term results of cemented metal-backed glenoid components for osteoarthritis of the shoulder. J Bone Joint Surg Am. 2009;91-A:160–6.
13. Thomas SR, Wilson AJ, Chambler A, Harding I, Thomas M. Outcomes of Copeland surface replacement shoulder arthroplasty. J Shoulder Elb Surg. 2005;14:485–91.
14. Schwartz BE, Savin DD, Youderian AR, Mossad D, Goldberg BA. National trends and perioperative outcomes in primary and revision total shoulder arthroplasty. Int Orthop. 2015;39:271–6.
15. Hollatz MF, Stang A. Nationwide shoulder arthroplasty rates and revision burden in Germany: analysis of the national hospitalization data 2005 to 2006. J Shoulder Elb Surg. 2014;23(11):e267–74.
16. Ankem HK, Blaine TA. Revision shoulder arthroplasty. Tech Should Elbow Surg. 2005;6(4):189–98.
17. Cofield RH, Edgerton BC. Total shoulder arthroplasty: complications and revision surgery. Instr Course Lect. 1990;39:449–62.
18. Cofield RH. Revision procedures in shoulder arthroplasty. In: Morrey BF, editor. Reconstructive surgery of the joints. 2nd ed. New York: Churchill Livingstone; 1996. p. 789.
19. Hassan SS, Leith JM, Campbell B, Kapil R, Smith KL, Matsen FA 3rd. Characteristics of unsatisfactory shoulder arthroplasties. J Shoulder Elb Surg. 2002;11:431–41.
20. Kalandiak SP, Wirth MA, Rockwood CA. Complications of shoulder arthroplasty. In: Williams Jr GR, Yamaguchi K, Ramsey ML, Galatz M, editors. Shoulder and elbow arthroplasty. Philadelphia: Lippincott Williams and Wilkins; 2005. p. 229–50.
21. Wirth MA, Rockwood CA Jr. Complications of total shoulder-replacement arthroplasty. J Bone Joint Surg Am. 1996;78:603–16.
22. Saltzman BM, Chalmer PN, Gupta AK, Romeo AA, Nicholson GP. Complication rates comparing primary with revision reverse total shoulder arthroplasty. J Should Elb Surg. 2014;23:1647–54.

23. Wall B, Nove-Josserand L, O'Connor DP, Edwards TB, Walch G. Reverse total shoulder arthroplasty: a review of results according to etiology. J Bone Joint Surg Am. 2007;89:1476 95.
24. Deutsch A, Abboud JA, Kelly J, et al. Clinical results of revision shoulder arthroplasty for glenoid component loosening. J Shoulder Elb Surg. 2007;16:706–16.
25. Melis B, Bonnevialle N, Neyton N, Walch G, Boileau P. Aseptic glenoid loosening or failure in total shoulder arthroplasty. In: Walch G, Boileau P, Mole D, Favard L, Levigne C, Sirveaux F, editors. Shoulder concepts 2010: the glenoid. Paris: Sauramps Medical; 2010. p. 299–312.
26. Walker M, Willis MP, Brooks JP, Pupello D, Mulieri PJ, Frankle MA. The use of the reverse shoulder arthroplasty for treatment of failed total shoulder arthroplasty. J Should Elb Surg. 2012;21:514–22.
27. Werner CM, Steinmann PA, Gilbart M, Gerber C. Treatment of painful pseudoparesis due to irreparable rotator cuff dysfunction with the Delta III reverse-ball-and-socket total shoulder prosthesis. J Bone Joint Surg Am. 2005;87:1476–86.
28. Boileau P, Watkinson DJ, Hatzidakis AM, Balg F. Grammont reverse prosthesis: design, rationale, and biomechanics. J Shoulder Elb Surg. 2005;14:147S–61S.
29. Dines JS, Fealy S, Strauss EJ, Allen A, Craig EV, Warren RF, Dines DM. Outcomes analysis of revision total shoulder replacement. J Bone Joint Surg Am. 2006;88:1494–500.
30. Antuna SA, Sperling JW, Cofield RH, et al. Glenoid revision surgery after total shoulder arthroplasty. J Shoulder Elb Surg. 2001;10.217–24.
31. Carroll RM, Izquierdo R, Vazquez M, et al. Conversion of painful hemiarthroplasty to total shoulder arthroplasty: long-term results. J Shoulder Elb Surg. 2004;13:599–603.
32. Cheung EV, Sperling JW, Cofield RH. Revision shoulder arthroplasty for glenoid component loosening. J Shoulder Elb Surg. 2008;17:371–5.
33. Petersen SA, Hawkins RJ. Revision of failed total shoulder arthroplasty. Orthop Clin North Am. 1998;29:519–33.
34. Strickland JP, Sperling JW, Cofield RH. The results of two-stage re-implantation for infected shoulder replacement. J Bone Joint Surg Br. 2008;90:460–5.
35. Topolski MS, Chin PY, Sperling JW, Cofield RH. Revision shoulder arthroplasty with positive intraoperative cultures: the value of preoperative studies and intraoperative histology. J Shoulder Elb Surg. 2006;15(4):402–6.
36. Wang B, Toye B, Desjardins M, Lapner P, Lee C. A7-year retrospective review from 2005 to 2011 of Propionibacterium acnes shoulder infections in Ottawa, Ontario, Canada. Diagn Microbiol Infect Dis. 2013;75:195–9.
37. Sonnaband D, Mohammed KD. Revision shoulder arthroplasty. J Shoulder Elb Surg. 1999;8:553.
38. Moeckel BW, Warren RF, Dines DM, et al. The unstable shoulder arthroplasty. In: Freedman RJ, editor. Arthroplasty of the shoulder. New York: Thieme; 1994. p. 254–63.

Management of Large Glenoid Defects: Bone Grafts and Augmented Components

17

Peter N. Chalmers

Introduction

There were over 100,000 shoulder arthroplasties in the United States from 2011 to 2012 [1]. Shoulder arthroplasty is becoming more common [2]. As it becomes more common and as experience and comfort with the procedure grow, rates of revision arthroplasty are increasing [3]. These procedures often involve substantial bone loss and often require either structural bone grafting or an augmented component [4]. For instance, although baseplate loosening is uncommon [5], when it does occur, deltoid tension leads to proximal migration of a fixed angle construct that cuts through the glenoid vault before compromising baseplate stability and is thus associated with challenging loss of glenoid bone stock [6]. Glenoid bone defects must be addressed to achieve optimal component position and stability and to avoid issues postoperatively [7–10]. For instance, superior glenoid component malpositioning may contribute to inferior impingement, notching, and instability [11], while medial glenoid component malpositioning may contribute to inadequate soft tissue tensioning[10] with reverse total shoulder arthroplasty (RTSA). Shoulder surgeons must therefore be familiar with the evaluation and treatment of glenoid bone defects in the setting of shoulder arthroplasty.

Preoperative planning is crucial in the setting of a glenoid bone defect. A thorough preoperative assessment is crucial to identify the best treatment option. This includes a full history to understand prior traumas, prior non-operative treatments, and prior operative treatments. If possible, prior operative reports should be obtained to determine prior implants and the dimensions of these prior failed implants. In particular, TSA has increasingly incorporated flanged central peg glenoid components that require drilling a larger central hole that can be the beginning of a cavitary defect. In RTSA the central post/screw is typically 8–9 mm but increasingly contains a shoulder section that is up to 15 mm in diameter. Many RTSA components also involve a large central screw that is up to 9.5 mm in diameter. Removal of these components can leave a substantial defect (Fig. 17.1). As glenoid components have evolved to improve fixation, their ease of revision may be worsening. A full examination should be performed including inspection of prior incisions, range of motion, strength, neurovascular testing, palpation for tenderness, and provocative tests. In all patients with prior surgical procedures, the possibility of infection should be considered and appropriately evaluated. Chapter 5 reviews the diagnosis of infection in the setting of shoulder arthroplasty. Infection is

P. N. Chalmers (✉)
Shoulder and Elbow Surgery, Department of Orthopaedic Surgery, University of Utah, Salt Lake City, UT, USA
e-mail: peter.chalmers@hsc.utah.edu

R. Z. Tashjian (ed.), *Complex and Revision Shoulder Arthroplasty*,
https://doi.org/10.1007/978-3-030-02756-8_17

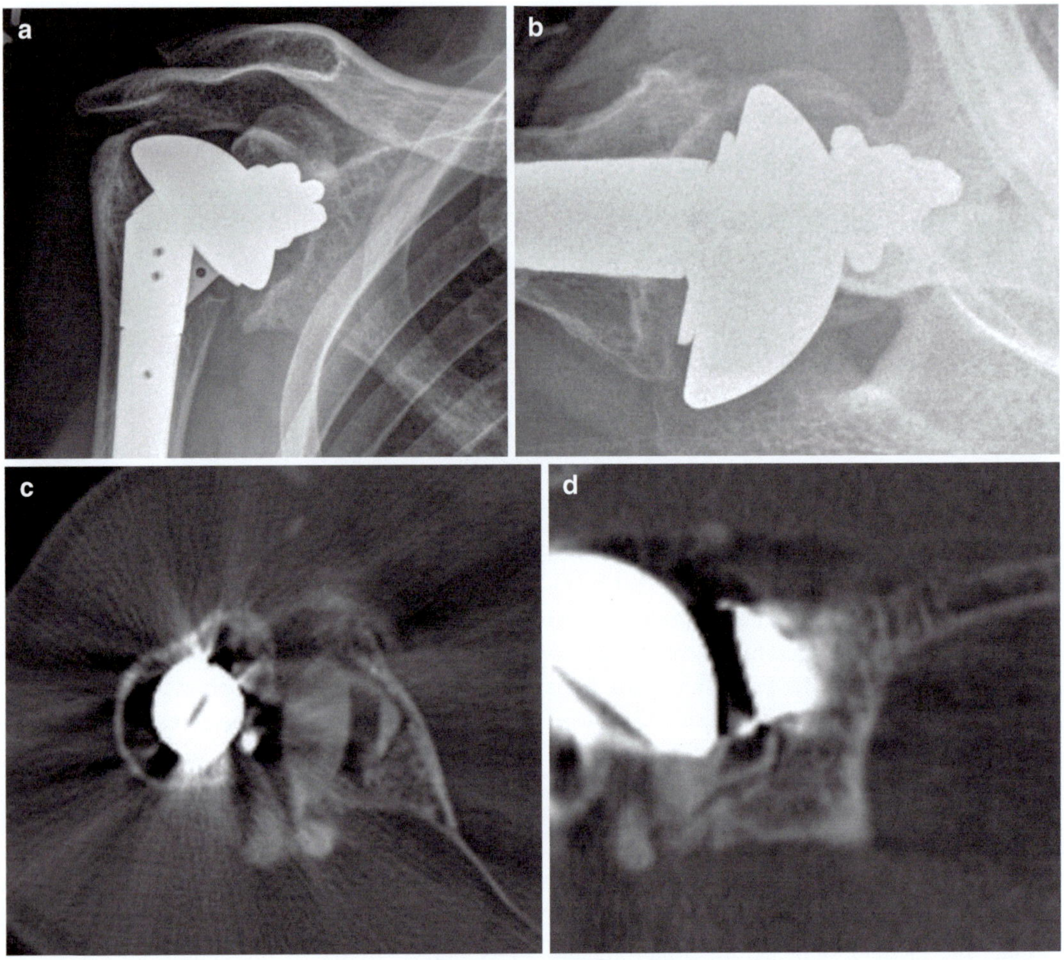

Fig. 17.1 These anteroposterior (**a**) and axillary (**b**) radiographs and axial (**c**) and coronal (**d**) computed tomographic arthrogram images demonstrate the severity of bone loss frequently encountered in the setting of glenoid loosening and TSA

an absolute contraindication to most glenoid reconstruction options.

The evaluation of these defects is complex and usually requires a three-dimensional computed tomographic scan in addition to high-quality triple-orthogonal plain radiographs. Often the deformity is biplanar, and the surgeon must use the remaining native anatomy to determine the pre-deformity anatomy (Fig. 17.2). Existing software allows the virtual implantation of components for preoperative planning [12], and future software will likely produce an estimate of the pre-deformity anatomy based upon statistical

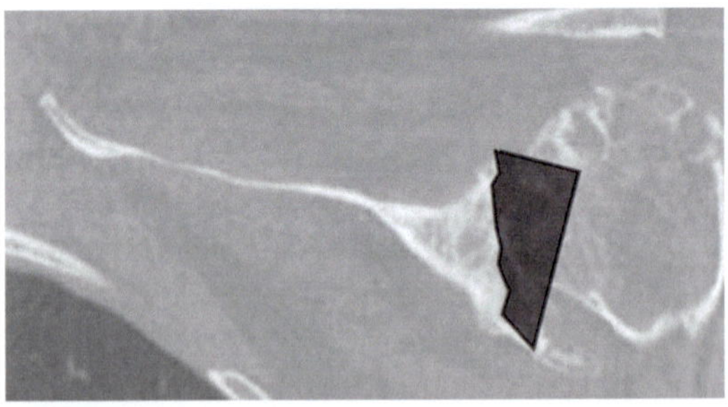

Fig. 17.2 This coronal computed tomographic image demonstrates a substantial superior bone defect in the setting of a primary RTSA. The triangle demonstrates the likely defect

Table 17.1 Advantages and disadvantages of each technique

Option	Advantages	Disadvantages
Femoral head allograft BIORSA	Ease and speed of graft sculpting Readily available graft Easily customizable	Allograft Nonstructural Baseplate does not rest on native scapula
Iliac crest autograft BIORSA	Structural Autograft	Donor-site morbidity Baseplate does not rest on native scapula
Femoral neck Allograft/cancellous autograft	Autograft Structural	Cortical allograft Baseplate does not rest on native scapula Less customizable
Structural grafting	Center point with native landmarks Autograft Structural Baseplate can rest on native scapula	Technically challenging Time-consuming
Augmented baseplate	Obviates graft-related issues Purpose-designed instrumentation Baseplate rests against native scapula	Does not restore native bone stock Less customizable Potentially biomechanically inferior Increased cost

BIORSA bony increased offset reverse shoulder arthroplasty

shape modeling [13]. These advances will be crucial as glenoid bone loss implies an alteration of the normal glenohumeral spatial relationship and a likely resultant soft tissue imbalance [7–10]. However, with a distortion of CT images by metal artifact, preoperative glenoid deformities in revision arthroplasty can be difficult to fully assess.

A variety of options exist to reconstruct osseous glenoid deficiencies, including eccentric reaming [14], augmented glenoid components [8, 15, 16], and bone grafting techniques [6, 9, 10, 15, 17–29]. There remains substantial controversy regarding the optimal technique (Table 17.1) [18, 25–27, 29]. The shoulder surgeon must master each of these options as glenoid reconstruction is often the most difficult and least forgiving portion of shoulder arthroplasty as bone stock is limited, exposure is challenging, and landmarks can be difficult to reliably identify. Glenoid exposure is covered in depth in Chap. 9 and thus will not be addressed in this chapter. However, most of the techniques discussed require excellent glenoid exposure. This usually requires a full view of the anterior, posterior, and especially inferior glenoid rims as well as exposure of the scapular spine and the ability to finger palpate along the anterior surface of the vault. Without sufficient exposure and hemostasis, none of the techniques described below are possible.

Anatomic Total Shoulder Arthroplasty

Historically, bone grafting techniques were used in the setting of revision to an anatomic TSA. The results of glenoid bone grafting in the setting of revision anatomic shoulder arthroplasty have been disappointing [20], with subsidence rates ranging from 20% [28] to nearly 50% [22]. Many surgeons have thus abandoned glenoid bone grafting in revision TSA in favor of RTSA, and thus these techniques will not be discussed here [20, 22, 28]. In primary TSA, the most common deformity is glenoid retroversion, posterior humeral subluxation, and wear of the posterior glenoid into a double concavity. In this deformity, the surgeon uses the original, pre-deformity "paleoglenoid" to reconstruct the new, post-deformity "neoglenoid" to the same level as the "paleoglenoid." Both bone grafting [30] and augmented component strategies [16, 31–35] are available to address this pathology. These are discussed in depth in Chap. 4.

Reverse Total Shoulder Arthroplasty

Glenoid bone defects are common in the setting of revision to RTSA. For instance, in one of the largest published series of revision RTSAs, 78% underwent glenoid bone grafting [6]. These defects vary in their extent and location, and the optimal reconstruction technique may be defect-dependent [18, 36, 37]. Prior surgeons have classified these defects as either central or peripheral and either as contained and uncontained [38]. Revision to RTSA is often associated with more global defects [17, 18, 27]. The most common indication for revision to RTSA from TSA is loosening of the glenoid component [6] which is also frequently associated with rotator cuff insufficiency, superior migration, and superior-predominant bone loss. In the setting of a native glenoid, most surgeons will aim for 10° of inferior inclination relative to the glenoid to avoid adduction impingement and to minimize notching and instability. In the setting of revision RTSA, superior glenoid bone loss is common; therefore if the baseplate is oriented in the plane of the glenoid, the baseplate will be superiorly inclined, which can lead to compromised range of motion, impingement, instability, and notching. Alternatively, in revision to RTSA, the inferior glenoid rim may have been compromised and may thus not provide optimal baseplate support. In this setting, the surgeon can consider the alternate center line method, which seeks to place the central post/screw within the scapular spine [25]. However, surgeons must be wary with this technique as it can increase the risk for adduction impingement, notching, and instability, and thus this technique may only be appropriate with a lateralized baseplates or glenosphere. In addition, fixation into the spine with a post may lead to a compromise of the scapular spine with scapular spine fractures or scapular body fractures (Fig. 17.3), which can lead to secondary loss of fixation of the baseplate, and thus this technique may only be appropriate with a central screw. Ultimately, baseplate position is a compromise as the surgeon seeks to achieve both initial stability and to minimize the long-term risk loosening while maximizing range of motion and minimizing impingement, instability, and notching.

Bone Grafting

Although largely abandoned in the setting of revision anatomic TSA, the results of glenoid bone grafting in the setting of RTSA have been encouraging, likely because of the stability of the initial glenoid component fixation [18, 25–27, 29]. These results have led to expanded indications for RTSA [6, 17, 18, 39]. However, substantial controversy remains about how best to apply this technique, and midterm survival of the glenoid component in the setting of bone grafting is likely inferior to when bone grafting is not necessary [18]. Potential graft sources include humeral head autograft (which is usually not available in revision arthroplasty settings) [10, 27], iliac crest autograft [6, 26, 27], cancellous autograft [6, 9], cancellous allograft [20], femoral neck allograft [9, 36], and femoral head allograft [19, 25]. Cancellous allograft is only appropriate with a contained defect, and it has been the author's experience that most defects in revision to RTSA are uncontained defects that necessitate structural grafts. The optimal graft choice may be host- and defect-dependent – in particular, when the biology of the remaining native bone is questionable, such as with failure of incorporation of a prior graft, history of nonunion, or prior radiation, consideration could be given to the use of autograft [6].

A variety of techniques exist for glenoid bone grafting. The ideal technique would allow the surgeon to address both contained and uncontained defects while providing good initial stability, optimizing graft incorporation, easing future revisions, minimizing cost, and minimizing donor-site morbidity. One of the most commonly utilized techniques is Boileau's bony increased offset reverse shoulder arthroplasty (BIORSA)

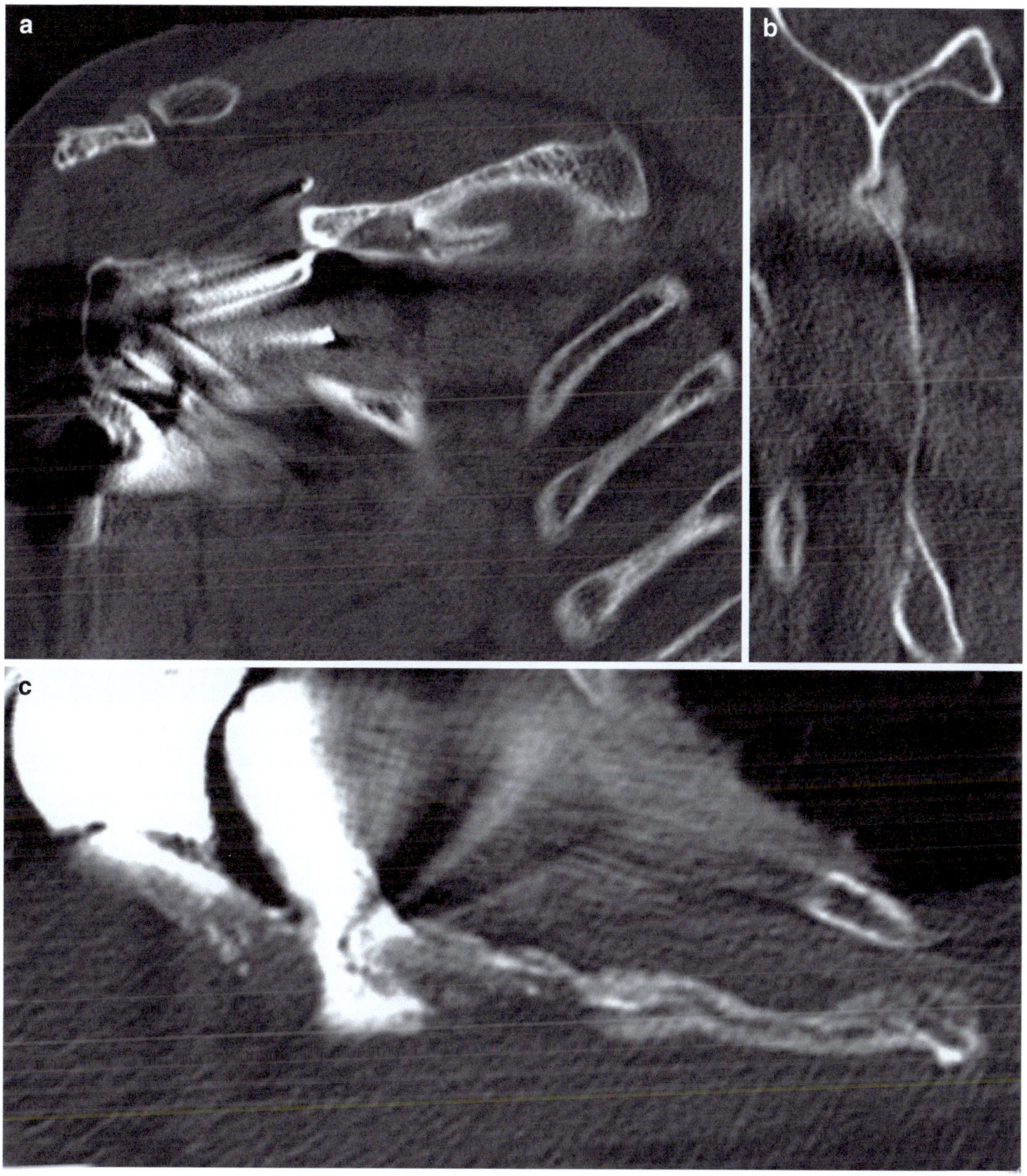

Fig. 17.3 These coronal (**a**), sagittal (**b**), and axial (**c**) computed tomographic cuts demonstrate a postoperative scapula fracture with placement of the central peg within the scapular spine

technique (Fig. 17.4) [10]. While this technique was originally described using humeral head autograft, it can also be applied using a femoral head allograft. In this technique, purpose-designed instrumentation is available. First, a pin is placed centrally in the allograft head using a centering guide. A combined reamer/bell saw assembly is then utilized to create a 1-cm-thick donut-shaped graft. A central hole is created using the same dimension as the central peg for the baseplate. The graft is then separated from the remainder of the femoral head using a side-cutting guide. If a thicker graft is desired, the slot created by the bell saw can be used as a template for an oscillating saw before the undercut is created. The graft can then be shaped to meet the

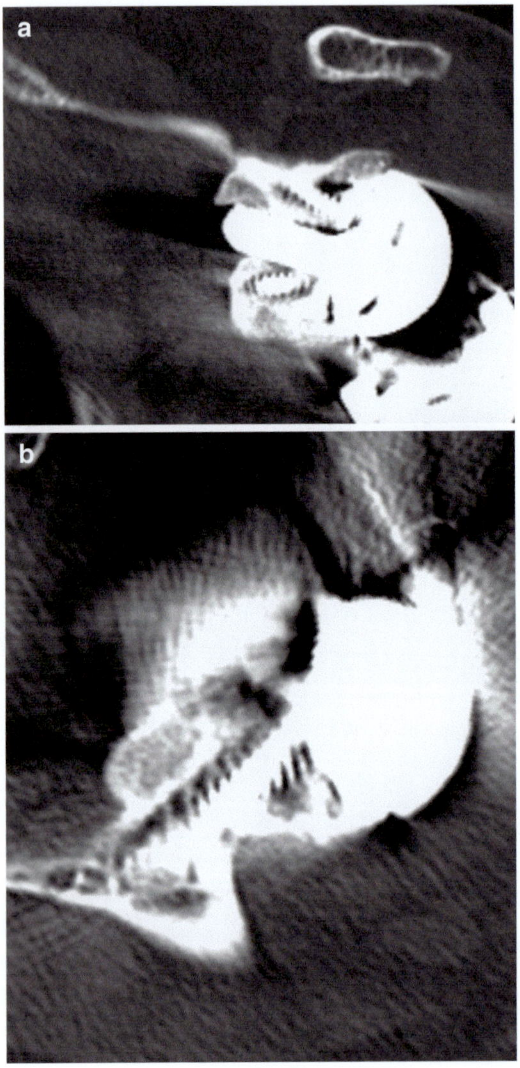

Fig. 17.4 These coronal (**a**) and axial (**b**) computed tomographic images demonstrate a completely incorporated femoral head allograft placed using a BIORSA technique

defect. Because the graft is entirely cancellous, it often undergoes some deformation during impaction to allow it to better conform to the deformity. This graft can then be loaded into the central post of the baseplate and implanted en bloc. Baseplate screws then fixate graft, baseplate, and hose bone together because the graft underlies the screw holes within the baseplate. Advantages of the technique include the relative speed and ease of creation of the graft because of the available instrumentation, the ease of implantation because the graft can be implanted with the baseplate, the readily available graft, and the customizability of the technique. Disadvantages of the technique include the use of allograft and the nonstructural nature of the graft. Finally, unless the donut graft is aggressively trimmed into a "U" shape, with this technique no portion of the baseplate rests on native glenoid.

A roughly similar technique of en bloc implantation can be applied with iliac crest autograft. First, the outer table of the crest is approached. It is then prepared for ba0seplate implantation as though it were a glenoid by drilling for the central post/screw and reaming. The baseplate is then implanted, and then the crest/baseplate construct is harvested using an oscillating saw [17]. After harvest, the graft backside (i.e., the inner table of the crest) must then be carefully shaped to match the defect with a burr. Because the graft is cortical, this process is time-consuming and challenging. Advantages of this technique include the use of structural graft and the use of autograft. Disadvantages include that, again unless the graft is aggressively trimmed into a "U" shape, no portion of the baseplate rests on native scapula and that this technique introduces donor-site morbidity.

Another option is to utilize the femoral neck portion of the allograft instead of the femoral head portion. This technique was initially described for global defects in which all rims of the glenoid are missing [9]. In this technique, the central pin is placed, and the remaining native glenoid is reamed at the desired angle. The femoral neck is cut from the head and is slid down over the central pin. The central cavity is then packed with cancellous autograft. The baseplate is then implanted such that the central peg/screw reaches native glenoid and compresses the graft between the baseplate and native glenoid. Advantages of this technique include the unique utilization of allograft and autograft, the ability to determine graft and baseplate position based upon the native anatomy, and the structural nature of the graft. Disadvantages include the use of cortical allograft with questionable ability to incorporate, that no portion of the baseplate rests on the native glenoid, and the relative inflexibility of the technique. In particular in cases with severe defect eccentricity, a graft centered around the baseplate may not be optimal.

The final option is to use free structural femoral head allograft or iliac crest autograft. In the described technique [40], the defect is first decorticated with a high-speed burr and perforated with a Kirschner wire (K-wire) multiple times. The central pin is then placed in the optimal location to achieve neutral version and 10° of inferior inclination relative to the pre-deformity anatomy. The graft is then cut with an oscillating saw to roughly match the defect. A slot is then created in the graft so that it can be slide down over the pin. The graft is then painstakingly sculpted to match the defect. The graft is then placed over the pin and secured with multiple K-wires around its borders. The glenoid-graft construct is then reamed, and a central hole for the post/screw is drilled. The baseplate is then placed such that a portion of the baseplate rests on the native scapula and such that a minimum of 5 mm of the central post/screw is fixated into the native scapula. The baseplate and graft are then secured with multiple screws. Advantages of this technique include that the center point can be selected prior to graft implantation before native landmarks are obscured, that is, it can use autograft, that it can employ a structural graft, that a portion of the baseplate can rest on native glenoid, and that the technique has the flexibility to address a wide variety of defects. Disadvantages of this technique include the technical challenge it presents to the surgeon and the time-consuming nature of graft sculpting (Fig. 17.5).

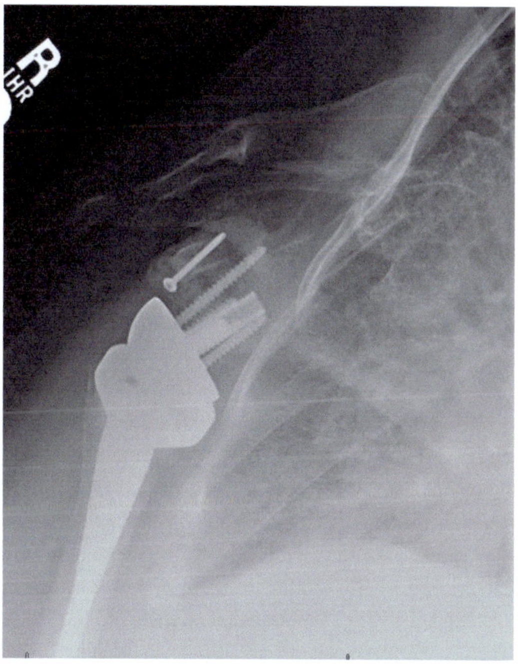

Fig. 17.5 This postoperative radiograph demonstrates a fully incorporated structural autograft with supplemental superior fixation

Results

Relatively few published outcomes are available for glenoid bone grafting. Those generally demonstrate remarkably high rates of graft incorporation between 76% [6] and 98%, [10] although incorporation may not be possible to accurately judge radiographically [41]. In the largest published series to date, Wagner et al. reported upon 40 patients who underwent glenoid bone grafting as part of revision RTSA with a mean follow-up of 3.1 years with an 18% revision rate and only 76% survival at 5 years, although these patients still had significant pain relief, improved range of motion, and increased satisfaction with their shoulders. In their series risk factors for loosening included increased body mass index, lateralized center of rotation, prior TSA (vs. hemiarthroplasty), and smoking status. Of note, these authors also categorized their grafts as either structural or corticocancellous and noted that 75% of their failures are corticocancellous [18], suggesting that structural bone grafting may be preferable to achieve baseplate stability [37]. In the second largest series published to date, Melis et al. reported upon 29 patients followed for a minimum of 2 years who revision from a TSA to an RTSA with a glenoid bone graft with either iliac crest autograft or femoral head allograft. These authors reported a low 8% glenoid loosening rate but found their clinical results to be disappointing with a mean final Constant score of 55 [6]. Kelly et al. reported 12 patients who underwent revision to RTSA with iliac crest autografting with a minimum of 2-year follow-up with only a single case of loosening related to failure of the graft to incorporate and significant improvements in patient-reported outcomes, although with a "considerable" complication rate [17]. Bateman et al. reported upon ten patients with a minimum of 2-year follow-up who underwent revision RTSA with femoral neck allograft with 100% graft incorporation and baseplate survival [9]. To date, the free structural head allograft technique described above has only been reported in the setting of primary RTSA with humeral head autograft but with the ability to achieve correction over up to 35° with a 93% chance of baseplate survival and a 100% chance of graft incorporation at 2-year minimum follow-up and with significant improvements in active forward elevation, pain, and function with a low complication rate [40].

Augmented Components

The alternative to bone grafting for the restoration of glenoid bone loss is to use an augmented component [15]. Very few published outcomes are currently available regarding these components. Only two systems currently have augmented baseplates available in the United States, and one was released within the past year. Currently, these are available as either fully angled or only half-angled depending upon the system. In addition, lateralization wedges are available. Finally, only combined two-plane deformity wedge is available for posterosuperior defects. These implants offer several potential improvements over glenoid bone grafting. First, because no graft is necessary, these components obviate graft-related issues such as disease transmission with allografts, donor-site morbidity with autograft, and incorporation with both allograft and autograft. Even if the graft does incorporate at the graft-host junction, it remains unclear whether a large allograft ever becomes completely replaced with host osteocytes via creeping substitution in an elderly individual. Second, because these implants are available with purpose-designed instrumentation to machine the glenoid to match the implant, they may be more easily implanted. Certainly they avoid the operative time and potential complications related to graft harvest, graft shaping, and graft fixation. Third, in many bone graft techniques, the baseplate does not rest against native bone, which may compromise stability until the graft incorporates. However, augmented baseplates also have several theoretical disadvantages. First, bone grafts have the potential to restore native bone stock and ease future revisions, while augmented base plates do not and may thus make future revisions more challenging. Second, while bone graft sizes can be customized to fit the defect, augmented baseplates are only offered in a limited variety of shapes and sizes, and thus intraoperatively native bone must be removed until the native defect matches the baseplate instead of vice versa with a bone graft. Third, bone grafts may be biomechanically superior. Once a graft incorporates, then stresses are dissipated at the bone-implant junction instead of the graft-bone junction, and thus forces are reduced as the length of the lever arm from the center of rotation is reduced. However, with an augmented baseplate, these torques are permanently increased. Fourth, augmented baseplates come at an increased cost as compared to autograft.

The surgical technique for implantation for an augmented baseplate is implant specific. While to date only two augmented baseplates are available, within the coming years, likely many manufacturers will develop and release similar components, and the instrumentation and technique will likely differ for each. Generally, regardless of the instrumentation and specific implant, the surgeon must respect similar concepts to glenoid bone grafting regarding component positioning to maximize initial stability and long-term biomechanics while minimizing impingement and instability.

To date, only two series have described the results of augmented baseplates, and both are in the setting of primary RTSA. In 39 patients followed for a mean of 28 months, the patients reported significant improvement in functional outcome scores with no complications [15]. In the second series, 39 patients who underwent primary RTSA with an augmented baseplate were followed for a minimum of 2 years, with significant improvements, although with significantly better outcome scores and elevation motion with posterior as compared to superior augments [8]. Likely in the future as the use of these components becomes more widespread, multiple outcome series will become available.

Postoperative Protocol

If initial baseplate stability is solid intraoperatively, the author's postoperative protocol does not differ between revision RTSA with a bone graft and primary RTSA without a bone graft. Patients are immobilized in a sling for the first 2 weeks postoperatively. At 2 weeks they discontinue sling use and begin to use the arm in their daily lives. They begin a home exercise program with pulleys. Patients are instructed not to put more than three to five pounds on the arm with either push or pull for the first 6 weeks. At 6 weeks, if radiographs demonstrate a stable baseplate, restrictions are lifted, and patients begin wall climbs, Jackins' exercises, passive external rotation exercises, and passive internal rotation exercises. At 3 months patients incorporate bands into their Jackins' exercises and begin hitch hiker's exercises, progressing to a resistance band as tolerated. For those patients who require physical therapy, they progress from passive to active assisted to active range of motion as tolerated with a goal of 120° of active forward elevation and 30° of active adducted external rotation by 6 weeks postoperatively. Isometric gentle strengthening begins at 6 weeks with concentric, closed chain anterior deltoid strengthening, open chain external rotator strengthening, and scapular stabilization exercises. However, patients are instructed to hold off on bands and weights until 3 months postoperatively. Patients can generally begin light athletic activities at 3 months and higher-level activities at 4 months. In cases where baseplate stability is uncertain, the author generally immobilizes patients in a sling for 6 weeks postoperatively and then begins the protocol above in a delayed fashion.

Complications

Generally, complications with revision to RTSA are extremely frequent, [42] with major complications occurring in 33% of cases. When all complications, including minor medical complications, are carefully measured, rates are as high as 70% [43]. The most frequently encountered complications include humeral or scapular fracture, infection, failure of graft incorporation, component impingement and instability, and baseplate loosening. While most of these complications are treatable, patients should be counseled preoperatively regarding the high frequency of perioperative complications. In addition, patients must be counseled that even a minor trauma such as a fall in the acute postoperative period can be catastrophic for a complex reconstruction.

Conclusions

Revision to RTSA with a concomitant glenoid bone defect is becoming increasingly common, and thus surgeons should be familiar with the evaluation and treatment options for these defects. A variety of bone grafts have been utilized, and each has advantages and disadvantages. These procedures are technically challenging, the complication rate is high, and the results are inferior to shoulder arthroplasty performed in the setting of normal glenoid bone. However, these procedures still lead to significant improvements in pain and function as compared preoperatively, and most patients are satisfied with the outcome if appropriately counseled preoperatively.

References

1. Sivasundaram L, Heckmann N, Pannell WC, Alluri RK, Omid R, Hatch GFR. Preoperative risk factors for discharge to a postacute care facility after shoulder arthroplasty. J Shoulder Elbow Surg. 2015; https://doi.org/10.1016/j.jse.2015.07.028.
2. Kim SH, Wise BL, Zhang Y, Szabo RM. Increasing incidence of shoulder arthroplasty in the United States. J Bone Joint Surg Am. 2011;93:2249–54.

3. Wagner ER, Houdek MT, Schleck C, Harmsen WS, Sanchez-Sotelo J, Cofield R, Elhassan BT, Sperling JW. The role age plays in the outcomes and complications of shoulder arthroplasty. J Shoulder Elbow Surg. 2017;26:1573. https://doi.org/10.1016/j.jse.2017.01.020.
4. Black EM, Roberts SM, Siegel E, Yannopoulos P, Higgins LD, Warner JJP. Failure after reverse total shoulder arthroplasty: what is the success of component revision? J Shoulder Elbow Surg. 2015; https://doi.org/10.1016/j.jse.2015.05.029.
5. Bacle G, Nové-Josserand L, Garaud P, Walch G. Long-term outcomes of reverse total shoulder arthroplasty: a follow-up of a previous study. J Bone Joint Surg Am. 2017;99:454–61.
6. Melis B, Bonnevialle N, Neyton L, Levigne C, Favard L, Walch G, Boileau P. Glenoid loosening and failure in anatomical total shoulder arthroplasty: is revision with a reverse shoulder arthroplasty a reliable option? J Shoulder Elbow Surg. 2012;21:342–9.
7. Laver L, Garrigues GE. Avoiding superior tilt in reverse shoulder arthroplasty: a review of the literature and technical recommendations. J Shoulder Elbow Surg. 2014;23:1582–90.
8. Wright TW, Roche CP, Wright L, Flurin P-H, Crosby LA, Zuckerman JD. Reverse shoulder arthroplasty augments for glenoid wear. Comparison of posterior augments to superior augments. Bull Hosp Jt Dis (2013). 2015;73(Suppl 1):S124–8.
9. Bateman E, Donald SM. Reconstruction of massive uncontained glenoid defects using a combined autograft-allograft construct with reverse shoulder arthroplasty: preliminary results. J Shoulder Elbow Surg. 2012;21:925–34.
10. Boileau P, Moineau G, Roussanne Y, O'Shea K. Bony increased-offset reversed shoulder arthroplasty: minimizing scapular impingement while maximizing glenoid fixation. Clin Orthop Relat Res. 2011;469:2558–67.
11. Kohan EM, Chalmers PN, Salazar D, Keener JD, Yamaguchi K, Chamberlain AM. Dislocation following reverse total shoulder arthroplasty. J Shoulder Elbow Surg. 2017;26:1238. https://doi.org/10.1016/j.jse.2016.12.073.
12. Walch G, Vezeridis PS, Boileau P, Deransart P, Chaoui J. Three-dimensional planning and use of patient-specific guides improve glenoid component position: an in vitro study. J Shoulder Elbow Surg. 2015;24:302–9.
13. Plessers K, Vanden Berghe P, Van Dijck C, Wirix-Speetjens R, Debeer P, Jonkers I, Vander Sloten J. Virtual reconstruction of glenoid bone defects using a statistical shape model. J Shoulder Elbow Surg. 2017;27:160. https://doi.org/10.1016/j.jse.2017.07.026.
14. Sears BW, Johnston PS, Ramsey ML, Williams GR. Glenoid bone loss in primary total shoulder arthroplasty: evaluation and management. J Am Acad Orthop Surg. 2012;20:604–13.
15. Jones RB, Wright TW, Roche CP. Bone grafting the glenoid versus use of augmented glenoid baseplates with reverse shoulder arthroplasty. Bull Hosp Jt Dis (2013). 2015;73(Suppl 1):S129–35.
16. Stephens SP, Spencer EE, Wirth MA. Radiographic results of augmented all-polyethylene glenoids in the presence of posterior glenoid bone loss during total shoulder arthroplasty. J Shoulder Elbow Surg. 2016;26:798. https://doi.org/10.1016/j.jse.2016.09.053.
17. Kelly JD, Zhao JX, Hobgood ER, Norris TR. Clinical results of revision shoulder arthroplasty using the reverse prosthesis. J Shoulder Elbow Surg. 2012;21:1516–25.
18. Wagner E, Houdek MT, Griffith T, Elhassan BT, Sanchez-Sotelo J, Sperling JW, Cofield RH. Glenoid bone-grafting in revision to a reverse total shoulder arthroplasty. J Bone Joint Surg Am. 2015;97:1653–60.
19. De Biase CF, Ziveri G, De Caro F, Roberts N, Delcogliano M. Reverse shoulder arthroplasty using a "L" shaped allograft for glenoid reconstruction in a patient with massive glenoid bone loss: case report. Eur Rev Med Pharmacol Sci. 2014;18:44–9.
20. Elhassan B, Ozbaydar M, Higgins LD, Warner JJP. Glenoid reconstruction in revision shoulder arthroplasty. Clin Orthop Relat Res. 2008;466:599–607.
21. Garofalo R, Brody F, Castagna A, Ceccarelli E, Krishnan SG. Reverse shoulder arthroplasty with glenoid bone grafting for anterior glenoid rim fracture associated with glenohumeral dislocation and proximal humerus fracture. Orthop Traumatol Surg Res. 2016;102:989–94.
22. Hill JM, Norris TR. Long-term results of total shoulder arthroplasty following bone-grafting of the glenoid. J Bone Joint Surg Am. 2001;83-A:877–83.
23. Iannotti JP, Frangiamore SJ. Fate of large structural allograft for treatment of severe uncontained glenoid bone deficiency. J Shoulder Elbow Surg. 2012;21:765–71.
24. Jones RB, Wright TW, Zuckerman JD. Reverse total shoulder arthroplasty with structural bone grafting of large glenoid defects. J Shoulder Elbow Surg. 2016; https://doi.org/10.1016/j.jse.2016.01.016.
25. Klein SM, Dunning P, Mulieri P, Pupello D, Downes K, Frankle MA. Effects of acquired glenoid bone defects on surgical technique and clinical outcomes in reverse shoulder arthroplasty. J Bone Joint Surg Am. 2010;92:1144–54.
26. Mizuno N, Denard PJ, Raiss P, Walch G. Reverse total shoulder arthroplasty for primary glenohumeral osteoarthritis in patients with a biconcave glenoid. J Bone Joint Surg Am. 2013;95:1297–304.
27. Neyton L, Boileau P, Nové-Josserand L, Edwards TB, Walch G. Glenoid bone grafting with a reverse design prosthesis. J Shoulder Elbow Surg. 2007;16:S71–8.
28. Neyton L, Walch G, Nové-Josserand L, Edwards TB. Glenoid corticocancellous bone grafting after glenoid component removal in the treatment of glenoid loosening. J Shoulder Elbow Surg. 2006;15:173–9.

29. Werner BS, Böhm D, Abdelkawi A, Gohlke F. Glenoid bone grafting in reverse shoulder arthroplasty for long-standing anterior shoulder dislocation. J Shoulder Elbow Surg. 2014;23:1655–61.
30. Klika BJ, Wooten CW, Sperling JW, Steinmann SP, Schleck CD, Harmsen WS, Cofield RH. Structural bone grafting for glenoid deficiency in primary total shoulder arthroplasty. J Shoulder Elbow Surg. 2014;23:1066–72.
31. Pinkas D, Wiater B, Wiater JM. The glenoid component in anatomic shoulder arthroplasty. J Am Acad Orthop Surg. 2015;23:317–26.
32. Allred JJ, Flores-Hernandez C, Hoenecke HR, D'Lima DD. Posterior augmented glenoid implants require less bone removal and generate lower stresses: a finite element analysis. J Shoulder Elbow Surg. 2016;25:823–30.
33. Favorito PJ, Freed RJ, Passanise AM, Brown MJ. Total shoulder arthroplasty for glenohumeral arthritis associated with posterior glenoid bone loss: results of an all-polyethylene, posteriorly augmented glenoid component. J Shoulder Elbow Surg. 2016; https://doi.org/10.1016/j.jse.2016.02.020.
34. Lenart BA, Namdari S, Williams GR. Total shoulder arthroplasty with an augmented component for anterior glenoid bone deficiency. J Shoulder Elbow Surg. 2015; https://doi.org/10.1016/j.jse.2015.08.012.
35. Sandow M, Schutz C. Total shoulder arthroplasty using trabecular metal augments to address glenoid retroversion: the preliminary result of 10 patients with minimum 2-year follow-up. J Shoulder Elbow Surg. 2016; https://doi.org/10.1016/j.jse.2016.01.001.
36. Seidl AJ, Williams GR, Boileau P. Challenges in reverse shoulder arthroplasty: addressing glenoid bone loss. Orthopedics. 2016;39:14–23.
37. Tashjian R. No bone? No problem! Is bone-grafting at the time of revision to a reverse shoulder arthroplasty a reasonable option? Commentary on an article by Eric Wagner, MD, et al.: "glenoid bone-grafting in revision to a reverse total shoulder arthroplasty". J Bone Joint Surg Am. 2015;97:e68.
38. Antuna SA, Sperling JW, Cofield RH, Rowland CM. Glenoid revision surgery after total shoulder arthroplasty. J Shoulder Elbow Surg. 2001;10:217–24.
39. Chalmers PN, Keener JD. Expanding roles for reverse shoulder arthroplasty. Curr Rev Musculoskelet Med. 2016;9:40–8.
40. Tashjian RZ, Granger E, Chalmers PN. Structural glenoid grafting during primary reverse total shoulder arthroplasty using humeral head autograft. J Shoulder Elbow Surg. 2017;27:e1. https://doi.org/10.1016/j.jse.2017.07.010.
41. Ferreira LM, Knowles NK, Richmond DN, Athwal GS. Effectiveness of CT for the detection of glenoid bone graft resorption following reverse shoulder arthroplasty. Orthop Traumatol Surg Res. 2015;101:427–30.
42. Wall B, Nové-Josserand L, O'Connor DP, Edwards TB, Walch G. Reverse total shoulder arthroplasty: a review of results according to etiology. J Bone Joint Surg Am. 2007;89:1476–85.
43. Saltzman BM, Chalmers PN, Gupta AK, Romeo AA, Nicholson GP. Complication rates comparing primary with revision reverse total shoulder arthroplasty. J Shoulder Elbow Surg. 2014; https://doi.org/10.1016/j.jse.2014.04.015.

Management of Large Humeral Defects: Bone Grafts and Augmented Components

18

William R. Aibinder and Joaquin Sanchez-Sotelo

Introduction

Revision shoulder arthroplasty can be particularly challenging in the presence of substantial proximal humeral bone loss. Bone deficiency of the proximal humerus after arthroplasty may occur due progressive osteolysis or stress shielding, uncontrolled bone loss or fracture at the time of component removal, or infection. It may have also been present at the time of the index failed shoulder arthroplasty, especially when performed for oncologic indications or sequels of trauma [1–5].

Management of extensive bone loss in the setting of revision shoulder arthroplasty is challenging due to several factors. First, there is an absence of metaphyseal bone for component fixation, which leads to an increased reliance on diaphyseal support. In these circumstances, the surgeon may feel tempted to implant the humeral component deeper, which will effectively shorten the overall length of the reconstruction and potentially facilitate dislocation. Second, the attachment sites for the rotator cuff, and in longer defects the deltoid and the pectoralis, may be compromised; poor active motion in all planes and instability may be the result. Finally, the lack of bulk of the proximal humeral metaphysis (and in particular the greater tuberosity) may contribute to loss of the wrapping effect on the deltoid [2, 4, 6, 7].

In the primary setting, proximal humeral bone loss is known to compromise stability at the time of reverse arthroplasty. Raiss et al. reported a 34% dislocation rate in 32 primary RSA performed for proximal humeral nonunion [4]. Intraoperative humeral head and tuberosity resection was a statistically significant risk factor for prosthetic dislocation. In the revision setting for failed hemiarthroplasty for fracture with tuberosity failure, Levy et al. reported a trend toward improved functional outcomes with proximal humerus allograft reconstruction with RSA compared to RSA alone [6].

Currently, the majority of the revision procedures performed for shoulders with proximal humeral bone loss are performed using reverse components, since anatomic hemiarthroplasty or total shoulder arthroplasty has an unacceptably high rate of a failure. This chapter will summarize a few concepts related to the management of large humeral defects at the time of revision reverse arthroplasty using one of two techniques: a proximal humerus allograft-prosthetic component

W. R. Aibinder
Department of Orthopedic Surgery, Mayo Clinic, Rochester, MN, USA
e-mail: Aibinder.william@mayo.edu

J. Sanchez-Sotelo (✉)
Department of Orthopedic Surgery, Mayo Clinic, Rochester, MN, USA

Mayo Clinic and Mayo College of Medicine, Rochester, MN, USA
e-mail: Sanchesotelo.joaquin@mayo.edu

R. Z. Tashjian (ed.), *Complex and Revision Shoulder Arthroplasty*,
https://doi.org/10.1007/978-3-030-02756-8_18

(APC) or proximal humeral prostheses with large metal replacement humeral bodies.

Options for Massive Proximal Humeral Bone Loss and Reported Outcomes

Oftentimes, moderate proximal humerus deficiencies may be reconstructed using *standard reverse arthroplasty components* at the time of revision surgery. When restoration of substantial length is anticipated, the glenoid baseplate is implanted flush with the inferior glenoid rim, and an eccentric larger-diameter glenosphere may be implanted with as much eccentricity as possible facing inferiorly in order to restore extra length on the glenoid side. In addition, humeral length may be gained by using the thickest possible humeral bearing; certain reverse systems provide more limited thickness of the humeral bearing, but some provide up to 22 mm. In addition, the humeral component may be cemented proud intentionally in order to restore some length. However, when humeral bone loss is beyond the ability of current standard implant systems, three main options exist to address massive proximal humeral bone loss: (1) osteoarticular allografts [8–11], (2) allograft-prosthetic composites (APCs) [1, 3, 12–14], and (3) large modular proximal humeral prostheses [7, 10, 15–19].

Osteoarticular allografts were originally developed for the management of proximal humeral bone loss as a consequence of resection of malignancies. They were particularly appealing for younger patients with an intact glenoid, and they provide the ability to reattach the deltoid and cuff musculature [11]. Unfortunately, the articulating portion of the humeral head collapses over time in a number of individuals. Other reported complications include nonunion, instability, and allograft fracture [8–10]. This reconstructive technique is seldom used for revision surgery.

Allograft-prosthetic composites (APCs) provide several perceived benefits, such as the ability to use standard implants, restore the length, offset an overall geometry of the proximal humerus, and attach the patient's native tissues to allograft tendon stumps in the bone in an effort to improve stability and function (Fig. 18.1). Potential complications and concerns with APCs include graft incorporation and resorption as well as the potential for disease transmission and infection. Chacon et al. reported on 25 shoulders with an average of 5.4 cm of humeral bone loss that were treated using an RSA with an APC [3]. The authors reported a 21% rate of incomplete graft incorporation with 17% resorption.

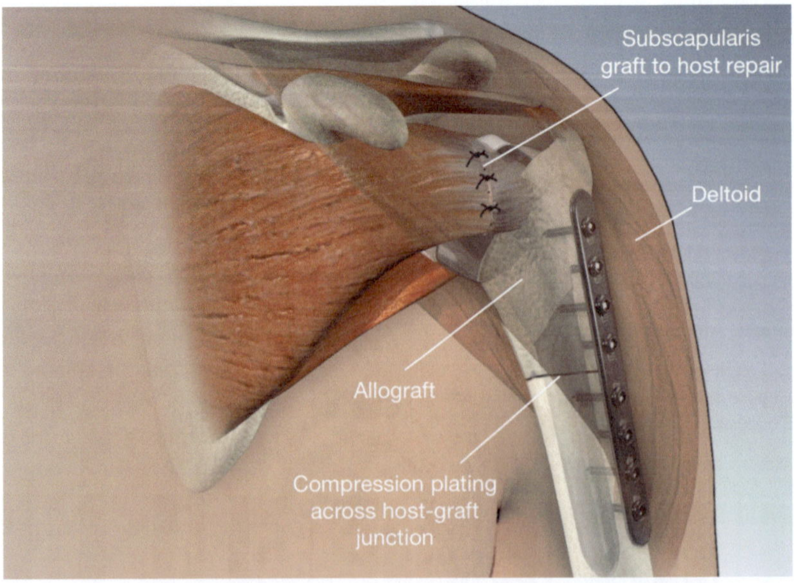

Fig. 18.1 Schematic drawing demonstrating the use of an APC with the use of standard implants, restoration of the normal anatomy and geometry of the proximal humerus, and attachment of native tissue to the allograft tendon stumps

Nonetheless, the literature has proven that host-allograft union is achievable [5, 20]. In a recent study, the senior author (J.S.S.) reported on 26 reverse shoulder arthroplasties implanted with a proximal humerus allograft in an APC fashion [14]. The cohort included 8 primary cases and 18 revisions. At a mean follow-up time of 4 years, there were significant improvements in pain and range of motion, with an overall postoperative active elevation of 98° (114° in primary cases). The mean time to graft-to-host union was 7 months. There were 2 (8%) asymptomatic non-unions in the revision setting and 2 (8%) cases of graft resorption and fragmentation, 1 of which occurred in the setting of infection.

Modular segmental proximal humeral replacement is another attractive option (Fig. 18.2). Historically, these prostheses were largely used in the setting of tumor resection and implantation of an anatomic tumor endoprosthesis [7, 10, 15–18]. The primary goal was often to preserve hand, wrist, and elbow function, with the humerus serving as a stable platform with limited active motion. Due to the absence of proximal soft tissue attachment sites in early implants, there was a high rate of instability with limited shoulder function. Bos et al. reported instability in 10 of 18 (56%) cases with either subluxation or frank dislocation [15]. Cannon et al. reported proximal migration of the prosthesis in 22 of 83 (27%) cases [16]. Additionally, the authors noted that function was limited with a mean forward elevation of only 41°. Kumar et al. reported on 100 patients, 47 of which were alive at final follow-up, with most patients unable to perform overhead activities [17].

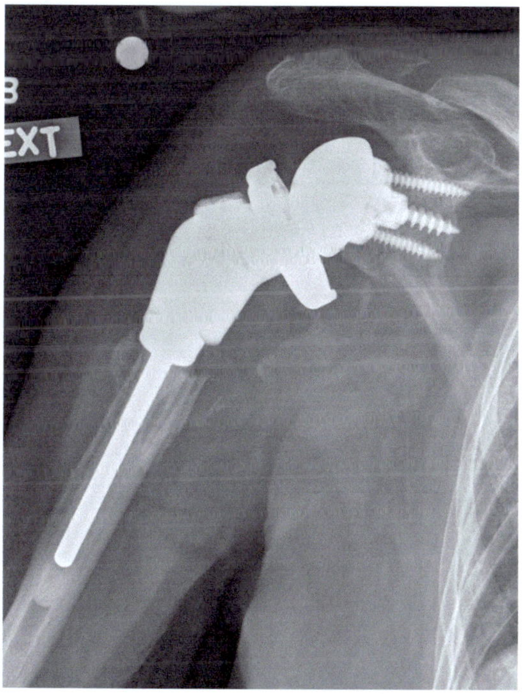

Fig. 18.2 A modular segmental proximal humeral replacement in a 77-year-old female with a failed anatomic total shoulder arthroplasty and proximal humeral bone deficiency

The advent of reverse shoulder arthroplasty designs that allow the use of metal modular segmental proximal humerus replacement has led to improved clinical shoulder function. Streitbuerger et al. reported on the use of a reverse design proximal humeral replacement [19]. When the axillary nerve function could be preserved, the mean active forward elevation was 84°, which is better than that reported for anatomic implants. However, the improved range of motion did not correlate with overall improved functional scores. We recently reviewed our outcomes using a modern proximal humeral metal replacement reverse system (SRS, Zimmer-Biomet, Warsaw, IN, USA). This particular system allows for the use of plates with ingrowth surfaces for the attachment of host soft tissues to metal segments, although the rate at which soft tissues heal to these metal surfaces is largely unknown. The study reviewed 23 consecutive primary and revision SRSs with a minimum of 2-year follow-up. The mean postoperative forward elevation was 109° with statistically significant improvement in pain scores. Instability was rare, with dislocation occurring only in one shoulder. There were, however, 4 cases (17%) of humeral component loosening, 3 of which had already required revision surgery at the time of the review (Fig. 18.3). Two additional shoulders were complicated by a periprosthetic fracture. The average amount of proximal humeral bone replaced by metal augmentation was 47 mm (range, 42–62 mm).

There remains a paucity of data to help guide decision-making between the use of modular segmental metal proximal humerus implants and allograft-prosthetic components in the management of proximal humeral bone deficiency. Comparative studies, in particular, are lacking (Table 18.1). We continue to use both options in our practice, and—as mentioned previously—we favor modular segmental metal prosthesis for shorter defect and patients with associated comorbidities that compromise allograft healing, whereas reverse APC is selected for shoulders with longer defects and substantial need for associated soft tissue reattachments. Other considerations for the selection of one modality over the alternative are summarized in Table 18.2. The general indications and contraindications for revision shoulder arthroplasty apply when performing a revision procedure using either one of these techniques.

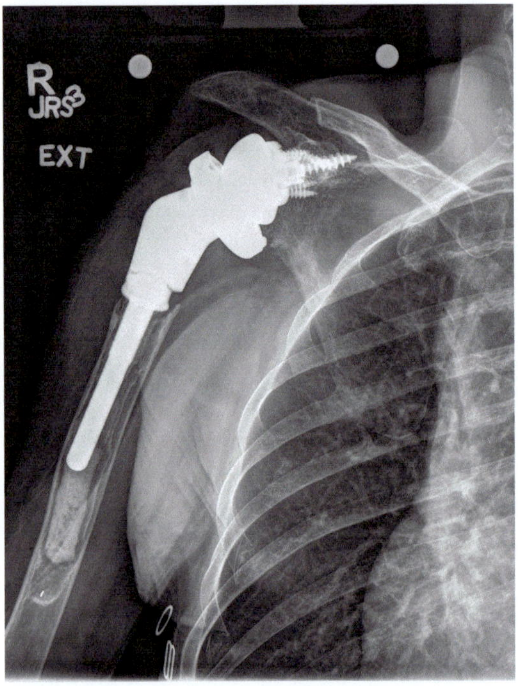

Fig. 18.3 Radiograph of a loose humeral SRS stem in a patient who was revised to a reverse APC

Allograft-Prosthetic Composite

Preoperative Planning

Preoperative planning aids with anticipating the correct length of the allograft needed to restore appropriate humeral length. A well-centered, full-length humerus radiograph with a magnification marker is extremely useful. A radiograph of the opposite intact humerus with magnification markers should be considered, although in revision procedures with associated soft tissue

Table 18.1 Comparative analysis of reverse APC and modular segmental metal replacement reverse in primary and revision cases: reported Mayo Clinic experience

	Reverse APC [14]	Reverse modular segmental metal replacement (currently unpublished)
Shoulders	26	34
Primary vs. revision	8 vs. 18	17 vs. 17
Elevation	98°	109°
External rotation	31°	34°
Reoperations	Five Revision APC for allograft fracture following trauma Larger glenosphere and thicker polyethylene bearing for periprosthetic dislocation Irrigation and debridement for infection Internal fixation for periprosthetic fracture Autogenous bone grafting of host-graft junction for delayed union	Eight Humeral body lengthening for periprosthetic dislocation Irrigation and debridement for infection (2 shoulders) APC for periprosthetic fracture (2 shoulders) APC for humeral component loosening Revision SRS with cemented humeral stem for humeral component loosening (2 shoulders)
Additional complications	Postoperative hematoma (1)	Minimally displaced periprosthetic fracture treated nonoperatively (1) Humeral loosening (1)

Table 18.2 Factors that favor allograft-prosthetic composite or modular segmental metal replacement prostheses

	Reverse APC	Reverse modular segmental metal replacement
Graft availability	–	+
Implant availability	Can be done with any standard implant	Needs dedicated implant system available
Length of deficiency	Longer defects	Shorter defects
Need to reattach major muscle-tendon structures	+++	+
Compromised bone healing (radiation, chemotherapy, others)	–	+
Ability to accommodate bulk under deltoid	Ample Need to recreate deltoid wrapping	Limited Contracture Narrow body frame
Duration/complexity of surgery	Longer More difficult	Shorter Simpler
Distal exposure	+++	+

contractures, it may not be possible to restore the length of the arm to normal. The final length of the allograft will need to be determined at the time of trialing.

Exposure

The exposure for performing a revision reverse shoulder arthroplasty with a proximal humerus allograft often requires an extensile approach. Our preference is to utilize the deltopectoral interval proximally and split the brachialis distally. It is important to mobilize the deltoid laterally, not only to gain adequate exposure but also to allow space for the bulk of the proximal humerus allograft. Throughout the exposure, care must be taken to protect the axillary, musculocutaneous, and radial nerves. Based on the site of the humeral defect, the distal third of the humeral shaft may need to be exposed for plate fixation. Ideally, five to six screws are preferred to achieve good purchase in the distal segment for secure plate fixation. If that is the case, the radial nerve is isolated and protected. The radial nerve can be identified at the interval between the brachialis and brachioradialis muscles. The brachialis is then divided with 20% of the muscle width remaining laterally.

Soft tissue structures are identified and tagged if intact, including the subscapularis and pectoralis major tendons and posterior rotator cuff (infraspinatus and teres minor tendons). If indicated, the latissimus dorsi and teres major tendons are identified, divided, and tagged for later transfer to provide active external rotation. The long head of the biceps tendon, if present, is tagged for tenodesis at the end of the procedure. Once the exposure is finalized, failed implants are removed according to the techniques described in other chapters of this book, and tissue samples are obtained for pathologic analysis and cultures.

Glenoid Component Implantation

Once all soft tissue structures are appropriately tagged, neurovascular structures are protected, and adequate humeral exposure is achieved, attention is directed at the glenoid. Exposure is generally straightforward in the presence of massive humeral bone loss. Surgeon preference dictates retractor placement. The inferior rim of the glenoid is identified while protecting the axillary nerve. The glenoid baseplate is implanted with slight inferior tilt and flush with the inferior rim, after reaming to allow adequate contact with healthy cancellous bone. Care should be taken when reaming following tumor resection and in the treatment of post-traumatic sequelae, as the absence of subchondral sclerosis often results in soft glenoid bone stock. Similarly, following failed arthroplasty and component removal, bone grafting procedures or the use of augmented components may be required as well. The glenosphere is then placed with diameter and offset based on surgeon preference, need for lateralization, and system-specific determinations.

Humeral Allograft Preparation

The proximal humerus allograft is prepared on the back table. An osteotomy of the proximal humerus is performed along the anatomic neck. This may be performed with a freehand technique or the use of either an intramedullary or extramedullary cutting guide in the appropriate amount of version. System-specific reamers and broaches are then used to prepare the humeral canal. It is imperative to preserve enough cancellous bone to allow for optimal cementation technique. The medial bone near the neck region is removed to prevent impingement with adduction. The tendon stumps from the graft are preserved if they are to be used for soft tissue attachment to native tissue; otherwise, they are sharply excised (Fig. 18.4).

The allograft is then cut to the correct length based on the preoperative plan and intraoperative trialing. Several techniques can be utilized for intraoperative trialing. The allograft with a trial broach and humeral bearing is reduced to the glenosphere in the surgical field. The deltoid is draped over the allograft. The resection level is determined based on the overlap with the native remaining humerus with traction applied. Alternatively, a long-stem broach and humeral bearing can be loosely placed into the distal canal, the joint is reduced, and the amount of proximal exposed broach is measured with an appropriate amount of traction applied to the extremity. In the setting of tumor surgery, the length of the allograft may be determined based on the resected specimen measured intraoperatively. The distal portion of the humeral allograft is resected. The remaining bone is saved in the event that strut grafting is required. When there is a short distal segment of remaining host bone, an intussusception technique may be performed to increase the stability of the construct. This typically requires widening the canal of the graft while thinning the proximal end of the remaining host bone, although occasionally it is best to intussuscept the allograft into an enlarged native humerus.

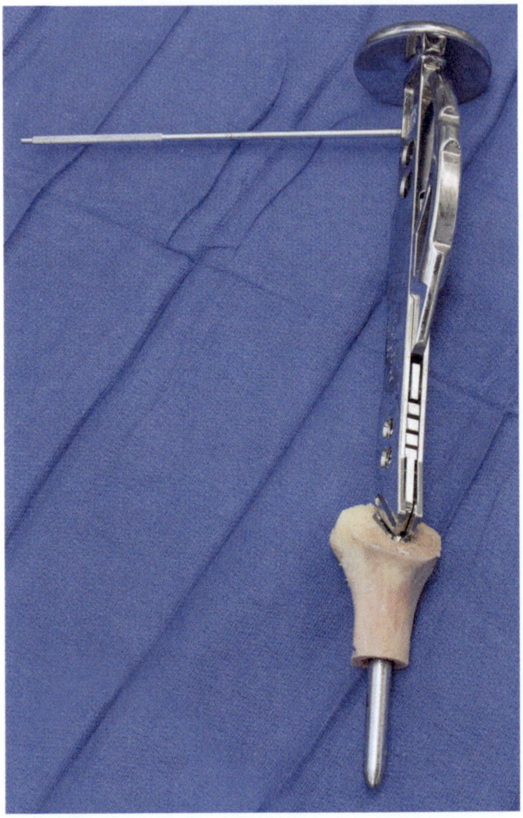

Fig. 18.4 Trial broach and a prepare proximal humeral allograft with all soft tissue removed

Humeral Component Implantation and Graft-to-Host Fixation

We believe it is critical to achieve excellent contact, compression, and stability between the graft and host in order to reliably obtain healing. A cement restrictor is placed into the canal of the host bone if the humeral stem will bypass the graft-host junction. This level of insertion of the cement restrictor is determined based on intraoperative trialing.

The graft and host bone ends are modified with the use of burrs and saws to create perfectly opposing surfaces. Once perfect apposition has been

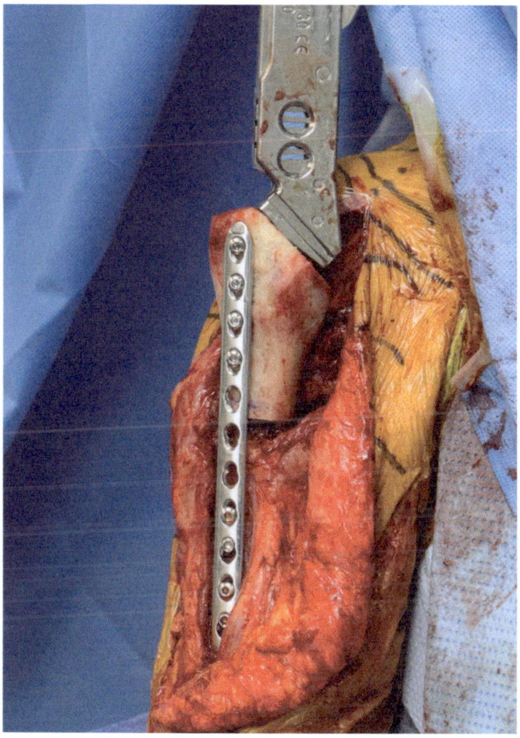

Fig. 18.5 Plate and screw fixation of the graft-host junction in compression mode with the trial broach in place

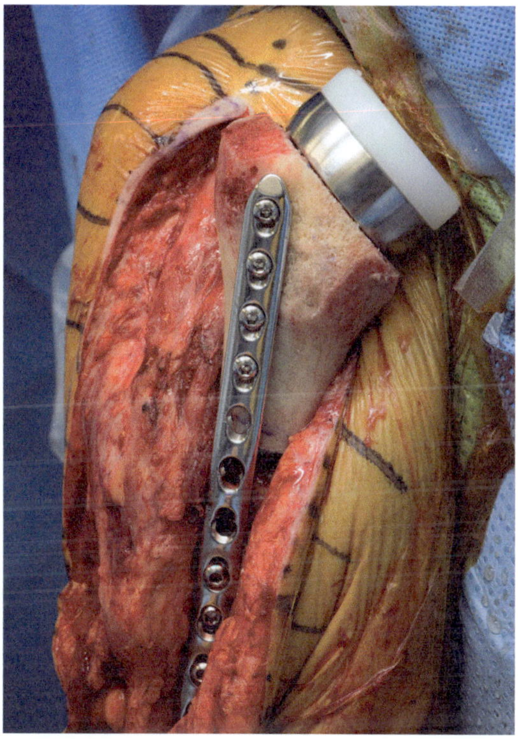

Fig. 18.6 Intraoperative photograph demonstrating implantation of the real humeral component with the humeral bearing polyethylene after compression plating of the graft-to-host interface

achieved, a 3.5 mm large fragment locking-compression plate is applied, with the goal of 5–6 holes distal to the graft-host interface. A trial broach is generally left in place in order to avoid any screws placed into the canal in positions that might and impede later component implantation (Fig. 18.5). The plate is pre-bent at the interface to optimize compression and avoid deforming forces. Clamps maintain plate positioning. Fully threaded cancellous screws are preferred in the allograft segment. A screw is loosely placed into the most proximal hole in compression mode. A nerve hook is used to pull the plate distally, and a screw is placed distally in compression mode, as well. Both screws are sequentially tightened, and compression is confirmed at the interface. The remaining holes are then filled with locking and non-locking screws, as indicated. If the broach prevents screw placement proximally, a circumferential wire through the plate may be used at that level instead.

The real humeral component is then cemented in the appropriate version, usually 30° of retroversion. Trialing of the humeral bearing is performed once the cement is cured. Humeral bearing thickness is determined based on appropriate soft tissue tension, ease of relocation, and range of motion. If a glenosphere trial has been used, the real glenosphere is then impacted. The humeral polyethylene bearing is then inserted as well (Fig. 18.6).

When the remaining distal humerus bone stock is severely compromised, it may be necessary to consider replacement of the whole humerus. This can be done using either a whole humerus graft with a reverse arthroplasty on the shoulder side and a total elbow arthroplasty on the elbow side, or alternatively it can be done using a modular segmental metal prosthesis that articulates with the glenosphere on the shoulder side and articulates with the ulnar component of an elbow arthroplasty on the elbow side. This is only considered in our practice if the remaining distal bone stock will not allow secure plate fixation using one or two plates with a minimum of three or four screws in native bone.

Tendon Repairs or Transfers

Once the real components are in place, attention is then turned to the soft tissue repairs. Prior to relocating the joint, multiple nonabsorbable sutures are placed into the native posterosuperior rotator cuff and the posterosuperior allograft tendon if needed (Fig. 18.7). If native rotator cuff tissue is absent, consideration is given to transferring the latissimus dorsi and teres major tendons to the posterosuperior allograft tendon. The joint can then be relocated, and these posterior sutures are tied with the arm in abduction and external rotation. If native subscapularis tendon tissue remained and can be repaired to the allograft tissue, our preference is to perform a repair with the goal of improving stability and strength in internal rotation. If the native tendon is absent, consideration is given to transferring the pectoralis major tendon to the subscapularis allograft stump. This is primarily important in this cohort of patients where proximal humeral bone loss leads to an increased risk of dislocation [4]. In large humeral defects or tumor resections where the insertion of the deltoid muscle is involved, the native deltoid tendon can be approximated to the allograft deltoid tendon. Lastly, the long head of the biceps tendon, if present, is tenodesed to the conjoined tendon.

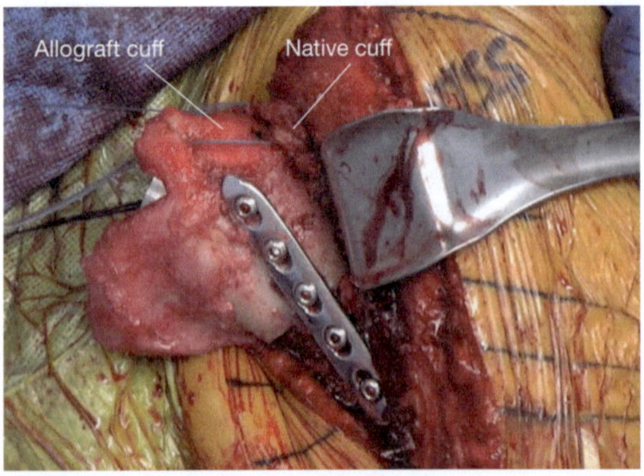

Fig. 18.7 Sutures are placed in the native posterosuperior cuff tissue and in the allograft tendon stump prior to joint relocation

Rehabilitation

Our preference is to immobilize these shoulders using a sling with a small abduction pillow and the arm in about 30° of internal rotation. Most shoulders are immobilized for 6 weeks. At that time, a program of passive- followed by active-assisted range of motion is initiated. Isometrics are added at week 10 and elastic band strength training at week 12. Progress through physical therapy is slowed in patients with an anticipated higher risk of postoperative instability (very large defects, need for deltoid repair to the allograft, lack of anterior soft tissue-restraining structures, poor patient compliance).

Potential Pitfalls

When performing an RSA with an APC, either in the primary or revision settings, it is imperative to avoid iatrogenic neurovascular injury. This is particularly relevant for the axillary and radial nerves to optimize function postoperatively [19].

Determining the appropriate humeral length is crucial. Meticulous care is taken during preoperative planning and during intraoperative trialing to perform an appropriate resection length. This optimizes lateral deltoid tension which leads to better stability and function. Care must be taken not to overlengthen the arm in patients with compromised soft tissue envelopes, since a permanent stretch of the brachial plexus can become a complication extremely difficult to overcome.

Additionally, it is imperative to precisely shape the graft-host interface to create perfect end-to-end bony contact. This helps facilitate excellent compression and a stable construct (Fig. 18.8). Nonetheless, historically, plate fixation of allograft in the humerus has had a higher rate of failure compared to intramedullary fixation [3, 20]. Prebending the plate, confirming excellent bony contact, utilizing multiple points of fixation (5–6) on either side of the interface,

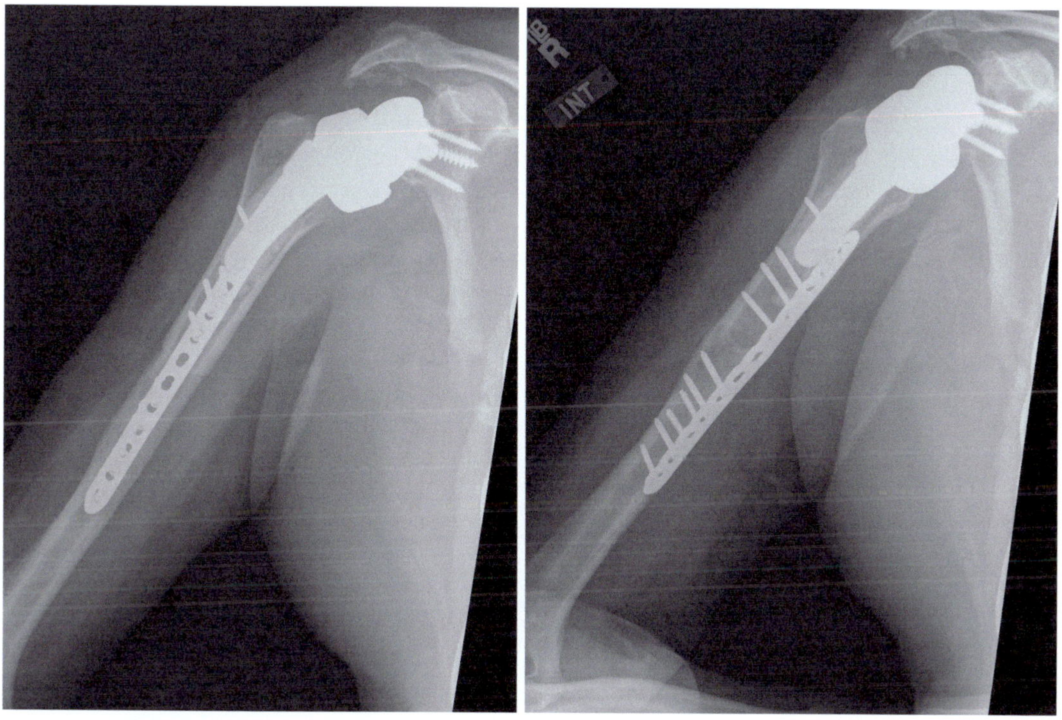

Fig. 18.8 Two-year postoperative anteroposterior and lateral radiographs of a 69-year-old male treated with a reverse shoulder arthroplasty with an APC

and using large modern compression plates improve the likelihood of union [14].

Failure to repair the soft tissues or perform tendon transfers may lead to an unstable shoulder with a risk of dislocation and decrease expected clinical outcomes, especially in terms of active motion and strength.

Modular Proximal Humerus Segmental Prosthesis

Preoperative Planning

A thorough understanding of the expected humeral bone defect helps formulate an effective operative plan. The use of templates allows the surgeon to determine the various combinations of proximal bodies and intercalary segments that may be required to restore humeral length. As mentioned in the section on APC, full-length bilateral humeral radiographs with magnifier markers are extremely useful to restore length and avoid instability.

Exposure

An extended deltopectoral approach is usually sufficient for exposure when performing a proximal humeral replacement. As only the proximal end of the remaining native humeral canal needs to be exposed, the extent of the distal dissection is limited to exposing the upper 1–2 centimeters of remaining native humerus. Care is taken to protect adjacent neurovascular structures through the exposure.

Similar to when performing an APC, detached soft tissue structures are tagged for later attachment. These may include the subscapularis, posterosuperior rotator cuff, pectoralis, and latissimus/teres major. Occasionally, the deltoid insertion is compromised by the magnitude of the bone defect and must therefore be reattached to the either the implant or the remaining bone if possible at the end of the procedure. The long head of the biceps tendon is tagged for tenodesis at the end of the procedure as well.

Humeral Preparation

Controversy remains about the use of cemented or cementless fixation for modular segmental metal humerus prosthesis. The stems of the system we use are textured for ingrowth, so that cementless application may be considered. However, we have had a relatively high loosening rate with cementless implantation and thus have a low threshold to cement this prosthesis. Cemented fixation is particularly recommended when revising a failed previously cemented humeral component, for very large defects where the length of the body will exceed the length of the implanted stem, as well as in patients with poor bone quality. For cementless application, the medullary canal of the native humerus is reamed sequentially until slight cortical chatter is felt. When planning for cement fixation, similar to with the technique described for an APC, some cancellous endosteal bone should ideally be preserved if present to facilitate cement interdigitation. Some systems provide reamers to create a perfectly flat bone surface to allow the metallic body to rest on and load the entirety of the bone. Broaching is then performed to finalize the preparation of the native humerus. In our practice using only one implant system, we have experienced a higher failure rate with cementless fixation, so our preference has become to cement most of these implants; this may not apply to alternative implant systems. Our preference is to use a stem length that will be equal or longer than the modular metal replacement segment.

Glenoid Component Implantation

Glenoid preparation is identical to that described in the section on APC technique.

Humeral Component Trialing and Implantation

The length and offset of the modular segments of the prosthesis is then selected based on preoperative planning and intraoperative trialing. In our preferred system, the humeral broach will accept the modular bodies and intercalary segments. Bodies of several lengths and offsets may be used for trialing; if a body with the desired offset and maximum length is not enough to restore the overall length, segmental intercalary modules are added (Fig. 18.9). Trial reduction is performed to assess stability, soft tissue tension, range of motion, impingement, and ease of closure.

Once the desired combination of modules has been selected, the real modules are opened and assembled on the back table (Fig. 18.10). The real humeral component is then implanted with or without cement at the same height and version as selected through trialing. Most of the times, the humeral component is implanted in 30° of retroversion, which is the version we prefer for the majority of reverse shoulder arthroplasty procedures in our practice. Once the humeral component has been implanted (and the cement is hard

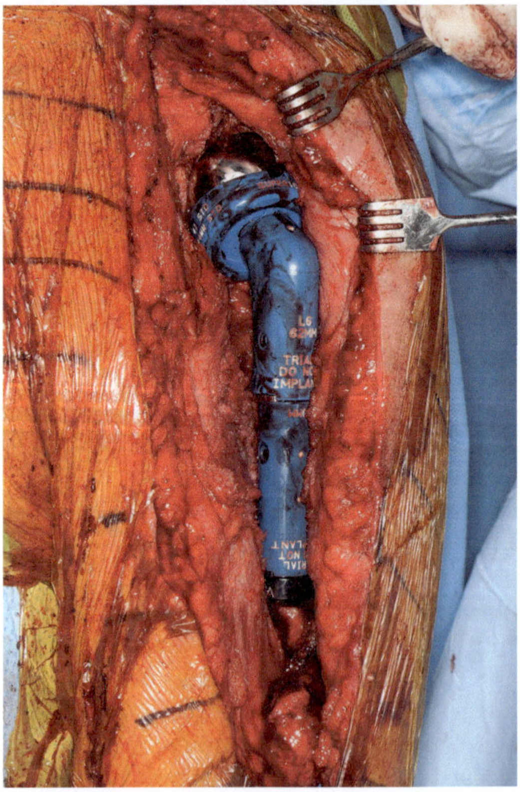

Fig. 18.9 Intraoperative photograph demonstrating trialing of the large proximal body and intercalary segments to assess the length and stability of the shoulder

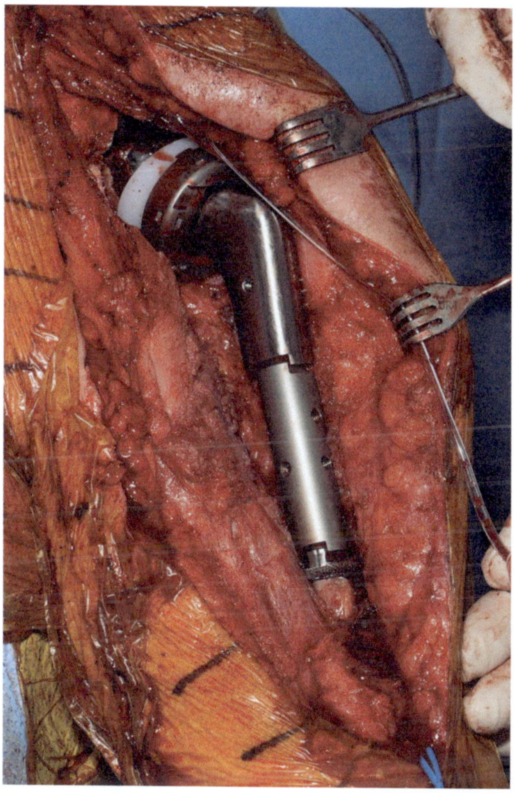

Fig. 18.10 Intraoperative photograph demonstrating the use of a proximal body and larger intercalary segment to restore humeral length with the use of a modular segmental proximal humeral replacement. Note the lateralization to allow for an effective wrapping of the deltoid

in cases of cemented fixation), the humeral bearing thickness may be changed to fine tune soft tissue tension. Once satisfactory, the real component is impacted and the shoulder is reduced.

Tendon Repairs or Transfers

Some newer modular implants allow for tissue attachment augments that can be secured to the proximal body or intercalary segments (Fig. 18.11). In these instances, the subscapularis and posterosuperior cuff can be attached through suture holes in these augments (Fig. 18.12). The latissimus and pectoralis can also be utilized to augment stability and rotation of the humerus if indicated. It is imperative to repair the deltoid tendon if it was detached during the procedure.

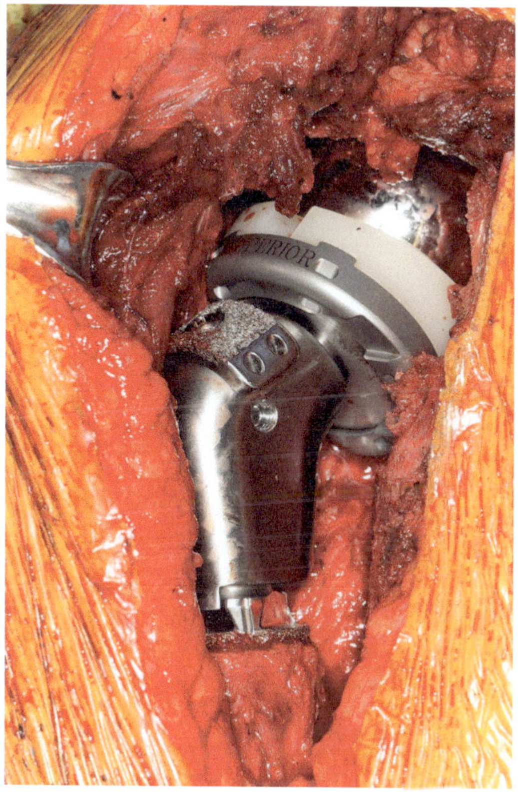

Fig. 18.11 Tissue attachment augments can be secured to the proximal body to allow for soft tissue repair

In our aforementioned series, soft tissue reconstruction was performed in 12 shoulders, 2 of which required reattachment of the deltoid tendon. The ability to repair soft tissue, however, did not correlate with the function or complications in our series of patients, and the ability of the soft tissues around the shoulder to reliably heal to these metal surfaces remains largely unknown.

Rehabilitation

The rehabilitation of these shoulders follows the same general lines described on the section on reverse APC.

Potential Pitfalls

When performing an RSA with a large metal augment for significant proximal humeral bone

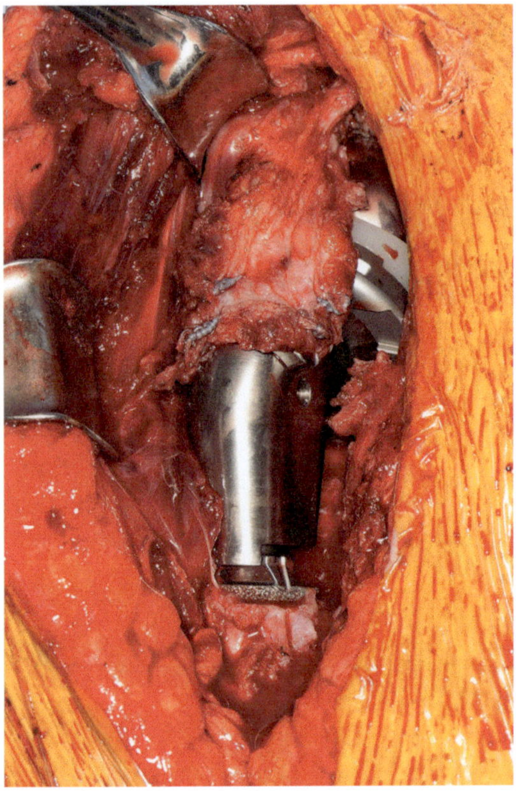

Fig. 18.12 Intraoperative photograph demonstrating attachment of the posterosuperior rotator cuff to the augment on the proximal body of an SRS implant

deficiency, it is important to use effective and accurate preoperative templating to anticipate the appropriate implant sizes needed to restore humeral length. All potential complications related to poor restoration of length described for reverse APC (dislocation if too short, poor motion and brachial plexopathy if too long) also apply to the proximal humeral modular metal replacements. As with any revision arthroplasty procedure, preserving axillary nerve function is key as well.

Given the absence of the bulk of the proximal humerus to assist in the draping effect of the deltoid, appropriate lateral offset must be achieved with the combination of a lateralized glenosphere if needed, a proximal body with the correct offset, and possibly a thicker humeral bearing. A scrutinized assessment of the stability of the shoulder is essential.

Lastly, secure stem fixation is necessary. Any evidence of substantial osteoporosis, metabolic disorders impairing bone formation, osteomalacia, or any other condition that affects bone quality should caution the surgeon, especially when utilizing larger proximal body segments. In these instances, consideration should be given to the use of cement fixation.

Conclusion

Revision shoulder arthroplasty in the presence of substantial proximal humeral bone loss can be challenging. Reverse implants are almost universally selected currently in these circumstances, since stability and function are extremely difficult to restore with anatomic components. The absence of proximal humeral bone translates into poor implant support, risk of humeral shortening, lack of attachment sites for crucial soft tissue structures, and loss of the wrapping effect of the greater tuberosity on the deltoid.

Moderate bone loss can occasionally be managed with implantation of a large glenosphere with substantial inferior eccentricity, combined with an ultra-thick humeral bearing or proud implantation of the humeral component. Larger defects require specialized reconstructive techniques. Allograft-prosthetic composites are favored for larger defects in situations where soft tissue reattachment is critical (Fig. 18.13). Proximal modular metal segmental replacements are favored for smaller defects, patients with impaired bone healing, and patients with a narrower body frame or severe contracture. Cemented fixation is recommended for the majority of APCs and modular segmental metal replacements. Rehabilitation must compromise motion for stability. Reasonable outcomes have been reported with both techniques; the complication rate is substantial but acceptable for salvage procedures of difficult reconstructive shoulder problems.

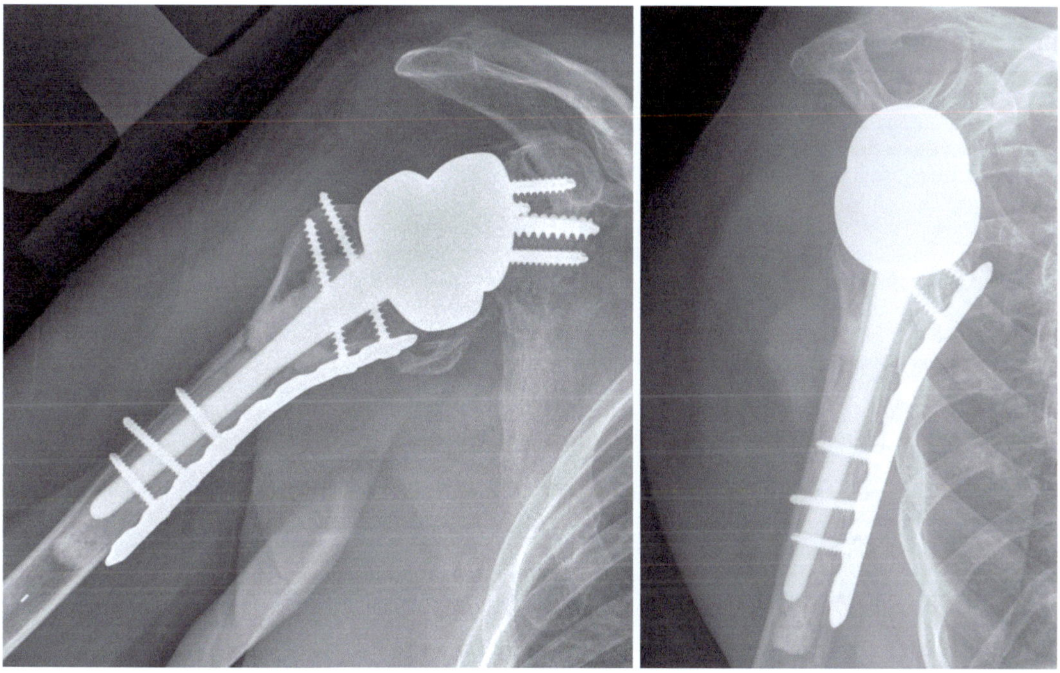

Fig. 18.13 Anteroposterior and lateral radiographs demonstrating graft-to-host union, adequate fixation, and stability of the humeral component with good restoration of proximal arm anatomy following a reverse APC

References

1. Abdeen A, Hoang BH, Athanasian EA, Morris CD, Boland PJ, Healey JH. Allograft-prosthesis composite reconstruction of the proximal part of the humerus: functional outcome and survivorship. J Bone Joint Surg Am. 2009;91(10):2406–15. https://doi.org/10.2106/JBJS.H.00815.
2. Budge MD, Moravek JE, Zimel MN, Nolan EM, Wiater JM. Reverse total shoulder arthroplasty for the management of failed shoulder arthroplasty with proximal humeral bone loss: is allograft augmentation necessary? J Shoulder Elbow Surg. 2013;22(6):739–44. https://doi.org/10.1016/j.jse.2012.08.008.
3. Chacon A, Virani N, Shannon R, Levy JC, Pupello D, Frankle M. Revision arthroplasty with use of a reverse shoulder prosthesis-allograft composite. J Bone Joint Surg Am. 2009;91(1):119–27. https://doi.org/10.2106/JBJS.H.00094.
4. Raiss P, Edwards TB, da Silva MR, Bruckner T, Loew M, Walch G. Reverse shoulder arthroplasty for the treatment of nonunions of the surgical neck of the proximal part of the humerus (type-3 fracture sequelae). J Bone Joint Surg Am. 2014;96(24):2070–6. https://doi.org/10.2106/JBJS.N.00405.
5. Cheng EY, Gebhardt MC. Allograft reconstructions of the shoulder after bone tumor resections. Orthop Clin North Am. 1991;22(1):37–48.
6. Levy J, Frankle M, Mighell M, Pupello D. The use of the reverse shoulder prosthesis for the treatment of failed hemiarthroplasty for proximal humeral fracture. J Bone Joint Surg Am. 2007;89(2):292–300. https://doi.org/10.2106/JBJS.E.01310.
7. Ross AC, Wilson JN, Scales JT. Endoprosthetic replacement of the proximal humerus. J Bone Joint Surg Br. 1987;69(4):656–61.
8. Getty PJ, Peabody TD. Complications and functional outcomes of reconstruction with an osteoarticular allograft after intra-articular resection of the proximal aspect of the humerus. J Bone Joint Surg Am. 1999;81(8):1138–46.
9. Potter BK, Adams SC, Pitcher JD Jr, Malinin TI, Temple HT. Proximal humerus reconstructions for tumors. Clin Orthop Relat Res. 2009;467(4):1035–41. https://doi.org/10.1007/s11999-008-0531-x.
10. Rodl RW, Gosheger G, Gebert C, Lindner N, Ozaki T, Winkelmann W. Reconstruction of the proximal humerus after wide resection of tumours. J Bone Joint Surg Br. 2002;84(7):1004–8.
11. Gebhardt MC, Roth YF, Mankin HJ. Osteoarticular allografts for reconstruction in the proximal part

of the humerus after excision of a musculoskeletal tumor. J Bone Joint Surg Am. 1990;72(3):334–45.
12. Black AW, Szabo RM, Titelman RM. Treatment of malignant tumors of the proximal humerus with allograft-prosthesis composite reconstruction. J Shoulder Elbow Surg. 2007;16(5):525–33. https://doi.org/10.1016/j.jse.2006.12.006.
13. Hartigan DE, Veillette CJ, Sanchez-Sotelo J, Sperling JW, Shives TC, Cofield RH. Reconstruction of the proximal humerus for bone neoplasm using an anatomic prosthesis-bone graft composite. Acta Orthop Belg. 2012;78(4):450–7.
14. Sanchez-Sotelo J, Wagner ER, Sim FH, Houdek MT. Allograft-prosthetic composite reconstruction for massive proximal humeral bone loss in reverse shoulder arthroplasty. J Bone Joint Surg Am. 2017;99(24):2069–76. https://doi.org/10.2106/JBJS.16.01495.
15. Bos G, Sim F, Pritchard D, Shives T, Rock M, Askew L, et al. Prosthetic replacement of the proximal humerus. Clin Orthop Relat Res. 1987;(224):178–91.
16. Cannon CP, Paraliticci GU, Lin PP, Lewis VO, Yasko AW. Functional outcome following endoprosthetic reconstruction of the proximal humerus. J Shoulder Elbow Surg. 2009;18(5):705–10. https://doi.org/10.1016/j.jse.2008.10.011.
17. Kumar D, Grimer RJ, Abudu A, Carter SR, Tillman RM. Endoprosthetic replacement of the proximal humerus. Long-term results. J Bone Joint Surg Br. 2003;85(5):717–22.
18. Raiss P, Kinkel S, Sauter U, Bruckner T, Lehner B. Replacement of the proximal humerus with MUTARS tumor endoprostheses. Eur J Surg Oncol. 2010;36(4):371–7. https://doi.org/10.1016/j.ejso.2009.11.001.
19. Streitbuerger A, Henrichs M, Gosheger G, Ahrens H, Nottrott M, Guder W, et al. Improvement of the shoulder function after large segment resection of the proximal humerus with the use of an inverse tumour prosthesis. Int Orthop. 2015;39(2):355–61. https://doi.org/10.1007/s00264-014-2560-2.
20. Vander Griend RA. The effect of internal fixation on the healing of large allografts. J Bone Joint Surg Am. 1994;76(5):657–63.

19 Humeral Windows, Osteotomies, and Episiotomies

Michael Charles and Gregory P. Nicholson

Introduction

Shoulder arthroplasty has seen a rapid increase over the last two decades in both inpatient and outpatient procedures [1] to nearly 50,000 cases a year [2]. The annual growth of primary total shoulder arthroplasty cases (9.4%) was only exceeded by the growth in revision cases (12.4%) [2]. Revision arthroplasty cases present the surgeon with several challenges that often lead to increased complication rates [3–5]. One particular challenge in revision arthroplasty is the management of the humeral component. A retrospective study of 1112 total shoulder arthroplasties (TSA) found that 75% of the revision cases were related to glenoid wear/loosening and instability, while the humeral component was the primary cause in 0.3% of cases [6]. Despite that primary humeral loosening varies from 0% to 1.6% [7] in the literature, the humeral implant must be addressed in many revision cases whether to address malposition (version and height), conversion from anatomic to reverse prosthesis, or glenoid exposure [3, 8–11]. Extensive bone ingrowth and stable cement mantles with humeral implants can make extraction difficult. Humeral fracture rates in revision arthroplasty range from 2.4% to 24% [3–5, 12, 13]. Risk factors for intraoperative fractures include female sex, history of instability, and a prior hemiarthroplasty [3, 13]. A majority of these occur during the removal of the previous humeral prosthesis. Despite recent trends of using shorter stem and stemless implants, which theoretically allows an easier revision [14], the majority of stems still extend beyond the metaphysis. This chapter is designed to highlight the current treatment strategies to remove a well-fixed humeral implant through either (1) humeral osteotomy/episiotomy or (2) humeral window.

General/Universal Proximal Techniques

As in any revision case, infectious workup including laboratories, aspirations, and cultures are performed when appropriate. The approach is an extensile approach of the previous incision. Most commonly, the deltopectoral approach is used as this can be easily extended into the anterolateral approach to the midshaft and distal humerus as needed. Extensive release of any adhesions in the subacromial and subdeltoid spaces is performed. Treatment of the subscapularis is per the surgeon's preference; our senior

M. Charles
Shoulder/Elbow Surgery and Sports Medicine, Orthopaedic Surgery, UCSF Fresno, Fresno, CA, USA

G. P. Nicholson (✉)
Department of Orthopedic Surgery, Rush University Medical Center, Chicago, IL, USA
e-mail: Gregory.nicholson@rushortho.com

R. Z. Tashjian (ed.), *Complex and Revision Shoulder Arthroplasty*, https://doi.org/10.1007/978-3-030-02756-8_19

author prefers a tenotomy, allowing for possible lengthening in contracted patients. Adequate capsular releases are performed to allow dislocation of the humerus.

Preparing the humeral implant for extraction should begin with removal of residual soft tissue or fibrosis along prosthetic head/neck junction. After removal of the humeral head in modular implants, one can use standard and flexible osteotomes and curettes to loosen the most proximal aspects of the stem. It is preferred to use ¼ inch standard osteotomes around the proximal prosthesis in a circular fashion. This "de-bonds" the implant from the proximal cancellous bone. It is very helpful to know the shape or geometry of the existing implant to facilitate this step. This initial step is very important to remove any adhesions connecting the stem to the tuberosities to avoid fracture. In shorter metaphyseal stems, this step can be all that is required to allow extraction of humeral prosthesis. In longer and flanged [15] stems, more distal strategies are required.

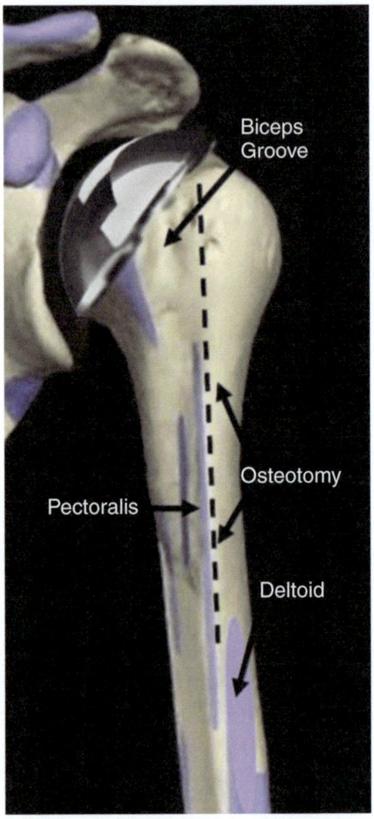

Fig. 19.1 Osteotomy is carried 10 cm distal sparing insertions of the deltoid and pectoralis major muscles

Humeral Osteotomy/Episiotomies

Humeral stem fixation can be achieved through cementing or press fit with and without coating for bone ingrowth [16]. In either case, the stability is reliant on hoop stresses and interdigitation of bone/cement/implant interfaces. Thus, the key to removing an implant is the disruption of the hoop stresses and "de-bonding" these interfaces. The simplest and least invasive approach is the vertical humeral osteotomy (VHO) [17] or humeral episiotomy and is the preferred technique of the senior author (GPN). The surgical steps are as follows:

1. Electrocautery is used to expose the proximal humerus from the neck cut beginning just lateral to the biceps groove and extending approximately 10 cm distal. This VHO does not go below the tip of the standard length stem. In this way a long stem implant is not required at revision implantation. The osteotomy path will be between the insertion of the pectoralis major medially and the deltoid insertion laterally. See Fig. 19.1.
2. A micro-oscillating saw is used to create the unicortical osteotomy. It is important that the bone and the cement mantle are perforated with this cut. If the implant is press fit and uncemented, the osteotomy is carried down to the implant.
   (a) A variation of this technique is to drill a 2.5 mm hole at the most distal aspect of the proposed osteotomy. This is to prevent the propagation of the osteotomy distally.
3. Successive osteotomes are inserted to "flex" open the osteotomy site. Recommended are the ½ and ¾ inch osteotomes to gently widen the gap and de-bond the implant. The osteotome is gently twisted to expand the osteotomy. This should result in a visible gap in both the bone and cement. See Fig. 19.2.

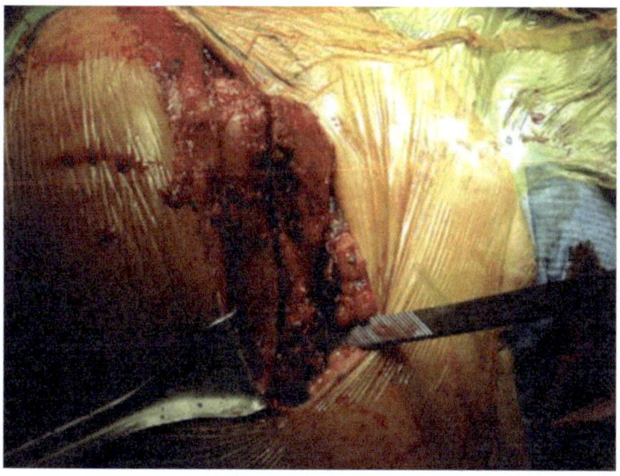

Fig. 19.2 Visible gap in bone and cement at the osteotomy site

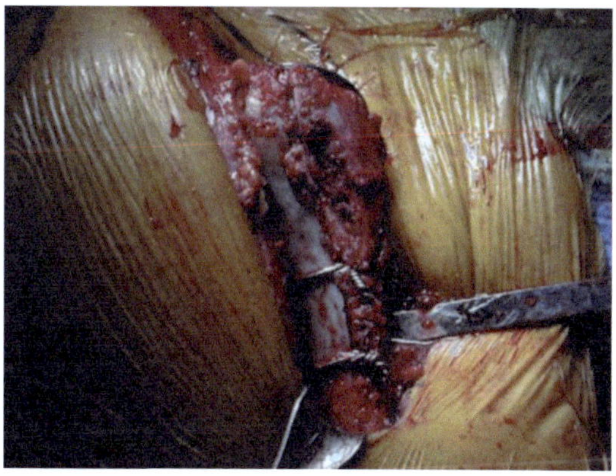

Fig. 19.3 Final stabilization of osteotomy with Luque wires

4. A footed impactor is placed at the medial aspect of the proximal neck of the prosthesis, and the implant is then malleted free. Make sure that as the implant moves, it does not impact or have residual attachments to the tuberosities. If the implant is not mobile, the osteotomy can be extended distally with the oscillating saw and the sequence repeated.
5. After removal of the implant, removal of residual cement can be performed through a combination of osteotomes, rongeurs, and ultrasonic devices. If it is not an infection case, incomplete removal of mantle is acceptable as you can still cement a smaller stem into the previous mantle.
6. Two looped 18 gauge Luque wires are then passed around the shaft and lightly tightened to re-create cortical apposition at osteotomy site.
   (a) In the cases of poor bone quality or bone stock, allograft struts can be added.
   (b) The latissimus dorsi tendon insertion is a safe area of the proximal humerus to pass cerclages around the humerus as it is distal to the axillary nerve and the radial nerve is still medial to the humeral shaft.
7. Ream the humeral canal and place trial stem with humeral head protector. This can protect the humerus during glenoid preparation and insertion.
8. As the new humeral stem is implanted, the Luque wires are tightened again and the final humeral stem position stabilized by cement or press fit. See Fig. 19.3.

In the larger series by our senior author, none of 23 patients who were available for final follow-up at 41 months had sustained perioperative or postoperative fractures [18]. The patients' average American Shoulder Elbow Society (ASES) score was 64.7 (contralateral was 76.9) but varied greatly due to a diverse etiology of the revision. There was no loosening of implants and no revision surgeries related to the humerus. Similar outcomes were found by Johnston et al. [19], with a 13-patient cohort followed up at an average of 30 months. In their study using the same technique, no intraoperative fractures occurred, and there was no evidence of non-union or implant loosening at final follow-up [19]. The lower ASES scores are on par with other publications that demonstrate, despite significant pain relief and improvement of function, revision arthroplasties have inferior results to primary cases [5, 9, 10].

Humeral Windows

Drawing from the success of femoral osteotomies, many early revision approaches included a more invasive bone window to allow greater exposure to the implant and cement mantle. Sperling and Cofield [12] best described the use of anterior and medial bone windows to loosen prosthesis.

1. The approach can be made through either a deltopectoral approach or anteromedial exposure (with partial deltoid release off the clavicle and acromion).
2. Size of the humeral window is determined by length of the implant and cement mantle.
3. Electrocautery is used to dissect out desired window site, and this could include partial release of muscle insertions.
   (a) Variations on this technique try to maintain tendinous insertions.
4. Unlike the VHO/episiotomy, the bone cuts are made vertically and horizontally to allow complete removal a rectangle of bone or creating a hinge to elevate the bone flap up. In this technique the window or bone flap will typically extend distal to the tip of the existing stem. This will require a longer stem implant to extend distally beyond this level at revision. See Fig. 19.4.
   (a) Medial windows involve the calcar of the humeral metaphysis. This should be avoided in cases with a metaphyseal-based stem.
5. The prosthesis is then removed again with either footed impactor, implant-specific backslap, or vice grip and backslap setup. After the window is completed and the stem remains well fixed, curve the osteotome can be used to circumferentially loosen the cement mantle/implant [15].
6. Additional cement is then removed. Provisional fixation and stabilization with trial stem are used to allow glenoid preparation and implantation.
7. The bone window is then stabilized with Luque wires, heavy sutures, or osteosynthesis. In the cases of poor bone quality or bone stock, allograft struts can be placed over the window site.
8. Final implantation can be done via press fit (with additional bone grafting) or cementing.

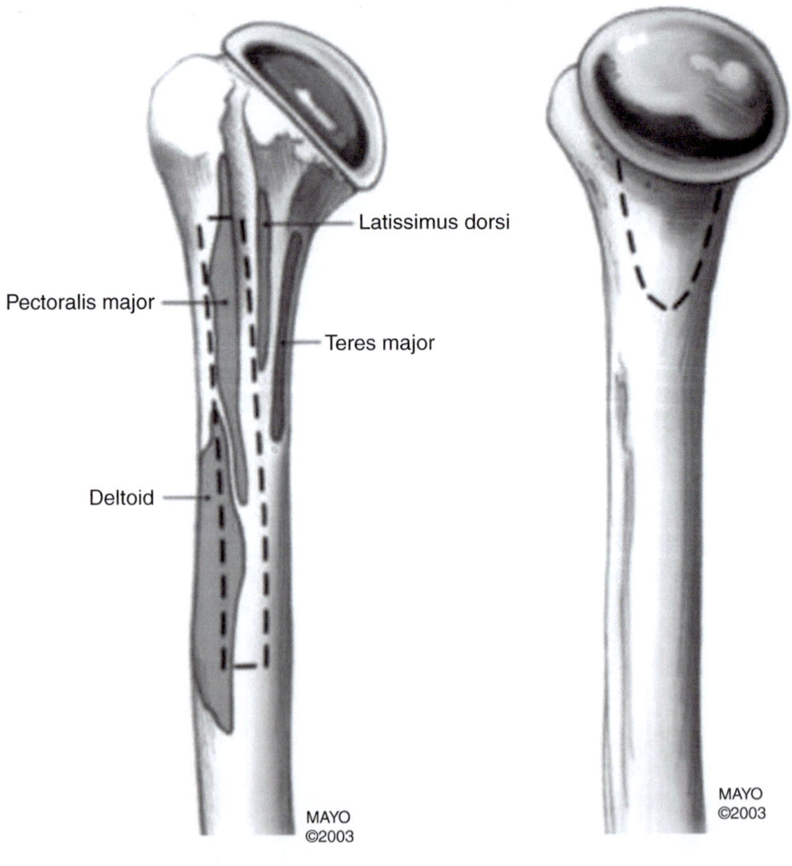

Fig. 19.4 Humeral window locations. (Courtesy of Sperling and Cofield [12])

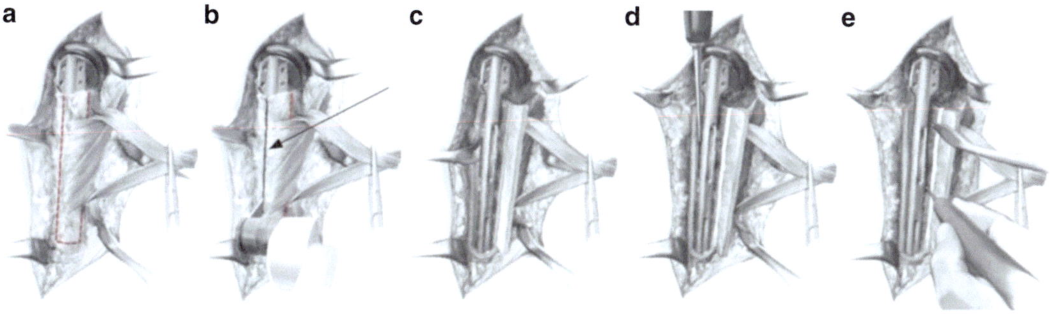

Fig. 19.5 Bone cuts for pectoralis major pedicled bone window. (Courtesy of Gohlke and Rolf [21])

The study by Sperling and Cofield [12] included 20 patients who required the bone windows (16 anterior, 3 medial, 1 required both) for revision arthroplasty. Four of their patients had intraoperative fractures related to implant removal despite the window. Three of their patients failed to heal their humeral window site. Despite these complications at an average of 3.3 years, there was no clinical loosening of implants. In a smaller cohort of flanged humeral implants undergoing revision arthroplasty, five of six patients required a window [15]. Of the 5 patients, 1 sustained an intraoperative fracture (20%) versus 3 fractures in the 37 non-flanged stem cohort (8.1%).

Vascularized windows are a variation of humeral windows that try to maintain soft tissue attachment and thus preserve blood supply to anterior bone. Wright [20] describes a technique in which a 3 mm strip of the anterolateral humerus is exposed distal to the standard deltopectoral approach. Drill holes about 5 mm apart are then placed just lateral to the bicep groove and medially 1–1.5 cm. The lateral and inferomedial holes are then connected with a saw or osteotome. This creates a vascularized hinge with the periosteum, pectoralis, and brachialis all attached to the flap of bone. The author reports of 25 cases, most healed within 8 weeks, but they had one fracture propagate distal to the window and 6 cases where the window became comminuted [20]. Another common vascularized window is the pectoralis major pedicled bone window described by Gohlke and Rolf [21]. In this variation the pectoralis is preserved to the bone window, and the deltoid insertion is spared. Again the size of the window is dependent on the size of the primary stem/mantle (Fig. 19.5) and is stabilized with cerclage wiring. In their cohort of 34 patients with an average follow-up of 31.5 months, there were no fractures, and age- and gender-adjusted Constant scores improved from 17.5% to 63% [21]. In longer-term follow-up, the same senior author (FG) demonstrated a concerning trend of 24 of 50 patients at a mean of 7 years had progressive humeral radiolucencies (6 were completely loose with migration) [22]. The cohort still had moderate outcomes with average adjusted Constant score of 56.7 ± 19.7.

Conclusion

Even when not the main cause of the revision, addressing the humeral stem remains a major challenge to the shoulder surgeon. The evolution of modular stems has allowed retention of humeral implant, which has decreased the time, blood loss, and intraoperative complications associated with humeral revision [23]. Despite the numerous publications regarding revision arthroplasty [5, 8, 10, 11, 13, 24, 25], especially the use of reverse prosthesis in revision [26], few publications discuss their surgical technique in humeral stem removal. A recent retrospective review compared the two major procedures used to revise stable humeral stems. Sahota et al. [27] compared 26 patients who were revised with bone windows to 19 patients revised with humeral osteotomy. There were a total of six intraoperative fractures in the window group, and one in the osteotomy group. Despite this difference, all the

Table 19.1 Summary of two major humeral revision techniques

	Advantages	Disadvantages
Humeral osteotomy/ episiotomy	Shorter technique Lower fracture risk More reliable healing rates Addresses bone and cement mantle No tendon/soft tissue releases	Smaller exposure More difficult to completely remove cement mantle
Humeral windows	Wider exposure of implant/ cement Increase ease of removal of cement	Higher fracture risk Higher non-union risk (though not clinically significant) Longer technique, more technically demanding

fractures healed, and there were no cases of malunion or loosening in either group. This study demonstrates that either technique can be used to safely remove a humeral prosthesis. Table 19.1 is a summary of the advantages and disadvantages of both major techniques in humeral stem revision.

References

1. Cancienne JM, Brockmeier SF, Gulotta LV, Dines DM, Werner BC. Ambulatory total shoulder arthroplasty: a comprehensive analysis of current trends, complications, readmissions, and costs. J Bone Joint Surg Am. 2017;99(8):629–37.
2. Day JS, Lau E, Ong KL, Williams GR, Ramsey ML, Kurtz SM. Prevalence and projections of total shoulder and elbow arthroplasty in the United States to 2015. J Shoulder Elb Surg. 2010;19(8):1115–20.
3. Ingoe HM, Holland P, Cowling P, Kottam L, Baker PN, Rangan A. Intraoperative complications during revision shoulder arthroplasty: a study using the National Joint Registry Dataset. Shoulder Elbow. 2017;9(2):92–9.
4. Saltzman BM, Chalmers PN, Gupta AK, Romeo AA, Nicholson GP. Complication rates comparing primary with revision reverse total shoulder arthroplasty. J Shoulder Elb Surg. 2014;23(11):1647–54.
5. Wall B, Nove-Josserand L, O'Connor DP, Edwards TB, Walch G. Reverse total shoulder arthroplasty: a review of results according to etiology. J Bone Joint Surg Am. 2007;89(7):1476–85.
6. Cil A, Veillette CJ, Sanchez-Sotelo J, Sperling JW, Schleck CD, Cofield RH. Survivorship of the humeral component in shoulder arthroplasty. J Shoulder Elb Surg. 2010;19(1):143–50.
7. Raiss P, Edwards TB, Deutsch A, Shah A, Bruckner T, Loew M, et al. Radiographic changes around humeral components in shoulder arthroplasty. J Bone Joint Surg Am. 2014;96(7):e54.
8. Deutsch A, Abboud JA, Kelly J, Mody M, Norris T, Ramsey ML, et al. Clinical results of revision shoulder arthroplasty for glenoid component loosening. J Shoulder Elb Surg. 2007;16(6):706–16.
9. Dines JS, Fealy S, Strauss EJ, Allen A, Craig EV, Warren RF, et al. Outcomes analysis of revision total shoulder replacement. J Bone Joint Surg Am. 2006;88(7):1494–500.
10. Carroll RM, Izquierdo R, Vazquez M, Blaine TA, Levine WN, Bigliani LU. Conversion of painful hemiarthroplasty to total shoulder arthroplasty: long-term results. J Shoulder Elb Surg. 2004;13(6):599–603.
11. Levy JC, Virani N, Pupello D, Frankle M. Use of the reverse shoulder prosthesis for the treatment of failed hemiarthroplasty in patients with glenohumeral arthritis and rotator cuff deficiency. J Bone Joint Surg Br. 2007;89(2):189–95.
12. Sperling JW, Cofield RH. Humeral windows in revision shoulder arthroplasty. J Shoulder Elb Surg. 2005;14(3):258–63.
13. Wagner ER, Houdek MT, Elhassan BT, Sanchez-Sotelo J, Cofield RH, Sperling JW. What are risk factors for intraoperative Humerus fractures during revision reverse shoulder arthroplasty and do they influence outcomes? Clin Orthop Relat Res. 2015;473(10):3228–34.
14. Cisneros LG, Atoun E, Abraham R, Tsvieli O, Bruguera J, Levy O. Revision shoulder arthroplasty: does the stem really matter? J Shoulder Elb Surg. 2016;25(5):747–55.
15. Phipatanakul WP, Bowen JM, Jobe CM. Removal of well-fixed flanged humeral prostheses may require humeral expansion. J Shoulder Elb Surg. 2009;18(5):724–7.
16. Keener JD, Chalmers PN, Yamaguchi K. The humeral implant in shoulder arthroplasty. J Am Acad Orthop Surg. 2017;25(6):427–38.
17. Van Thiel G, Piasecki D, Nicholson GS. Vertical humeral osteotomy for revision of well-fixed humeral components: case report and operative technique. Am J Orthop (Belle Mead NJ). 2009;38(2):67–71.
18. Van Thiel GS, Halloran JP, Twigg S, Romeo AA, Nicholson GP. The vertical humeral osteotomy for stem removal in revision shoulder arthro-

plasty: results and technique. J Shoulder Elb Surg. 2011;20(8):1248–54.
19. Johnston PS, Creighton RA, Romeo AA. Humeral component revision arthroplasty: outcomes of a split osteotomy technique. J Shoulder Elb Surg. 2012;21(4):502–6.
20. Wright TW. Revision of humeral components in shoulder arthroplasty. Bull Hosp Jt Dis (2013). 2013;71(Suppl 2):77–81.
21. Gohlke F, Rolf O. Revision of failed fracture hemiarthroplasties to reverse total shoulder prosthesis through the transhumeral approach: method incorporating a pectoralis-major-pedicled bone window. Oper Orthop Traumatol. 2007;19(2):185–208.
22. Werner BS, Abdelkawi AF, Boehm D, Hudek R, Plumhoff P, Burkhart KJ, et al. Long-term analysis of revision reverse shoulder arthroplasty using cemented long stems. J Shoulder Elb Surg. 2017;26(2):273–8.
23. Crosby LA, Wright TW, Yu S, Zuckerman JD. Conversion to reverse total shoulder arthroplasty with and without humeral stem retention: the role of a convertible-platform stem. J Bone Joint Surg Am. 2017;99(9):736–42.
24. Alentorn-Geli E, Clark NJ, Assenmacher AT, Samuelsen BT, Sanchez-Sotelo J, Cofield RH, et al. What are the complications, survival, and outcomes after revision to reverse shoulder arthroplasty in patients older than 80 years? Clin Orthop Relat Res. 2017;475(11):2744–51.
25. Cil A, Veillette CJ, Sanchez-Sotelo J, Sperling JW, Schleck C, Cofield RH. Revision of the humeral component for aseptic loosening in arthroplasty of the shoulder. J Bone Joint Surg Br. 2009;91(1):75–81.
26. Otto RJ, Nigro PT, Frankle MA. Reverse shoulder arthroplasty for chronic shoulder pathology. In: Nicholson GP, editor. Orthopaedic knowledge update: shoulder and elbow 4. 4th ed. Rosemont: AAOS; 2013. p. 379–96.
27. Sahota S, Sperling JW, Cofield RH. Humeral windows and longitudinal splits for component removal in revision shoulder arthroplasty. J Shoulder Elb Surg. 2014;23(10):1485–91.

Arthroscopic Treatment of the Failed Shoulder Arthroplasty

20

Ian A. Power and Thomas W. Throckmorton

Introduction

Since the introduction of Neer's shoulder prosthesis in the 1950s [1], the use of total shoulder arthroplasty (TSA) has steadily increased. One study indicated that since 1990, the use of TSA has increased more than 550% [2], with approximately 53,000 individuals having TSA in the United States [3]. Padegimas et al. [4] found an 8% increase in patients 55 years of age and younger between 2002 and 2011 and predicted that demand for TSA in younger patients will increase by more than 300% by 2030. Expanding indications for TSA have driven this increase, and current indications include arthritis, comminuted proximal humeral fractures, rotator cuff arthropathy, and osteonecrosis [5]. As the number of TSAs increases, the number of revision procedures also can be expected to increase.

Complications following shoulder arthroplasty fall broadly into categories of bone-related or soft-tissue pathology [6]. Pain and decreased range of motion are the two most common presenting symptoms [7]. Anatomic shoulder arthroplasty, specifically, has a reported complication rate of almost 23%, with 11% of patients requiring revision surgery [8]. Complications may manifest as pain, loss or limitation of range of motion, or instability. Patients may have symptoms following the initial surgery, or symptoms may occur after an initial period of improvement. Causes of failure include technical issues from the index procedure, pain, component loosening, rotator cuff tear, fracture, or a combination of problems [9]. Loosening of the glenoid component is one of the most common causes of failure, accounting for 12.4% of all complications and an average rate of 1.2% per year. Surgical revision occurs in two-thirds of these patients [10].

Traditionally, treatment of failed shoulder arthroplasty has been limited to open procedures; however, as experience and comfort with shoulder arthroscopy have evolved, there has been growing interest in adapting its use to management of problems that occur after shoulder replacement. Shoulder arthroscopy after shoulder arthroplasty was first described to evaluate glenoid component loosening in patients with pain and loss of motion [11]. It has since been demonstrated to be useful for other problems following shoulder arthroplasty, most commonly for diagnostic purposes. One review found that almost half of patients who had arthroscopy after shoulder arthroplasty eventually went on to have open revision surgery [7]. The most common indications for arthroscopy include evaluation for pain without loss of motion, soft-tissue biopsy to rule out infection, evaluation of the rotator cuff, or evaluation for loosening of the glenoid component. Several pathologies can

I. A. Power · T. W. Throckmorton (✉)
University of Tennessee-Campbell Clinic, Department of Orthopaedic Surgery & Biomedical Engineering, Memphis, TN, USA

R. Z. Tashjian (ed.), *Complex and Revision Shoulder Arthroplasty*,
https://doi.org/10.1007/978-3-030-02756-8_20

be treated successfully with arthroscopy, including rotator cuff impingement syndrome, loose bodies, rotator cuff tears, a loose glenoid component, and arthrofibrosis [6, 7].

Diagnostic Arthroscopy

Arthroscopy has been used after hip and knee arthroplasty for the diagnosis and treatment of infection, arthrofibrosis, and impinging hypertrophic synovitis. Arthroscopy is a useful diagnostic tool after shoulder arthroscopy, too, because artifact from the metal implants mitigates the utility of MRI and/or CT [7].

Hersch et al. [12] found that diagnostic arthroscopy was required in almost half of patients undergoing revision shoulder arthroplasty because of inconclusive radiographs and clinical examinations for motion and stability. Physical therapy and anti-inflammatory medications also had failed to relieve symptoms in these patients. Diagnostic arthroscopy can be helpful when arthrogram or ultrasound is normal and has been shown to demonstrate malpositioning, such as glenoid component malrotation, or loosening of the glenoid and/or humeral components [11, 12]. Several methods for determining loosening arthroscopically have been described, including movement of 2 mm or more of the glenoid and placement of a probe between the glenoid and the bone and lifting of the component [11, 13]. While arthroscopic examination may demonstrate glenoid loosening, it will not detect microscopic loosening or humeral component loosening. Additionally, there is a small risk of postoperative periprosthetic infection following arthroscopy [11, 12]. Garberina and Williams [14] used arthroscopy to identify dissociation of a polyethylene component in a reverse total shoulder arthroplasty; the definitive diagnosis allowed open revision in the same surgical setting.

The largest series of diagnostic arthroscopy for failed shoulder arthroplasty includes 29 patients [6]. In 15 patients, a preoperative diagnosis could not be made before arthroscopy. Seven patients were suspected to have arthrofibrosis, and arthroscopy was used to rule out any other cause of loss of motion. Six of these seven shoulders were successfully treated with arthroscopic lysis of adhesions, and the remaining patient was treated with an open procedure. Constant scores in this group improved, although they remained below the group mean score. Range of motion was significantly improved as well. In only 1 of the 29 patients could an identifiable pain source not be determined, although even this patient's pain resolved following diagnostic arthroscopy.

Glenoid Component Removal

Glenoid loosening is another common complication after total shoulder replacement and typically occurs after an asymptomatic period [8, 15]. O'Driscoll et al. [13] described arthroscopic removal of the glenoid component in five patients with implant loosening who were unable to have new components implanted or were unable to undergo open revision surgery. This method included the use of osteotomes to section the glenoid into pieces, which were then individually removed through arthroscopic portals. This allowed successful removal of the glenoid component and, therefore, a conversion to hemiarthroplasty. Three of the five patients had improved motion and complete pain relief, while the other two had relatively unchanged motion and modest pain relief. There were no reoperations or complications; however, there was damage to the articular humeral surface despite taking precautions, making a humeral head exchange necessary if future reimplantation of a glenoid is needed. The use of an arthroscopic burr also has been described to help remove the glenoid. Additionally, impaction bone grafting can be accomplished arthroscopically [16]. The concern with arthroscopic glenoid component removal is that residual microscopic debris may cause intra-articular inflammation [13].

A significant advantage of arthroscopic glenoid removal is the ability to obtain intraoperative cultures to rule out septic loosening at the same time. While reimplantation would remain a two-stage procedure, proponents of this approach cite the avoidance of an additional open exposure and relative preservation of the subscapularis tendon [17].

Periprosthetic Joint Infection

Periprosthetic shoulder infections may occur either early or late in the postoperative period, and patients often present with unexplained pain. Periprosthetic shoulder infections differ from infections after total hip and knee arthroplasty in that inflammatory indices and synovial cultures often are normal. Arthroscopic tissue biopsy has been shown to be useful in these situations. In particular, arthroscopic tissue biopsy has been advocated in patients presenting with a painful shoulder arthroplasty who have normal laboratory values, negative synovial aspirate cultures appropriately held for 14 days, and even negative intraoperative histology [18].

Arthroscopic tissue biopsy has been shown to be useful for the diagnosis of periprosthetic shoulder infections, specifically for identifying *P. acnes*. When cultures of arthroscopic tissue biopsy were compared to cultures of open tissue biopsy in a revision setting, cultures of the arthroscopic biopsies had 100% sensitivity, specificity, and positive and negative predictive values [19]. These results were significantly better than fluoroscopically guided shoulder joint aspirations, which had a sensitivity of 16.7%. Some of this difference may be explained by the intracellular and fastidious nature of *P. acnes*, which makes it difficult to culture. While the accuracy of arthroscopic biopsy is likely not 100%, it is superior to aspiration in determining septic arthritis before a revision and may help guide planning [19, 20].

In our practice, we believe arthroscopic tissue biopsy is reasonable in patients with no other identifiable cause for pain and limited motion, even in the setting of a normal infectious workup; however, the surgeon should have a high level of suspicion before performing diagnostic arthroscopy in these patients [21]. Periprosthetic shoulder infection remains very difficult to diagnose and define, and arthroscopic tissue biopsy, while potentially useful, should not be viewed as the ultimate diagnostic test in a painful shoulder arthroplasty. Other variables, including surgeon judgment, are still critical because the diagnosis of an infected shoulder arthroplasty remains primarily clinical.

Subacromial Impingement

Freedman et al. [22] were the first to describe arthroscopic acromioplasty for subacromial impingement following shoulder arthroplasty. They retrospectively reviewed six patients with a type II or III acromion with subacromial outlet narrowing and clinical impingement signs. These patients had diagnostic lidocaine injections, and 5 of 6 improved significantly, with pain scores decreasing from 7.5 to 1.6 and UCLA end-result scores of good or excellent following surgical debridement. Our experience with subacromial decompression in this setting without clear demonstration of rotator cuff pathology has not been satisfying. As such, we generally recommend workup with a CT arthrogram for evaluation of the rotator cuff to provide correlation with the clinical examination.

Rotator Cuff Repair

When rotator cuff deficiency develops following shoulder arthroplasty, it can lead to loss of motion, instability, and pain. TSA performed in the setting of isolated supraspinatus tears, and to a lesser extent subscapularis tears, may not affect postoperative outcome, while moderate to severe fatty degeneration of the infraspinatus is associated with poor results [23]. While anatomic shoulder arthroplasty may do well with repair of a small rotator cuff tear at the time of primary surgery, larger tears treated this way or tears that develop following arthroplasty often are symptomatic [24, 25]. When rotator cuff repairs are performed concominantly with TSA for partial and full-thickness tears, up to 31% may have a poor result, and patients with a preoperative acromiohumeral interval of less than 8 mm have been shown to have an increased rate of reoperation ($p = 0.003$) [26]. While repair of existing rotator cuff tears involving the supraspinatus at the primary arthroplasty may lead to good results, repair of tears following shoulder arthroplasty has been shown to have poor results, with difficulty regaining motion or improving pain. About half of patients undergoing repair also require humeral component exchange, further complicating recovery and rehabilitation [14, 23, 24].

Hersch and Dines [12] noted that most patients with failed shoulder arthroplasty who were treated with arthroscopy had full-thickness rotator cuff tears or subacromial impingement, as well as scarring of the long head of the biceps with tendonitis. While most of the rotator cuff tears were treated with open repair, all patients had significant improvements in range of motion and Hospital for Special Surgery (HSS) scores. Worse results occurred in patients with rheumatoid arthritis along with a rotator cuff tear or adhesive capsulitis. One complication, a periprosthetic fracture, was recognized and treated intraoperatively and healed with a good outcome. During diagnostic arthroscopy of 29 patients, Tytherleigh-Strong et al. [6] identified 4 rotator cuff tears, 3 of which had good results after treatment with debridement or subacromial decompression. At present, we prefer an arthroscopic repair for symptomatic small tears. For medium-sized tears, particularly in younger patients, we tend to favor an open repair with downsizing of the humeral head component. For large and massive tears, we typically manage this situation with conversion to reverse arthroplasty in most patients.

Biceps tenodesis at the time of the index TSA has been shown to improve treatment success (OR 2.97, CI 1.00–8.85, $p = 0.05$) [27], as well as improve pain relief and Constant scores [28]. For patients with anterior shoulder pain and persistent biceps pathology following shoulder arthroplasty in whom conservative treatment has failed, arthroscopic debridement of the remaining biceps tendon and arthroscopic or mini-open tenodesis have been shown to be successful at relieving these symptoms [29]. Because of this, our current practice is to routinely perform a biceps tenodesis at the time of primary arthroplasty.

Arthrofibrosis

Arthroscopic lysis of adhesions and capsular release have been advocated for postoperative stiffness following hemiarthroplasty for four-part proximal humeral fractures. Given the high likelihood of tuberosity migration (24%) and malunion or nonunion (53%) in these fractures, some prolonged immobilization has been recommended to improve healing, followed by arthroscopic treatment to regain motion if needed, especially in younger, more active patients, who may be relatively easily treated with arthroscopy rather than open revision surgery [30]. In addition to hemiarthroplasty, patients with TSA with adhesive capsulitis who failed to regain motion despite adequate rehabilitation and no evidence of rotator cuff tear may benefit from arthroscopic capsular release [6, 12]. Our experience with arthroscopic treatment for arthrofibrosis is that roughly one-third of patients make significant motion gains, but two-thirds are either unchanged or do not make significant improvements after capsular release and manipulation under anesthesia. It should be noted that many of these patients have an underlying collagen disorder, such as Sjögren syndrome, which may predispose to a more stubborn form of stiffness.

Instability

Instability also is a frequently reported complication of shoulder arthroplasty [10, 31]. Two case reports described success with arthroscopic treatment of instability after arthroplasty [32, 33]. One reported the treatment of atraumatic posterior shoulder instability following standard shoulder arthroplasty. The patient had good preoperative range of motion and no signs of complication or infection but exhibited posterior laxity and instability postoperatively, including several dislocations that required sedation and reduction. Arthroscopic examination confirmed a patulous posterior capsule, and suture anchors were used to perform a capsular imbrication. The patient had a good outcome with some decreased range of motion [33]. The second case report described the

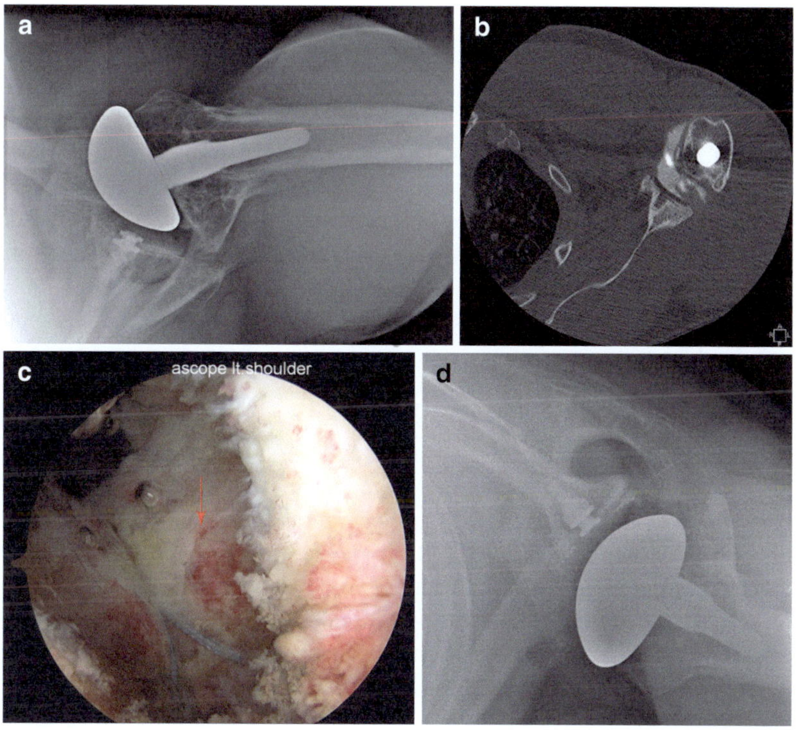

Fig. 20.1 A 43-year-old man with acute subscapularis failure following anatomic total shoulder arthroplasty resulting in anterior instability and loss of forward elevation. (**a**) Radiograph. (**b**) MRI. (**c**) Because of his young age, he had arthroscopic repair of the subscapularis (*arrow*) with clinical and radiographic (**d**) recompensation and restoration of forward elevation

use of arthroscopy to assist with reduction of a chronic traumatic dislocation of a reverse shoulder arthroplasty [32]. After a failed closed reduction, arthroscopic debridement of scar tissue allowed reduction, with a stable postoperative course. Aside from these case reports, arthroscopic treatment of instability following shoulder arthroplasty has been less successful [33].

Open approaches to address instability after anatomic shoulder arthroplasty also have been reported. One retrospective review [34] evaluated a cohort of 33 patients with instability, more than half of whom had anterosuperior or direct anterior instability, with the remaining patients having posterior instability. Of those eventually treated with open revision, two-thirds had soft-tissue imbalance, and one-third also involved component malpositioning. Only 28% of patients achieved a stable shoulder, and two-thirds had unsatisfactory results. Those with anterior instability had worse outcomes than those with posterior instability. The authors highlighted the importance of maintaining the subscapularis tendon for anterior instability and the role of posterior bone loss in posterior instability. Endres and Warner also described use of a coracoid transfer to address instability after anatomic TSA in a small series [35]. Given the results and high failure rate of solutions for post-arthroplasty instability, it may be appropriate to view open revision as a salvage procedure. In our practice, we rarely use arthroscopy in the treatment of instability following shoulder arthroplasty except in acute rotator cuff failure (Fig. 20.1).

Techniques

When performing arthroscopy in a shoulder joint with a prosthesis, there are several technical considerations. Before arthroscopy, a final aspiration under sterile conditions can be considered before administration of perioperative antibiotics [12]. If tissue cultures are to be obtained, antibiotics may be held until those are taken.

As is typical in shoulder arthroscopy, portal placement is paramount. The standard posterior portal is made blindly, with other portals made using an outside-in technique and blunt trocars to minimize iatrogenic damage [12]. For evaluation of reverse shoulder arthroplasty, the initial posterior portal should be made superior to the glenoid to avoid damage to the humeral bearing surface. Anterior and lateral portals are then established with an outside-in technique [14]. To minimize iatrogenic damage to the metallic and polyethylene components, the arm can be held internally rotated. The use of traction to distract the glenohumeral joint also is helpful.

Several other challenges arise when performing shoulder arthroscopy in the setting of arthroplasty. One of these is the glare and/or reflection of camera light from the highly polished prosthesis. This requires the surgeon to look away with the arthroscope from the humeral component. Additionally, postoperative scar tissue and arthrofibrosis limit the working area. This requires careful dissection with an electrocautery probe to release the capsule and allow improved visualization [6]. Maintaining relative hypotension and appropriate pump pressure also can be helpful in this regard.

We perform all of our standard arthroscopy and arthroplasty procedures with the patient in the beach chair position and use this for post-arthroplasty arthroscopy as well. Twelve pounds of traction is applied to the arm to distract the joint and allow better visualization (Fig. 20.2). This also typically avoids the need to work through the rotator interval to establish an intra-articular view and is useful to establish anterior and posterior portals to allow visualization from multiple angles. If biopsies are taken for culture, we use the protocol described by Dilisio et al. in which clean grasping instruments are used to take at least three specimens from tissue directly in contact with the arthroplasty components [19]. Any suspicious material in the subacromial space also is biopsied in the same way, and all cultures are sent for a 2-week incubation. We do not routinely obtain intraoperative pathologic consultation.

Arthroscopic glenoid component removal has been described by O'Driscoll and is indicated in our practice for an uninfected, loose, painful glenoid implant, preferably with an intact rotator cuff and a functional range of motion [13]. After adequate arthroscopic visualization is obtained, a small (4 mm) curved osteotome is advanced through the anterior portal to section the polyethylene component into three or four pieces (Fig. 20.3). These can then be retrieved with a grasper. Large cavitary defects can be bone grafted with crushed cancellous allograft as needed. Postoperative rehabilitation consists generally of sling immobilization for 2 weeks with gradual progression of active motion in the absence of any additional repairs.

Appropriate preoperative consideration must be given to the type of glenoid implant that is being removed. In particular, ingrowth components with anchor peg central posts often are not

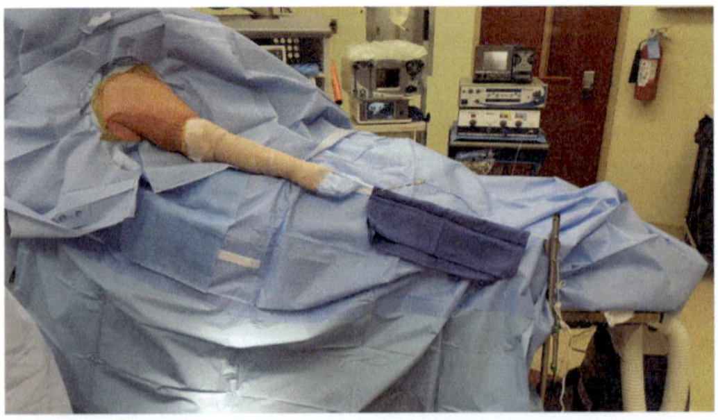

Fig. 20.2 With the patient in the beach chair position, 12 pounds of traction is placed on the arm for distraction of the glenohumeral joint to improve intra-articular visualization

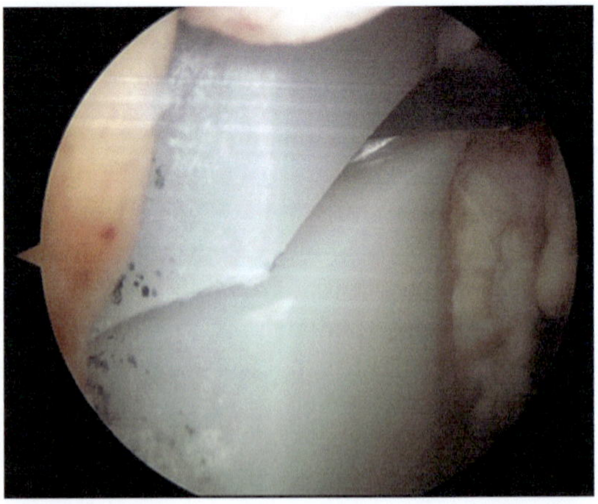

Fig. 20.3 Arthroscopic image showing a small osteotome being used through the anterior portal to cut the all-polyethylene glenoid component into several pieces to allow arthroscopic removal

suitable for this technique because the central post can be exceedingly difficult to remove arthroscopically. We have had better success with this procedure when it is reserved for radiographically loose, all-polyethylene glenoid components that have a clear shift in position or circumferential radiolucent line. Overall, when performed for this relatively narrow indication, this is a fairly reliable procedure that can potentially avoid future arthroplasty revision. However, the presence of any associated problems such as infection, component malposition, or rotator cuff failure generally obviates this procedure in favor of revision arthroplasty to fully address the patient's pathology [36].

Conclusion

Evaluation of the painful or stiff shoulder after arthroplasty should include clinical examination, laboratory tests, and radiographs to identify component loosening or malposition, infection, impingement, arthrofibrosis, loose bodies, rotator cuff tears, and instability. Additionally, advanced imaging, including CT, MRI, and ultrasound, should be obtained to rule out component loosening, malposition, or rotator cuff tearing. Despite these tests, there may be no conclusive diagnosis of a painful or dysfunctional shoulder arthroplasty. In these circumstances, diagnostic arthroscopy can be helpful to provide additional information to formulate a diagnosis, especially in ruling in or out a periprosthetic infection [7, 11, 12, 18, 19]. Glenoid loosening also can be diagnosed, and, in limited circumstances, it can be treated with arthroscopic glenoid component removal [13, 17]. In addition, loose bodies, subacromial impingement, arthrofibrosis, scarring of the long head of biceps tendon, and occasionally rotator cuff tears can be identified and treated [6, 22]. The main drawback of diagnostic arthroscopy in these situations is the possible need for additional surgery; however, this is countered by the minimal risk posed by the procedure and the avoidance of repeated violations of the subscapularis. Before diagnostic arthroscopy is done, the surgeon should have exhausted all nonoperative diagnostic measures and have a clear understanding of the treatment goals and must recognize the technical difficulties of arthroscopy in the setting of implanted prosthetic components.

References

1. Neer CS 2nd. The components of our global exchange on surgery of the shoulder. J Shoulder Elbow Surg. 1995;4:477–80.
2. Yu S, Mahure SA, Branch N, Mollon B, Zuckerman JD. Impact of race and gender on utilization rate of total shoulder arthroplasty. Orthopedics. 2016;39:e538–44.
3. Wiater JM. Shoulder joint replacement. OrthoInfo. Available at https://orthoinfo.aaos.org/en/treatment/shoulder-joint-replacement. Accessed 7 Dec 2017.
4. Padegimas EM, Maltenfort M, Lazarus MD, Ramsey ML, Williams GR, Namdari S. Future patient demand for shoulder arthroplasty by younger patients: national projections. Clin Orthop Relat Res. 2015;473:1860–7.
5. Wiater JM, Fabing MH. Shoulder arthroplasty: prosthetic options and indications. J Am Acad Orthop Surg. 2009;17:415–25.
6. Tytherleigh-Strong GM, Levy O, Sforza G, Copeland SA. The role of arthroscopy for the problem shoulder arthroplasty. J Shoulder Elbow Surg. 2002;11:230–4.
7. Horner NS, de Sa D, Heaven S, Simunovic N, Bedi A, Athwal GS, Ayeni OR. Indications and outcomes of shoulder arthroscopy after shoulder arthroplasty. J Shoulder Elbow Surg. 2016;25:510–8.
8. Gonzalez JF, Alami GB, Baque F, Walch G, Boileau P. Complications of unconstrained shoulder prostheses. J Shoulder Elbow Surg. 2011;20:666–82.
9. Wiater MP, Moravek JE Jr, Wiater JM. The evaluation of the failed shoulder arthroplasty. J Shoulder Elbow Surg. 2014;23:745–58.
10. Bohsali KI, Wirth MA, Rockwood CA Jr. Complications of total shoulder arthroplasty. J Bone Joint Surg Am. 2006;88:2279–92.
11. Bonutti PM, Hawkins RJ, Saddemi S. Arthroscopic assessment of glenoid component loosening after total shoulder arthroplasty. Arthroscopy. 1993;9:272–6.
12. Hersch JC, Dines DM. Arthroscopy for failed shoulder arthroplasty. Arthroscopy. 2000;16:606–12.
13. O'Driscoll SW, Petrie RS, Torchia ME. Arthroscopic removal of the glenoid component for failed total shoulder arthroplasty. A report of five cases. J Bone Joint Surg Am. 2005;87:858–63.
14. Garberina MJ, Williams GR. Polyethylene dissociation after reverse total shoulder arthroplasty: the use of diagnostic arthroscopy. J Shoulder Elbow Surg. 2008;17:e16–8.
15. Black E, Roberts S, Siegel E, Yannopoulos P, Higgins L, Warner J. Failure after reverse total shoulder arthroplasty: what is the success of component revision? J Shoulder Elbow Surg. 2015;24:1908–14.

16. Namdari S, Glaser D. Arthroscopically assisted conversion of total shoulder arthroplasty to hemiarthroplasty with glenoid bone grafting. Orthopedics. 2011;34:862–5.
17. Venjakob AJ, Reichwein F, Nebelung W. Arthroscopic removal of a polyethylene glenoid component in total shoulder arthroplasty. Arthrosc Tech. 2015;4:e149–52.
18. Morman M, Fowler RL, Sanofsky B, Higgins LD. Arthroscopic tissue biopsy for evaluation of infection before revision arthroplasty. J Shoulder Elbow Surg. 2012;20:e15–22.
19. Dilisio MF, Miller LR, Warner JJ, Higgins LD. Arthroscopic tissue culture for the evaluation of periprosthetic shoulder infection. J Bone Joint Surg Am. 2014;96:1952–8.
20. Tashjian RZ, Granger EK, Zhang Y. Utility of prerevision tissue biopsy sample to predict revision shoulder arthroplasty culture results in at-risk patients. J Shoulder Elbow Surg. 2017;26:197–203.
21. Sanchez-Sotelo J. Periprosthetic shoulder infections are less elusive to diagnostic arthroscopy: commentary on an article by Matthew F. Dilisio, MD, et al: "arthroscopic tissue culture for the evaluation of periprosthetic shoulder infection". J Bone Joint Surg Am. 2014;96:e197.
22. Freedman KB, Williams GR, Iannotti JP. Impingement syndrome following total shoulder arthroplasty and humeral hemiarthroplasty: treatment with arthroscopic acromioplasty. Arthroscopy. 1998;14:655–70.
23. Edwards T, Boulahia A, Kempf J, Boileau P, Nemoz C, Walch G. The influence of rotator cuff disease on the results of shoulder arthroplasty for primary osteoarthritis: results of a multicenter study. J Bone Joint Surg Am. 2002;84-A:2240–8.
24. Iannotti J, Norris T. Influence of preoperative factors on outcome of shoulder arthroplasty for glenohumeral osteoarthritis. J Bone Joint Surg Am. 2003;85-A(2):251–8.
25. Simone JP, Streubel PH, Sperling JW, Schleck CD, Cofield RH, Athwal GS. Anatomical total shoulder replacement with rotator cuff repair for osteoarthritis of the shoulder. Bone Joint J. 2014;96-B:224–8.
26. Livesey M, Horneff JG, Sholder D, Lazarus M, Williams G, Namdari S. Functional outcomes and predictors of failure after rotator cuff repair during total shoulder arthroplasty. Orthopedics. 2018;1:1–6.
27. Simmen B, Bachmann L, Drerup S, Schwyzer HK, Burkart A, Flury M, Goldhahn J. Usefulness of concomitant biceps tenodesis in total shoulder arthroplasty: a prospective cohort study. J Shoulder Elbow Surg. 2008;17:921–4.
28. Godeneche A, Boileau P, Favard L, Le Huec JC, Levigne C, Nove-Josserand L, Walch G, Edwards T. Prosthetic replacement in the treatment of osteoarthritis of the shoulder: early results of 268 cases. J Shoulder Elbow Surg. 2002;11:11–8.
29. Tuckman D, Dines D. Long head of the biceps pathology as a cause of anterior shoulder pain after shoulder arthroplasty. J Shoulder Elbow Surg. 2006;15:415–8.
30. Barth J, Andrieu K, Fotiadis E, Hannink G, Barthelemy R, Saffarini M. Critical period and risk factors for retear following arthroscopic repair of the rotator cuff. Knee Surg Sports Traumatol Arthrosc. 2017;25:2196–204.
31. Gallo R, Gamradt S, Mattern C, Cordasco F, Craig E, Dines D, Warren R. Instability after reverse total shoulder replacement. J Shoulder Elbow Surg. 2011;20:584–90.
32. Arriaza R, Couceiro G, Fernández HC. Arthroscopic reduction of a chronically dislocated reverse shoulder arthroplasty. Arthrosc Tech. 2013;2:e423–5.
33. Gee AO, Angeline ME, Dines JS, Dines DM. Shoulder instability after total shoulder arthroplasty: a case of arthroscopic repair. HSS J. 2014;10:88–91.
34. Sanchez-Sotelo J, Sperling JW, Rowland CM, Cofield RH. Instability after shoulder arthroplasty: results of surgical treatment. J Bone Joint Surg Am. 2003;85:622–31.
35. Endres NK, Warner JJ. Anterior instability after total shoulder replacement: salvage with modified Latarjet procedure. A report of 2 cases. J Shoulder Elbow Surg. 2010;19:e1–5.
36. Hattrup SJ, Cofield RH, Cha SS. Rotator cuff repair after shoulder replacement. J Shoulder Elbow Surg. 2006;15:78–83.

Index

R. Z. Tashjian (ed.), *Complex and Revision Shoulder Arthroplasty*,
https://doi.org/10.1007/978-3-030-02756-8

MIX
Papier aus verantwortungsvollen Quellen
Paper from responsible sources
FSC® C105338

If you have any concerns about our products,
you can contact us on
ProductSafety@springernature.com

In case Publisher is established outside the EU,
the EU authorized representative is:
Springer Nature Customer Service Center GmbH
Europaplatz 3, 69115 Heidelberg, Germany

Printed by Libri Plureos GmbH
in Hamburg, Germany